FITNESS AND AGING

John Piscopo
State University of New York at Buffalo

John Wiley & Sons

New York Chichester Brisbane Toronto Singapore

Library of Congress Cataloging in Publication Data:

Piscopo, John, 1922–
   Fitness and aging.

   Includes index.
   1. Physical fitness for the aged.   2. Gerontology.
I. Title.

GV482.6.P57   1985   613.7′0880564   84-21988
ISBN 0-471-87425-6

Printed in the United States of America

10 9 8 7 6 5 4 3 2 1

This book is dedicated to my wife, Carolyn,
for all possible reasons.

Foreword

The rapid increase in number of elderly persons in our society, the escalating costs of their care and social support, and the increasingly eloquent demand, by the elderly and their families, for a parallel improvement in the quality of this care and support have made the care of the elderly a major national priority.

In ancient times, a considerable percentage of individuals died in infancy and many others during youth and middle life. By 1900, as the result of improved housing, sanitation, and the introduction of antiseptics, the number of neonatal deaths had fallen markedly and fewer people were dying in the early years of life. Similarly, as the century progressed, with the introduction of antibiotics, improved medical practice and nutrition, and health education, further advances were made. Biomedical breakthroughs between 1950 and 1960 resulted in more widespread use of modern antibiotics, the beginning of the intensive care unit, improved concepts of parenteral therapy, and improvements in clinical pharmacology. With the developments since 1960, including coronary bypass, renal transplantation and some of the most effective breakthroughs in cancer chemotherapy, the number of people surviving to the period of old age has further increased. Thus we now see a large population of elderly persons, many of whom suffer from multiple diseases and disabilities, requiring expanded programs of care and support.

Clearly, the continuing emphasis on the development of modalities of acute care must be paralleled by greatly increased emphasis on factors which will improve the quality of life for these elderly persons, and improve their ability to maintain independence outside the framework of long-term care institutions.

Thus, health maintenance and preventive medicine emerge as very important aspects of health care. Of the many approaches that will be taken, some are medical, some nutritional, some social and psychological, and some relate to an individual's ability to maintain normal physical functioning. All of these, however (with the possible exception of immunization), can be assembled under the heading of "fitness."

In this context, fitness and aging become an extremely important topic to students and practitioners in the caring professions, to families, to people looking forward to their own aging, and to elderly persons themselves.

This book provides a remarkably broad and understandable review of the many individual facets of fitness and aging. It is not intended to be a medical or research treatise nor does it attempt to provide a critical review of the recent research literature. On the other hand, the bibliography cites articles that, while understandable by a broad reading public, also contain the necessary references required for in-depth studies of individual topics.

As with any book of this size and scope, especially one written by a single author, individual readers may find certain statements to which they take exception. Nevertheless, the very fact that it has been written by a single person, and one who has a broad understanding and good ability to communicate, brings to the book a sense of unity and cohesiveness that will be welcome, especially to students who are beginning to "get their bearings" in the two related fields of fitness and aging. The numerous figures and illustrations also contribute greatly to the book's clarity. John Piscopo is to be commended for a fine job.

To the readers, especially those who are students in the broad range of health and caring professions, we who have committed ourselves to the exciting field of gerontology extend a warm hand of welcome. We need you!

EVAN CALKINS, M.D.
Professor and Head,
Division of Geriatrics—Gerontology
Department of Medicine
State University of New York at Buffalo

Preface

This book grew out of an urgent concern with providing a basic scientific and practical rationale for the development and maintenance of fitness, focusing upon persons past 50.

Fitness and Aging embraces the fundamental concept "What you do not use—you lose," and the firm conviction that the human form needs appropriate and sensible physical activity throughout the life span.

Although the book is focused upon fitness as central to human efficiency, I have attempted to present the subject matter from a multidisciplinary perspective, incorporating knowledge and understanding from the biological, psychological, and sociological disciplines.

I have endeavored to present each topic area in a scholarly, yet readable, fashion with the realization that many readers may not have completed courses in human anatomy and kinesiology. For example, whenever essential technical terms are used, such phrases are accompanied with supplemental explanations or defined in the glossary.

This text is written for upper-division undergraduate and introductory graduate courses. It should be useful for health, physical education, recreation, occupational therapy, therapeutic recreation, physical therapy, and nursing majors and other students in health-related professions. The book should also be of value to gerontologists from the various disciplines and field practitioners interested in physical activity and the aging process.

Fitness and Aging begins with an overview of aging, including demographic changes and the effect of aging upon society, followed by a presentation of myths, stereotypes, and the economic impact of fitness in reducing health cost inflation.

Chapters 2 and 3 deal with biological and psychosocial theories of aging, and the general structural and functional changes that occur in adult maturation. Intelligence, memory, personality, and human sexuality changes are considered in this section. Considerable attention is given to the human physique and functionality of the spine. Musculoskeletal, motor learning, balance and equilibrium, and sensory changes are discussed, with implications for human performance.

Chapter 4 concentrates upon specific fitness modalities with a comprehensive analysis of muscular strength, flexibility, cardiovascular-respiratory efficiency, balance and equilibrium, senior sports, exercise, and relaxation. The practicing professional in the field will find a set of indications and contraindications of activities particularly useful in establishing exercise prescriptions for older adults.

Chapter 5 contains principles and guidelines for the design and conduct of adult fitness programs in community settings. Emphasis is placed upon developing organizational and administrative practices that will enhance optimum fitness and recreational activities in noninstitutional environments.

Chapter 6 is concerned with special health and fitness problems commonly found among senior adults. Specific types of movement skills, based upon individual capacities and motor skill levels, are presented with adaptive guidelines. Arthritis, osteoporosis, sensory losses, nutrition, obesity, and special exercises for incontinence are discussed along with fitness activities for older persons with limited ambulatory capabilities.

I have devoted an entire chapter (7) to "Drugs and the Elderly," because the consumption of prescriptive and nonprescriptive medicines is exceedingly high among older adults. Thus, professionals involved in program development and implementation should be thoroughly acquainted with the characteristics and effects of drug agents, particularly as they relate to exercise and physical activity.

Chapter 8 contains principles, guidelines, and specifications for facilities and equipment for fitness and recreation programs. Consideration is given to essential and desirable outdoor and indoor structures for the conduct of physical, social, and intellectual activities.

Chapter 9 explores basic measurement and evaluation concepts germane to the application of fitness testing instruments, and the overall program elements presented in the preceding chapters. The discussion accents the necessity of selecting appropriate instruments and procedures commensurate with intended program goals and objectives.

The chapter summations and many illustrations included throughout the text should assist the reader to review, synthesize, and clarify the concepts discussed in this book.

ACKNOWLEDGMENTS

The writing and creation of a textbook is rarely the product of one person. Many people have contributed to the advancement of this book. It is my pleasure to acknowledge the cooperation and assistance of those persons and organizations who have directly or indirectly contributed to the text.

First and foremost, I am gratefully indebted to my wife, Carolyn, for her efficient typing of the manuscript, and for the performance of numerous other tasks which facilitated its preparation. The dedication of this book signifies my indebtedness to my wife for her unfailing support, encouragement, and understanding.

I especially thank the many senior adults who served as models from the following organizations: Ken-Ton YMCA, Town of Tonawanda, N.Y.; Town of Tonawanda Senior Citizen Center, N.Y.; Town of Amherst Senior Center, Williamsville, N.Y.; Niagara Falls YMCA, N.Y.; Nautilus Fitness Center, Williamsville, N.Y.; Episcopal Church Home, Buffalo, N.Y.; and the Senior Lifeline Program, University of Southern Maine, Portland.

Appreciation is expressed to Winston Barton and Deborah L. Morris for their photographic expertise, and to Joan Magin, Ellen Latham, Randi Edwards, James Kenney, and Kirsten Milbrath for their help in gathering essential photographs. I also wish to extend my thanks to Dr. James V. Sullivan and Robert E. Folsom for their assistance in securing illustrative program materials.

A special thanks is extended to the following persons for their creative art work: Catherine Limina Sullivan, for her anatomical illustrations; Deborah L. Morris, for exercise illustrations for the appendixes and court diagrams.

Appreciation is extended to Patricia Rice for her assistance with the index.

Finally, I thank the staff of the Health Science Library of the State University of New York at Buffalo for their splendid cooperation and help in securing the research materials and references used for this volume.

JOHN PISCOPO

Contents

3. Anthropometric and Kinesiologic Aspects of Aging

8. Facilities and Equipment for Activity Programs   322

CHAPTER 1

Aging: An Overview

DEMOGRAPHIC SHIFTS

The graying of society has begun. The combination of lower birthrates and reduced mortality is creating a rising proportion of older adults to younger people. In 1900, one of every twenty-five persons in the United States was over 65. Now, the ratio is one of every nine, and by 2020—when the baby boom becomes the senior boom—it is expected to be one of every six or possibly of every five.[1] The 25 million Americans over 65 now make up about 12 percent of the population, compared to 4 percent in 1900 (see Figure 1.1).

Specific increases within the aging population are anticipated, as well as numerical expansion of the group as a whole. The 75 to 84 age bracket is expected to increase rapidly in the next 30 years. It is anticipated that we will have almost five million people over 85 by the year 2010.[2] The expectation of life at birth in the United States reached an all-time high of 74.5 in 1982. Life expectancy for newborn males rose to 70.7 years, while for females it increased to 78.2 years.[3] According to Table 1.1, men aged 65 can look forward to another 14.5 years of life, and women of the same age can anticipate an additional 18.8 years.

Females continue to have a longevity advantage, outliving males by approximately eight years. Based upon current mortality data, about seven out of ten white women can expect to celebrate their 75th birthday, while only about one in two white men can do so. Among nonwhites, the chances

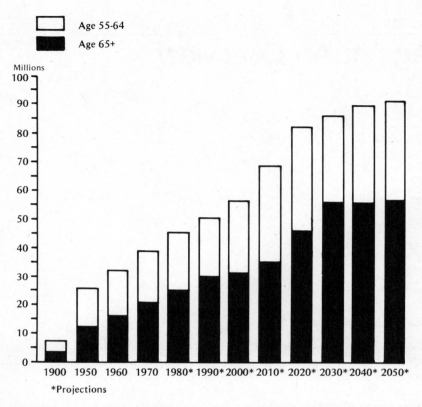

Figure 1.1 Number of persons aged 55 and over, from 1900 to 2050. (From U.S. Department of Commerce, Bureau of the Census, 1980 Census of the Population, vol. 1 [Washington, D.C.: USGPO, 1981].)

of surviving to age 75 are about three in five for women, and about one in three for men. Gains in longevity generally occur among white and nonwhite persons at each age; however, data indicate that longevity is higher for white men at earlier ages, but that after age 69, nonwhite men hold the advantage. A similar pattern holds for nonwhite women until age 72, while thereafter, the reverse is true.[4]

The phenomena of demographic shifts, reflecting increasing members of older people, point to two significant segments within the older population that will require different kinds of services and support systems. One group is composed of capable and self-sufficient seniors in reasonably good health. The other group, usually over 75, contains the "old-old," and is composed of persons with varying levels of illness, ranging from partial disability to complete dependence requiring skilled nursing facility care.

Table 1.1 Expectation of Life (in Years): United States, 1979–1982

Age	National Center for Health Statistics 1979	1980[a]	1981[a]	Metropolitan Life Insurance Company 1982[a]
Total				
Population				
0	73.9	73.8	74.1	74.5
1	73.9	73.7	74.0	74.3
15	60.3	60.1	60.4	60.7
25	50.9	50.8	50.9	51.2
35	41.5	41.4	41.6	41.8
45	32.4	32.2	32.4	32.6
55	24.0	23.8	24.0	24.2
65	16.7	16.5	16.7	16.8
75	10.7	10.5	10.7	10.8
Male				
0	70.0	70.0	70.3	70.7
1	70.1	69.9	70.2	70.6
15	56.5	56.4	56.7	57.0
25	47.4	47.3	47.5	47.8
35	38.2	38.1	38.3	38.6
45	29.2	29.1	29.3	29.5
55	21.1	21.0	21.2	21.4
65	14.3	14.2	14.3	14.5
75	9.1	8.8	9.0	9.1
Female				
0	77.8	77.7	77.9	78.2
1	77.7	77.5	77.7	77.9
15	64.1	63.9	64.0	64.2
25	54.4	54.2	54.3	54.6
35	44.8	44.6	44.7	44.9
45	35.4	35.2	35.3	35.5
55	26.7	26.4	26.6	26.7
65	18.7	18.5	18.7	18.8
75	11.9	11.6	11.9	11.9

[a] Provisional.
Source: Metropolitan Life Insurance Co., *Statistical Bulletin* 64, No. 1 (January-June 1983):13. Used with permission.

The well and vigorous group under 85 will likely seek out ways and means of preventing illness and maintaining health-fitness for as long as possible. At this point we cannot know how long the well-elderly can remain healthy and self-sufficient, given the rapid scientific gains in modern medicinal practice, nutrition, and exercise. It is conceivable that in the near future more elders past 85 will remain functionally able and independent.

At the opposite end of the spectrum, the number of seniors within the frail category also will increase. As the over-85 age group multiplies, the need for long-term care and support services will intensify, as such persons are most likely to become frail.[5] Sheer growth in numbers of persons over 85, with 1.4 million more old-old projected by 1999, will increase long-term care expenditures. Thus, in the years ahead, millions of elderly will require a variety of services and support systems sponsored by multiple agencies, both private and those under local, state, and federal government. Such services will include housing, transportation, public health insurance, long-term care, and programs in preventive medicine and desirable health practices. There is widespread agreement that no matter where the older adult falls within the health and wellness spectrum, each is entitled to an environment that allows him or her the right of independence in decision making and freedom in performing everyday living tasks, whether he or she is functioning in a home, community, or institutional setting.

The chapters that follow are based on the premise that maintaining health-fitness and vitality for as long as possible depends not only on genetic endowment, but also on active engagement in sound nutritional practices, appropriate physical exercise and activity, and participation in satisfying affairs of the mind and spirit.

Implications of Demographic Changes

The changing population phenomena point to the elderly as a significant force in shaping the political and social policies of the future. Our older adults of the 1980s and 1990s will demand more gerontology knowledge, information, and services. Consequently, lifestyles of older citizens will require myriad public organizations and private enterprises, including schools, colleges, universities, multipurpose senior centers, adult day care centers, adult residences, and skilled nursing facilities—each focusing upon one or more target groups within the senior population.

Pension plans, Social Security, Medicare, and Medicaid are contemporary public issues that are receiving priority attention at all government levels. Older adults vote consistently and in large numbers—a powerful motivator for politicians to respond on behalf of the elderly.

The educational level of older persons currently is rising. By 1990, half the population over age 65 will have had some college education.[6] Adult public education programs about pre-retirement and the aging process are multiplying in schools and colleges. More older students, from middle maturity through retirement, are attending colleges and universities.

The "Elderhostel" movement, whereby retired persons can enroll in summer college classes, is featured on campuses around the world. Courses are offered in a wide and diverse collection of subjects, including literature, art, health, fitness, political theory, music, leisure, finance, mental health, and other academic studies, as well as practical topic areas.

Our emerging older adult population is: (1) predominantly female, with a growing number of widows; (2) better educated, with more funds to purchase services; (3) less passive and more politically active; (4) less dependent on others for its living environments; and (5) diverse and heterogeneous.

AGING: INTERCONNECTIONS

The study of gerontology is based upon interdisciplinary subject matter embracing the disciplines of biology, psychology, and sociology. Any approach to improve the health and well-being of the older adult should focus upon a unified strategy applying valid precepts and concepts from these disciplines. For example, we know that certain structural and functional changes that occur in the aging process can create anxiety and stress. Specifically, for example, acuity of vision and hearing diminish and tolerance to heat and cold is lessened (see Chapter 6). These changes may threaten the security and comfort, subsequently upsetting the homeostatic balance and emotional coping mechanisms, of the senior adult (see Chapter 2). Thus, the prudent professional worker strives to develop a friendly atmosphere for the conduct of activities coupled with adaptations of facilities and equipment whereby participants can see and hear without discomfort. Such an operational process interconnects the effects of biological changes with the basic psychological principle of satisfying a fundamental safety and security need of the senior adult.

Maslow's hierarchy of human needs places high priority on the yearning for belonging and affiliation with others.[7] Modalities and programs that encourage activity participation and friendships reinforce social support systems and help to fulfill this need. This approach tends to strengthen membership, sharing, and mutual respect for one another—all compelling social needs that should be satisfied. Principles and guidelines that encourage participation in individual and group fitness programs will be examined in later chapters.

Perceptions of age, whether recognized as chronological or functional, vary among individuals and among cultures. Such differences are often rooted in folklore or legend, rather than substantiated by facts. The following section discusses contemporary definitions, interpretations, myths, and misunderstandings surrounding the biological and psychological components of aging—all of which affect the health and well-being of our senior adults.

DEFINITIONS AND INTERPRETATIONS

When is a person called *old? Old* is a relative term, which to youth may mean over 40, but among people past numerical mid-life may mean 70 or 80. Most people attach a chronological concept to aging, an unreliable criterion of a person's age index for either sex. People reflect a wide range of differences with the passage of time, demonstrating diverse biological, psychological, and social characteristics. Nevertheless, because of such widespread acceptance, the World Health Organization has developed a chronological classification of aging:

45 to 59—middle age

60 to 74—elderly

75 to 90—old

over 90—very old[8]

It may be surprising to some readers that this organization categorizes middle age as from 45 to 59. As we approach the year 2000, middle age may well move up to the present chronological classification of *elderly*.

A modern concept of aging places emphasis upon *functionality*—i.e., how well a person can perform physically, mentally, emotionally, and socially. Neugarten refers to the *young-old* and the *old-old*, basing her distinction upon health and social characteristics.[9] The young-old are those who are healthy and vigorous retirees—age is irrelevant, and they pursue a wide variety of lifestyles. The old-old, by contrast, are those persons with major physical and mental deterioration who need assorted services and support systems.

Other classifications that connote various levels of functional age are: well-aging, well-elderly, frail, ambulatory elderly, wheelchair elderly, and bedfast elderly. These terms are discussed in Chapters 5 and 6 in relation to developing fitness programs for specific target populations.

Functional aging has three general elements: biological, psychological, and sociological. *Biological age* refers to the slow and progressive structural and functional changes that take place in the cellular, tissue, and organ levels, ultimately affecting performance of all body systems.

Psychological age refers to the individual's adaptive capacities; that is, to how well he or she can cope with changing environmental demands. Such functions as memory, intelligence, learning, motivation, and emotion are involved in psychological aging. A basic requirement of successful psychological aging is healthy physiological aging, particularly in terms of the brain, with its neural-related mechanisms, and the cardiovascular system, which supplies essential oxygen-rich blood to cerebral cells.

Social aging refers to those changes with respect to the individual's role in society, and to his or her social patterns in relation to what is expected by members of a given culture.

British scientist Alex Comfort, who has made many contributions to gerontology, particularly in the biology of aging, categorizes two types of aging: physical and sociogenic.[10] The latter has no physical basis, but is a social role that folklore, prejudices, and misconceptions about age has imposed on the old.

Many falsehoods, negative stereotypes, and myths have developed about the conduct of senior adults. For example, it is not uncommon for senility, rigidity, debility, sickness, unintelligence, and unproductivity to be associated with elders. Comfort believes that such prejudices, founded on attitudes rather than on scientific evidence accounts for as much as 75 percent of the aging phenomenon in American society.

Biological aging is usually associated with life span; i.e., whether a person is younger or older connotes the quality of functioning organ systems and distance from death. Another operational method of defining aging is to separate the functioning process into *primary* and *secondary* aging.[11] Primary aging is related to the biological processes of decline rooted in heredity. These are inborn and inevitable detrimental changes that are time-related, but are independent of stress, trauma, or acquired disease. Secondary aging refers to those defects and disabilities caused by external environmental factors of trauma and disease.

Erickson, in dealing with life-span development, is considered by some gerontologists to have had the greatest impact of all ego psychologists in the field of aging.[12] His theory focuses upon healthy maturation and life adjustment. Erickson postulates that eight crises must be resolved throughout the life span: (1) trust versus mistrust; (2) autonomy versus shame; (3) initiative versus guilt; (4) industry versus infirmity; (5) identity versus role confusion; (6) intimacy versus isolation; (7) generativity versus stagnation; and (8) integrity versus despair.

The first four are psychological situations that are assigned to childhood. Identity versus role confusion is the task of adolescence. Intimacy versus isolation is resolved in young adulthood, followed by generativity versus stagnation in middle age. Integrity versus despair represents the final stage or crisis in the life cycle of personality.

According to Erickson, ego maturation requires this series of eight stages. Failure to resolve each aspect leads to incomplete or inappropriate development of some aspect of personality.[13]

The final stage (old age), which involves either the attainment of integrity or the manifestation of despair, depends upon the degree and quality of satisfaction and contentment in life review. Satisfaction and contentment throughout the life cycle enhances integrity, whereas loneliness and meaningless accomplishments foster despair.[14]

Most descriptions of aging refer to changes or decline in function after maturity. Some definitions accent the biological component. Others express the aging process in terms of psychosocial adaptation and coping with losses. The following interpretation offered by Birren and Renner presents a balanced perspective, which suggests incremental as well as decremental changes in function over the life span: "Aging refers to the regular changes that occur in the mature genetically representative organisms living under representative environmental conditions as they advance in chronological age."[15] Their definition does not apply exclusively to biological or psychosocial environments, but does suggest *all* changes that naturally take place over a time span.

Aging is a normal process, not a disease. Many of the conditions that cause disability—e.g., arthritis, cancer, arteriosclerosis, diabetes, and organic brain syndromes—stem from pathological sources and are the true bases of dysfunction, illness, and dependency in later life. Although aging does result in some slowing of speed, strength, endurance, and certain types of perception and motor skills, the process does not imply deterioration only—it also means growth and accomplishment of maturity.

MYTHS AND MISUNDERSTANDINGS

Many myths and stereotypes surround the process and effects of aging. For example, many people persist in believing that old people are all alike; old people are senile; old people cannot learn new skills; old people are not interested in sex; old people are rigid and set in their ways; and old people are sick and depressed. Such clichés and negative attitudes, unsupported by fact and applied solely on the assertion of chronological age, exemplify what is termed *ageism*.[16]

Some of these perspectives are rooted in folklore and tales of past centuries which continue to linger in contemporary society. Other misunderstandings stem from studies of institutionalized elderly, where the majority of residents are ill and disabled. Although only 5 percent of the elderly are found in nursing home–type institutions, many continue to identify older adults with ill health, dull personalities, and contrary temperaments.

Intellectual, social, and health myths can be self-destructive. That is, if older adults perceive themselves as losing their ability to function well, they may actually perform below their real capacities and abilities. For example, if older persons are continually told that memory loss is a sign of senility, their retreat from intellectual activities may follow. If elders are repeatedly informed that their sexual capacities are defunct, older males may become impotent and females frigid.

The following myths about aging are discussed in greater detail in other chapters. The intent of this section is to point out the fallacies and false-hoods of common stereotyped notions about older people.

Myth of Senility

The term *senility* is often loosely interpreted to mean "losing one's mind" or applied to any eccentric form of behavior of the old, such as defective memory, disorientation, or dementia. The majority of older people are not senile. In fact, only about 2 to 3 percent of persons aged 65 or over are institutionalized as a result of psychiatric illness.[17] The mental deterioration associated with senility usually is caused by a specific pathological dysfunction or disease, not advanced age. For example, depression, confusion, and disorientation may be caused by improper nutrition, drug reactions, or meta-

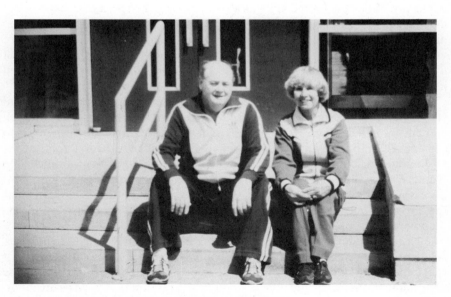

Figure 1.2 Refuting the myth of ill-health and disability.

bolic derangements. Often brain disease is mimicked by depression, alcoholism, paranoid conditions, or common everyday emotional states, and sometimes passed off as the product of aging.

Butler refers to "the senile write-off" of patients labeled too old to treat or simply "disposition problems."[18] Thus, many treatable medical problems in the elderly are assumed to be the inevitable consequences of aging and nothing is done for them.

Actual senile dementias, such as Alzheimer's disease, of unknown etiology, and organic brain syndromes, caused by hardening of the arteries, indeed exist (see Chapter 7). However, even though some three to four million Americans suffer from Alzheimer-type dementias, it is the consensus of the biomedical community that such brain dysfunctions are not necessarily part of growing old.[19] Thus, the assumption that old people "forget," become depressed, and suffer from intellectual deterioration because of senility is an erroneous generalization.

Myth of Homogeneity

The notion that older adults are alike in health, character, personality, and functional performance is another common negative stereotype. Despite the reality that approximately 95 percent of the elderly live in the community and exhibit the same diversity of traits found among young people, older adults are often considered alike as a group: isolated, sick, and unhappy. Yet most older people are not separated from family members. Although most older people prefer to live in their own households, the sicker or more vulnerable an older person becomes, the more likely it is that he or she will live in a home of a child, usually a daughter. Old persons are not dumped into mental hospitals or nursing homes by cruel and indifferent children.[20]

Although it is true that the incidence of acute and chronic illness increases among persons past 65, the vast majority of elders function well enough into their 70s and 80s—even with illnesses and impairments—to sustain self-sufficiency and independence. Many elderly do have some activity limitations, but a severe decline does not become prevalent until age 85. Numerous studies show that chronological aging from 60 to 85 does not necessarily diminish an individual's interests and activities. The fact is that the overwhelming majority of old people are well and living normally, and on the average they spend less than 14 days in bed a year due to illness.[21]

Nor are older people necessarily unhappier than younger population segments. Although short episodes of depression occur among the elderly, it is estimated that clinical depressions develop in only about 10 percent of the 65 + population.[22] Chronic or longstanding depression is viewed as an abnormal state, which should not be considered part of normal aging. Studies have

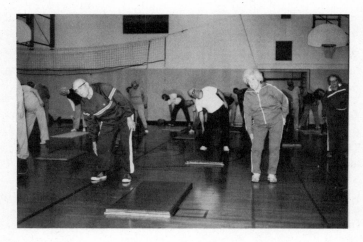

Figure 1.3 A nonagenarian man (95) and octogenarian woman (87), enjoying and maintaining fitness in a group setting.

shown that greater satisfaction and happiness are reflected in the young and older populations compared to middle-aged persons.[23]

Other data from the Duke Longitudinal Studies on Aging indicate little or insignificant decline in happiness or life satisfaction.[24] Thus, the notion that most older persons are isolated, sick, and unhappy simply represents another example the negative stereotyping imposed upon seniors without scientific evidence.

Myth of Decline in Sexuality

The topic of sexuality and aging with regard to sexual interests, normal physiological changes, and special problems is discussed in chapter 2. The focus here is on several persistent myths and stereotypes about sexuality and aging.

Although greater openness and accessibility of information about sexual matters is common among adolescents and youth, such is not the case concerning elders. For example, phrases such as "that dirty old man" or "she is an old biddy" tacitly imply that older men are impotent and elder women are sexless. Such so-called humor gives rise to the inaccurate assumption that sexual activity belongs to youth and is a deviation from normal in older adults. Butler asserts that sexual negativism stems from *ageism*.[25] Another reason for such sexual negativism relates to the lack of correct information about the normal changes that occur with aging. The following statements represent common fallacies held by society:

- Sexual desire and interest cease with the onset of old age.
- Sexual capacity in men and women ends after the age of 70.
- Sexual activity hastens "the wearing out" process.
- Sexual feelings and activity are undignified past 60.
- Menopause ends a woman's sexual desire and attractiveness.
- Prostatectomy ends the male's sex life.
- The likelihood of a sudden heart attack during sexual intercourse is high.
- Sexual activity is physically dangerous for older people.
- Chronic impotency is primarily due to physical causes rather than psychological origins.
- In most cases, the older person should refrain from sex after a heart attack.

Sexual expression is a normal need throughout the life cycle. An important step in breaking down cultural myths and stereotypes is to arm older people with accurate information about sexuality in the overall context of successful aging (see Chapter 2).

Myth of Rigidity and Inflexibility

The majority of older people are not set in their ways but can indeed change. There is some evidence that older people tend to become more stable in their attitudes, but it is clear that most older people do change and successfully adapt to the many major events that occur in old age: e.g., death of a spouse, moving to a new home, children leaving home, and serious illness.[26]

The notion of rigidity and inflexibility implies resistance to change. Such a supposition, broadly conceived, suggests that behavioral responses may be neatly identified as flexible or inflexible, rigid or obstinate.

People, young or old, are seldom resilient to change in all personal and social situations. Studies on rigidity show that this characteristic is not a unitary trait, but is composed of a variety of rigidities. A person can be rigid in one area of endeavor and not in another.[27]

Expressions of rigid behavior patterns, whether manifested in motor skills, intellectual, or emotional domains, largely depend upon the basic personality and temperamental patterns that have been established in earlier life. In some cases rigid behavior may stem from brain damage and illness; however, when rigidity is seen, it usually is a form of continuing behavior that has extended into the mature years, as diverse in older adults as in the total population. A more detailed discussion of personality and aging is presented in Chapter 2.

Myth of Unproductivity

The notion that older adults cannot produce on the job, and that retirement is a time for rest and complete disengagement from professional and social activities, is another popular misconception. Although some retirees elect to disengage from societal group affairs and restrict their activities to home and family (see the discussion of the disengagement theory in Chapter 2), many seniors are active and productive in personal, community, and professional activities. Studies of older workers in the workforce show a positive relationship between productivity and age in the following ways:

- Older workers have better attendance records than workers under 35.
- Older workers have fewer disabling and nondisabling injuries.
- Older workers have relatively low unemployment rates.
- Frequency of accidents and illnesses tends to decrease with age—though time needed for recovery tends to increase.[28]

Thus, the widespread belief that older adults are less productive, less reliable, and more prone to accidents and absenteeism than are younger people is grounded upon myth and stereotyping. Professional and creative talent does not disappear at 60 or 70. The following individuals are only a small sample of the many seniors who have achieved greatness after 70:

- *Pope John XXIII*—chosen Pope at 77.
- *Golda Meir*—named prime minister of Israel at 71.
- *Pablo Picasso*—completed his portraits of "Sylvette" at 73 and continued to draw into his 90s.
- *Arthur Rubinstein*—performed a recital at Carnegie Hall at 89.
- *Frank Lloyd Wright*—completed the Guggenheim Museum at 89.
- *Robert Frost*—continued to write poetry well into his 80s.
- *"Grandma Moses"*—began her art career at 72.
- *Giuseppi Verdi*—wrote *Otello* at 74, and *Falstaff* at 78.

As we come to the end of the century, older people continue to demonstrate more vigor and involvement in a myriad of productive activities, from health regimens of jogging to complex computer management tasks. The idea of uselessness and unproductivity among elders is a contradiction of fact.

Myth of Inability to Learn New Skills

Contrary to popular belief, learning ability (in the absence of brain disease) does not significantly decline with age. In fact, certain types of mental skills, such as vocabulary and conceptual ability, may improve after the age of 60 (see Chapter 3). It is true that older persons often require somewhat longer to learn new material, but given extra time, they can learn as well as younger persons.[29]

The cliché, "You can't teach an old dog new tricks" is a distorted adage. Much of what is to be learned depends upon motivation, nature of learning material, and conditions under which the learner is functioning. For example, because older persons generally need more time to encode and assimilate information, speed tests of any kind tend to obscure the true mental powers of persons past 60.

Several studies have demonstrated that subjects with advanced education and superior ability, working without time pressure, show little or no deterioration with age.[30] Another important condition that significantly influences the learning process of elders (and of the young as well) is the relevance or meaningfulness of information presented. The more meaningful the material, the better it can be processed and absorbed. Irrelevant information, particularly in abstract form, is difficult for older persons to grasp.

Older people retain high performance in tests of verbal meaning, reasoning power, and word fluency, and in some cases perform better with advancing age.[31] The capacity and ability to learn new motor skills is retained well into the sixth and seventh decades, provided adequate levels of motivation and health-fitness are maintained. Reaction and movement time decline slowly: however, in many older persons, reaction and response to stimuli are equal to that of the average young person (see the discussion of Spirduso's research in Chapter 3).

The myths and fallacies discussed in this chapter represent a few common prejudices imposed upon the elderly. Others include:

- Old people are poor.
- Old people are alone.
- Old people are sad and dependent.
- Old age is a disease.
- Old people are grouchy.
- Old people are not innovative and dislike new ideas.

The realities of life contradict each of the above expressions. Aging is an individual experience that shows great diversity among people. Although certain common changes and tendencies do exist, the quantitative and qualitative rate of decremental and incremental alterations in the aging extends from the extremely frail and bedfast to the vigorous and high-energy senior inventor, business person, community worker, artist, writer, lawyer, or teacher.

ECONOMICS OF FITNESS AND PREVENTIVE MEDICINE

Health care expenditures have been rising rapidly since 1960. A total of $255 billion was spent for personal health care in 1981, an increase of 16 percent over 1980. The 1981 figures represented $1090 per capita, a 15 percent increase compared to $947 per person in 1980.[32] These expenditures are incurred in a variety of areas, including: hospitalization; outpatient clinical service; nursing home care; services of physicians, specialists and health professionals; and drugs and drug sundries.

Circulatory diseases (heart disease, stroke, and hypertension), digestive diseases, and mental disorders head the list of health care expenditures, with a combined cost of $85.3 billion.[33] Health expenses continue to rise, and with the burgeoning number of middle-aged and older adults, health professionals forecast higher costs in the years ahead. The prospect of continuing growth in health care spending makes it a major economic issue for both the public and private sectors of our society.

The major theme of this book stresses the importance of good nutrition, exercise, and an active lifestyle as preventive medicine, not only for life enrichment, but also as a sensible strategy for reducing health inflation.

The 1981 White House Conference on Aging recommended a number of resolutions aimed directly at the promotion of fitness and maintenance of wellness. The following resolutions would be particularly important in helping to deflate the health care cost balloon and in contributing to the total health and well-being of our middle-aged and senior population:

1. Tax incentives should be given to companies who sponsor pre-retirement and post-retirement programs which include the promotion and maintenance of wellness.
2. A governmental plan should be established whereby individuals are reimbursed for expenses paid for preventive care and the maintenance of wellness.[34]

The first recommendation would offer a real inducement for corporations and business establishments to sponsor professional health and fitness programs. Such legislation would allow private enterprise to write off grants as tax incentives. Membership allowances paid by employers to YM/YWCAs and community health-fitness centers reinforce the preventive concept of good health.

The second recommendation offers a personal incentive for individuals to participate in preventive health and fitness programs. Our health care system is primarily designed to assist individuals after they have become ill or functionally incapacitated. This philosophical stance contributes to the exorbitant cost of health services. For example, it is not unusual for heart bypass surgery—a procedure related to atherosclerosis and obesity—to cost in excess of $20,000. Such surgery can be avoided, in many cases, by changes in lifestyle, cessation of smoking, nutrition adjustments, and proper systematic exercise.

Each of these recommendations is a sound and logical approach to reducing the cost of illness. The preventive initiative can be built into the Medicare disbursement system to allow participation in bona fide community fitness program. These programs would be based on interdisciplinary education about the benefits of the right mix of nutrition, exercise, and an active lifestyle. Appropriate physical activity lessens the need for drastic treatment of heart disease, obesity, hypertension, diabetes, musculoskeletal problems, stress, anxiety, and depression—each of which is discussed in subsequent chapters.

REFERENCES

1. Bernice L. Neugarten, "Older People—A Profile," in Neugarten, ed., *Age or Need* (Beverly Hills, Calif.: Sage Publications, 1982), p. 33.
2. U.S. Department of Commerce, Bureau of the Census, *1980 Census of the Population,* vol. I (Washington, D.C.: USGPO, 1981).
3. Metropolitan Life Foundation, "Life Expectancy in the United States," *Statistical Bulletin* 64, no. 1 (1983):12.
4. Ibid., p. 16.
5. U.S. Department of Health and Human Services, "Final Report: The 1981 White House Conference on Aging—A National Policy on Aging," vol. I (Washington, D.C.: USGPO, 1981), pp. 84–86.
6. Neugarten, "Older People," pp. 7–8.
7. Abraham Maslow, *Toward a Psychology of Being* (Princeton, N.J.: Van Nostrand, 1962).
8. Margaret Hawker, *Geriatrics for Physiotherapists and the Allied Health Professions* (London: Faber & Faber, 1974), p. 15.
9. Neugarten, "Older People," pp. 21–22.
10. Alex Comfort, "Age Prejudice in America," in H. Cox, ed., *Aging,* 3 ed. (Guilford, Ct.: Dushkin Publishing Group, 1983), pp. 73–74.
11. Ewald W. Busse and Dan Blazer, "The Theories of Aging," in Busse and Blazer, eds., *Handbook of Geriatric Psychiatry* (New York: Van Nostrand Reinhold, 1980), p. 4.
12. Margurite D. Kermis, *The Psychology of Aging: Theory, Research and Practice* (Boston: Allyn & Bacon, 1984), p. 68.
13. Ibid., p. 225.
14. Ibid., p. 69.
15. J. E. Birren and V. J. Renner, "Research on the Psychology of Aging," in Birren and K. W. Schaie, eds., *Handbook of the Psychology of Aging* (New York: Van Nostrand Reinhold, 1977), p. 4.

16. Robert N. Butler, "Ageism," in Cox, *Aging,* pp. 66–71.
17. Erdman Palmore, "Facts on Aging," *The Gerontologist* 17, no. 4 (1977): 315–320.
18. Robert N. Butler, "The Doctor and the Aged Patient," *Hospital Practice* 13, no. 3 (1978): 99–106; and Butler, "Ageism," p. 67.
19. U.S. Department of Health and Human Services, "Final Report," p. 112.
20. Neugarten, "Older People," p. 44.
21. U.S. Department of Health and Human Services, "Final Report," p. 9.
22. Neugarten, "Older People," p. 50.
23. Erdman Palmore and George L. Maddox, "Sociological Aspects of Aging," in E. W. Busse and E. Pfeiffer, eds., *Behavior and Adaptation in Later Life,* 2d ed. (Boston: Little, Brown, 1977), p. 44.
24. Erdman Palmore, "The Social Factors in Aging," in Busse and Blazer, *Handbook of Geriatric Psychiatry,* p. 231.
25. Robert N. Butler, "Sex after 65," in L. E. Brown and E. O. Ellis, eds., *Quality of Life* (Acton, Mass: Publishing Sciences Group, 1975), pp. 129–143.
26. Palmore, "Facts on Aging," p. 317.
27. Jack Botwinick, *Aging and Behavior* (New York: Springer Publishing, 1978), p. 97.
28. Palmore and Maddox, "Sociological Aspects of Aging," p. 42; and U.S. Dept. of Health and Human Services, "Final Report," p. 21.
29. Palmore, "Social Factors," p. 228–229.
30. Ibid.
31. Jack Botwinick, "Psychological Aspects of Aging" (Paper presented at the Fifth Annual Conference of *SAGE,* Buffalo, New York, October 1977).
32. U.S. Department of Health and Human Services, *Health: United States and Prevention Profile* (Hyattsville, Md.: Public Health Service, National Center for Health Statistics, DHHS Publication no. 84–1232, 1983), p. 157.
33. Ibid., p. 166.
34. U. S. Department of Health and Human Services, Summary of Committee Number 4, The 1981 White House Conference on Aging "Promotion and Maintenance of Wellness," (Washington, D.C.: USGPO, 1981), p. 100.

2

Biological and Psychosocial Aspects of Aging: Implications for Health and Fitness

OVERVIEW

Most biological and psychosocial changes in aging occur slowly over a period that begins after growth has been attained and continues its irreversible path of normal decline into the 70s and 80s with astonishing variations in degree and rate among people. Rates of aging are the product of the genetic background, environmental milieu, and personal lifestyle of the individual. Research has yet to define clearly the exact relationship of each of these elements to longevity or the state of functionality we label "quality of life."

Why do certain persons who defy accepted principles of good nutrition, or engage in lifestyles contrary to logical and sound practices, live longer and with fewer disabilities than those who follow the rules of healthful living? Part of the answer lies in the unique genetic makeup of each individual, which responds homeostatically (processes through which internal bodily equilibrium is maintained) according to the person's own inherited blueprint. In addition, however, environmental influences account for many of the structural, physiological, and mental patterns found among older persons.

Although senescence is a universal phenomenon, no single theory fully accounts for human differences that manifest themselves in the process of growing old. The following presentation discusses several well-known biological and psychosocial theories, and related topics that attempt to demystify the process of aging.

BIOLOGICAL THEORIES OF AGING

There are many theories of aging. Some are ancient, others are of recent vintage. The idea that the body simply "wears out," for example, can be traced to the time of Aristotle.[1] Newer biological theories include the notion that aging is caused by the formation of free radicals that alter the molecular structure and function of body cells. Others hypothesize that we lose our natural immunities as we age, and antibodies develop that react with normal cells in the body and destroy them. And other contemporary proposals advance cross-linking, stress, and cellular error theories.

Certain theories focus on the microscopic level (cellular), others deal with macroscopic research (at the organism level).

Why do human females live longer than males? Shock contends that since the primary factor that determines sex is the presence of XY chromosomes in males and XX chromosomes in females, the difference in longevity is due to the greater amount of X chromatin in females. He further believes that: (1) a genetic program sets the upper limits of life span in a species; (2) there is some familial characteristic that influences differences in life span among individuals of a single species; and (3) the expression of the basic genetic program can be altered by environmental factors.[2]

It is rational to conclude that longevity in the human species is determined by the interplay of one's personal genetic program (internal forces) and environment (external forces). The aging phenomenon thus begins with the genetic molecule that alters the function of the cell, eventually manifesting its effects at the organismic level.

Free Radical Theory

Free radicals are chemical elements produced during the metabolic processes, which are highly reactive and disruptive at the cellular level. Although they are ubiquitous in living substances, their highest concentration is found in the cytoplasm of cells (mitochondria), which contain the site of energy (adenosine triphosphate, ATP), and the extranuclear source of deoxyribonucleic acid (DNA).

In addition, free radicals are produced by external exposure to radiation and chemical toxins such as ozones and hydrogen peroxide. It is believed that excessive free radicals are damaging to DNA membrane, and that they play a role in the cross-linking of collagen. Damage to the DNA may alter the cell's ability to synthesize the proteins necessary to run the chemical machinery (enzymes) or to maintain its basic structure.

It is also theorized that free radicals generate the production of aging pigments, especially in the neurons, and myocardium (muscle tissue of the heart).[3] Proponents of the free radical theory, then, believe that degrading changes in connective tissue, skin, heart function, neurons, and musculo-skeletal characteristics all are due to DNA alterations or mutations brought about by the radical substances formed within the cell.

Wear-and-Tear Theory

This theory explains the aging process at the macroscopic or organismic level. It is based on the assumption that living organisms work as machines do; i.e., parts wear out with continued use and finally stop functioning.

All theories based upon "wear and tear" in neurons or other cells postulate a similar sequence: loss of regeneration power followed by me-chanical or chemical exhaustion.[4] Exponents of these theories believe that lowering the rate of metabolism delays the anatomical and physiological consequences of aging.

Shock questions the man-machine analogy, indicating that unlike ma-chines, which cannot repair themselves, living organisms have many mecha-nisms that permit self-repair.[5] For example, in tissues such as the skin, the lining of the gastrointestinal tract, and red blood cells, new cells are continu-ously formed to replace old ones.

Rate-of-living theorists point to small animals such as the rat and mouse that have relatively short life spans and high metabolic rates compared to larger animals such as the horse and man, which manifest the opposite—lower metabolism and longer lives.

While the concept of "taking it easy" is simplistic, aspects of the wear-and-tear theory probably have some merit. However, more than one theory is required to explain the many specific losses that are part of the aging process.

Cross-Linking (Collagen) Theory

Tissues contain a tough fibrous protein called *collagen* that holds cells to-gether (see Chapter 3). Collagen tends to become stiffer with age. The ten-dons and joints of the aged appear to be dry. For developing humans, the body water content in bone is about 60 percent; for old bone, it has dimin-ished to about 10 percent.[6]

Collagen appears to replace the water content of bones and also to deposit itself in a changed form within the blood vessels, neurons, and heart through a molecular process producing *cross-links* with DNA strands so that they no longer function in a normal fashion. Cross-links develop between the intertwined and adjacent strands of the collagen molecule. Such linkages result in loss of fibril flexibility, the permeability of material into and out of the blood vessels necessary for the functioning of surrounding tissues and organs. Arteries may become stiff, and passage of gases, nutrients, antibodies, and other life-sustaining chemicals is diminished.

Researchers who study the aging process have noted the similarities between the aged human skin and tanned leather. Chemical tanning of leather is actually a cross-linking of cells, which become bound to their neighbors—suggesting an analogy between tanning chemicals and the aging protein of skin.[7] Cross-linkage theorists believe that the life processes slow down with aging, and that retarding cross-linkage molecular formation may extend longevity. Some experiments show that caloric restriction in rats prolongs life, and delays the increase in collagen cross-linkage, but the causal sequence is not known.[8]

The cross-linking theory continues to be tested with various drugs aimed at slowing the collagen aging process. Although the theory may be viable, it remains hypothetical at this time.

Autoimmune Theory

Simply stated, the autoimmune theory of aging assumes that senescence results from a decline in the body's immune system. Antibodies develop that react with normal cells and destroy their structure and function.

Shock suggests that this condition may occur because of the failure of the new antibodies to recognize normal cells as normal, or the development of errors in the formation of antibodies so that they react against normal cells as well as the deviate ones.[9] The theory proposes that such diseases as maturity-onset diabetes, arteritis, rheumatoid arthritis, certain types of anemia, and certain cancers are a result of age-related cell changes that produce deviate antibodies. Most research about immune function decline has been with laboratory animals. However, several human population studies completed in Australia showed the presence of an autoantibody associated with cancer and vascular disease.[10]

While connections between certain age-related infections and diseases do exist, the evidence has yet to prove the causal relationship between the autoimmunity theory and the normal consequences or pathogenesis of aging.

Genetic Mutation Theory

According to this theory, somatic cells undergo mutational changes and accelerate aging. The somatic mutationist proclaims that the genetic structure of the cells in the chromosomes are damaged, allowing a possible synthesis of the wrong proteins and formation of mutated cells.[11]

Mutagenic agents are thought to damage the orderly process of cell function, ultimately resulting in the inability of the cell to manufacture essential enzymes necessary for maintaining cell life. The somatic mutation premise was developed through cancer research involving radiation when it was observed that radiation increased the mutation rate in rats and mice.[12] The mutation theory advances the position that radiation hastens cell mutation, thus speeding up the aging process. The evidence surrounding somatic mutation as a cause of aging is ambiguous. Scientific explanations of how and why mutants occur remain unresolved.

Cellular Error Theory

In general, the error theory of aging—which focuses on the cellular level— assumes that senescence and cell death result from errors that may happen at any step in the sequence of information transfer, resulting in the formation of a protein or enzyme that is not an exact copy, and, therefore, is unable to carry out its function properly.[13]

Orgel expanded on the error cellular theory, indicating that even infrequent errors in transcription of DNA would produce imperfect RNA molecules, any of which sequentially would code many faulty enzymes and other proteins. These proteins are thought to accumulate rapidly in the cell, imperil its function, and progressively lead to an "error catastrophe" producing age changes and death.[14]

The Orgel error theory expresses the concept that aging is due to faulty protein-forming mechanisms at the genetic level. Theories involving enzymes, protein alterations, and synthesis continue to be examined. Orgel's work serves as a base of information from which other investigations can be pursued.

The biological theories presented here represent a selection from many probable hypotheses, each of which contains various elements of merit. However, aging is neither strictly genetic nor exclusively environmental. The interplay of intrinsic and extrinsic forces profoundly affects the rate of human aging.

The possibility of one single theory to explain multiple anatomical, physiological, and psychological changes is improbable. Rather, an integrated assortment of biological, psychological and social theorems collectively interacting must be considered to explain the diverse nature of the senescence phenomena.

PSYCHOSOCIAL THEORIES OF AGING

Biological theories lean toward genetics and heredity. The psychosocial theories are premised, to a large extent, upon the factors of personality, temperament (which may, in part, be inherited), and the environmental milieu of the individual. It is probably more realistic at the present time to consider modifying personality and behavior than manipulating an individual's normal original blueprint or hereditary base. A central concept promulgated throughout this book subscribes to the premise that older adults are not a homogeneous group, but that heterogeneity is the rule, rather than the exception, both biologically and behaviorally. When expressing theoretical constructs and models, attention must be given to interpretations and generalizations about the merits or demerits of any single psychosocial approach because of the esoteric mix of each person's personality, experiences, and environmental background. Such factors are influenced by other variables, including health, economic status, level of intelligence, cognitive understanding, spiritual and religious persuasion, and education. This list is not exhaustive or exclusive, but typifies the array of factors that affect the basic tenets of behavioral and social theories.

The following perspectives represent three contemporary attempts to explain the psychosocial behavior of aging adults and their interactions with society.

Activity Theory

The central thesis of the activity theory is that successful aging requires a certain threshold of activity participation. Specifically, activity theorists hold that: (1) the majority of normal aging persons maintain certain levels of activity and engagements; (2) the amount of engagement or disengagement is more influenced by past lifestyles and socioeconomic forces than by any intrinsic inevitable process; and (3) maintaining or developing substantial levels of physical, mental, and social activity is usually necessary for successful aging.[15]

The terms *successful aging* and *activity* lend themselves to different interpretations, depending upon one's philosophical orientation. For purposes of our discussion, the person who is successfully aging is one who has achieved the minimum of actuarially based standard of chronological age, still possesses the abilities necessary for everyday living and leisure activities, and manifests a reasonable level of satisfaction and contentment.

Activity is viewed in its broadest sense: engagement in all types of experiences including individual or group activities and physical, mental, and social expressions. Peppers established a set of leisure types that lend themselves to the key concepts that may be applied to the activity theory:

1. *Active-social*—activities that require considerable physical effort and normally take place in a group (e.g., team sports).

2. *Active-isolate*—activities that require considerable physical effort and are normally performed by one person (e.g., jogging).
3. *Sedentary-social*—activities that require little physical effort and are normally performed in groups (e.g., bingo).
4. *Sedentary-isolate*—activities that require little physical effort and are normally performed by one person (e.g., reading).[16]

The optimum older adult, according to the activity theory, stays in the mainstream of economic, social, and cultural life, rather than withdrawing from environmental mores, stresses, and pressures. Perhaps the greatest threat to successful aging is gross engagement in sedentary-isolate type of activities, along with the complete avoidance of other forms of activities described by Peppers. The reader will quickly discover from the subsequent chapters of this text that gross inactivity and isolation lead to an inevitable breakdown of health and fitness of the human organism. Simply stated, "What you do not use—you lose." This concept is not new, and has been discussed since the Renaissance period of da Vinci.

Activities in which older persons engage are as varied as the individuals. Essentially, a selected activity should not be evaluated in terms of the activity itself, but in relationship to *what* and *how* the activity contributes to mental, emotional, and well-being of the participant. For example, playing cards may be one person's pleasure and another's boredom. Personality, interests, skill proficiency, and past experiences play a vital role in the selection and degree of activity participation by senior adults.

Although the selection of activity engagement is very personal, and should remain so, exclusive participation in passive individual or social experiences is incongruent with the mind/body needs of retaining good health, vigor, and vitality. Activity theorists generally recognize that involvement in physical motor activities on a regular basis is a central element of the activity theory model.

Palmore conducted a longitudinal predictive study of successful aging involving 155 persons, including males and females, both white and black, from ages 60 to 94. He found that two of the strongest predictors among men and women for successful aging were the physical function rating and happiness; and he concluded that individuals who engage in more physical activity are more likely to age successfully.[17]

Another study by Decarlo et al., involving 56 identical and fraternal subjects of both sexes from ages 79 to 91, showed that recreative activity involving motor, cognitive, and affective domains can satisfy physical health, mental health, and intellectual performance used as criteria for successful aging.[18]

An interesting review of age changes by Bortz calls attention to the striking similarity of biologic and cognitive decrements attributed to enforced physical inactivity and aging.[19] For example, the physiology of rest and weightlessness revealed by space medicine research demonstrated: (1) decreased sense of balance; (2) loss of red and white blood cell production; (3) loss of lean body mass and relative increase in body fat; (4) loss of calcium; and (5) increased levels of hormonal secretions (renin and aldosterone) associated with high blood pressure.

These changes were found among both young and older populations subjected to prolonged rest and inactivity. Bortz believes that at least some of the changes commonly attributed to aging are in reality caused by disuse; and he proclaims: "There is no drug in current or prospective use that holds as much promise for sustained health as a lifetime of physical exercise."[20] His research evidence, as well as that of others such as Maddox, and Lemon et al., lends credence to the view that older people should remain active as long as possible.[21]

Disengagement Theory

The disengagement view of aging was introduced in 1961, and in its extreme form incorporates the following principles: (1) the course of withdrawal from society is a typical and normal process between the aging adult and society; (2) the process is biologically and psychologically inherent and inevitable to the older adult; and (3) the disengagement mode is related to successful aging in the social system.[22] The withdrawal process is perceived as mutually satisfying to society and the individual because it allows the older adult release from societal pressures and permits younger persons who are more energetic to assume functional roles in a natural and orderly manner.

Gulbrium accents three defining characteristics of the disengagement view, which open the theory to criticism: mutuality, inevitability, and universality.[23] He questions each of these characteristics as standards or normative forms of behavior. First, retreating from society may or may not be mutually satisfying to both parties. Second, disengagement can be a matter of degree; for example, involvement with clubs, colleagues, or former employees may be replaced by social interactions with a smaller circle of family and friends. Third, disengagement is not universal; for example, satisfaction, good health, and longevity in Turkey are associated with high rates of physical and social engagement.[24] Most older people continue to participate in normal social and community affairs. Failure to account for the individuality of personality and the influence of cultural mores among people is a prime weakness of the disengagement theory. Complete withdrawal to a disengaged lifestyle is not inevitable or universal in our society. Thus, the disengagement perspective, in its extreme form, does not hold up as a model for producing the most agreeable psychological climate for older people.[25]

The consequences of disengagement when applied to physical inactivity is cogently expressed by Dr. Raymond Harris, geriatric physician and cardiologist:

> Physically inactive people past 50 perceive their bodies to be broader and heavier than they really are and they experience bodily activities as increasingly strenuous. Kinesthetic pleasures which young people derive from motor action are steadily reduced in habitually sedentary elderly subjects who eventually become reluctant to move at all. Inactive older people develop increased internal tensions and pent-up aggressions. Group exercise programs at all ages assist people to acquire new friends, new interests, and lead to better mental and physical health. The rationale of exercise and activity programs in geriatric day-care centers is based upon helping older people to rejoin society and thereby feel better mentally and physically. Ludotherapy (treatment by games) is useful to help the aged person who exhibits a tendency to disengage from the world and society.[26]

The disengagement theory as first proposed was later modified by Havighurst et al.[27] Disengagement was redefined as simply a process rather than a theorem of optional development, and as only one of many possible patterns of aging.

Four major personality types were identified: integrated, defended, passive-dependent, and disintegrated. Integrated personalities exhibit characteristics of successful aging, whereas disintegrated seniors are disorganized and show gross defects in thought processes.

Defended types are persons who are "armored," or "defended." These individuals are striving, ambitious, and achievement-oriented persons, who tend to drive themselves hard, as exemplified in the "holding-on pattern" ("I'll work until I drop!") and the "constricted sub-type," who defends himself or herself against aging, becoming preoccupied with losses and deficits. These personalities constrict their social interactions and shut out new experiences, taking few risks.

Passive-dependents are persons with strong dependency needs. Some function fairly well with the support of others, while others arrive at the "apathetic" stage, where life exhibits very few activities and social interactions.

Integrated personalities were also identified among the disengaged patterns, but with some activity present. These individuals tend to move away from organized societal role commitments, but to hold on to a relaxed life at home with family and some gardening and housework. Thus, the modified disengagement view was altered to account for personality differences and the concept of voluntary withdrawal, and to allow for some physical activity and social interaction at a low level of performance.

Continuity Theory

Another psychosocial view holds that maturity into old age is a phenomenon of continuity. The continuity theory advances the concept that the individual clings to habits, preferences, and dispositions that have been developing throughout the various stages of life development. In other words, rather than changing their lifestyles from one course to another, people show a consistent pattern of behaving, responding, and adjusting throughout the lifespan.

Vander Zyle reports several studies that suggest that the older person's behavioral adaptation can evolve in different directions, depending upon the individual's personality and developmental experiences:

- People become more like themselves as they age.
- Continuing life patterns and styles are measured in relation to each individual's own baseline behavior.
- Patterns of overt behavior are likely to become increasingly consonant with the individual's needs and desires.
- Aging does not destroy continuities between what a person has been—what is—and what will be as the individual grows to old age.[28]

The continuity theory proposes that the key to successful aging may be found in the person's past, which will determine what kind of physical, motor, and psychological characteristics are brought into old age; how well previous adjustment has been made will strongly influence (positively or negatively) adult maturity.

The continuity perspective has certain implications for program organizers in senior centers and health care facilities. Physical, mental, and social activities should be planned with due recognition of the diversity of personalities and backgrounds that affect motivations, desires, and activity interests of participants. Chapters 5 and 6 offer specific design and content protocols, using basic principles of continuity for maintaining fitness in senior centers and health-related facilities.

FUNCTIONAL AGE CHANGES

This section examines the anatomical, physiological, mental, and emotional changes that occur in most people past 50. Although cognitive and motor performance operate psychosomatically, affecting the mind and body as an integrated unit, we have organized our presentation under the broad categories of anatomical/physiological changes and mental/emotional/cognitive changes.

Anatomical/Physiological Changes

Intrinsic and extrinsic forces constantly act upon mental and physiological systems, slowly resulting in a subtle decline in human efficiency. However, the degree and rate of losses are diverse within and among people.

Intrinsic forces are those alterations that are typically age-specific and originate from some internal deviation within the body. Extrinsic forces are changes caused by external environmental conditions such as disease, toxic exposure, or physical and emotional trauma. Frequently, internal and external forces operate concurrently. For example, some older adults under multiple medications may lose their appetite because of simultaneous taste bud losses (intrinsic) and drug ingestion (extrinsic), which can result in malnutrition and the hastening of physical and mental dysfunctions. The following section presents a descriptive analysis of primary biological age changes that emanate from internal and external causes at the tissue and organ level.

Aging Skin. The skin is the largest organ of the body—and the most visible in detecting age changes, with facial wrinkling recognizable in the second decade in most individuals.[29]

Since skin is so visible, it has considerable psychologic and social value, as well as physiologic significance. Skin serves as a protective organ between the individual and environment, providing body defenses against extreme temperatures, injury, ultraviolet radiation, chemicals, bacteria, and other foreign pathogens. It also is a sensitive tactile organ, through which individuals receive pleasurable stimuli, pain, and initial activation of proprioception, which is related to balance and equilibrium (see Chapter 3). It should be remembered that not all skin dysfunctions associated with aging are caused by longevity alone. Skin that is continually exposed to sunlight wrinkles faster, and, in some cases, such overexposure triggers squamous cell carcinoma (skin cancer).

Each of the vital functions, e.g., protection, touch sensations, and temperature acuity, diminish with advancing age. Major appearance changes include dryness, wrinkling, uneven pigmentation, thinning, and loss of elasticity and plasticity. Such conditions follow normal morphological changes in the epidermis (outer skin layer) and dermis (inner skin layer).

The epidermis is composed of three layers: the deepest germ layer where new cells are produced; the actively growing layer that is nearest the surface, and the outermost layer where old discarded cells form a protective defense against the hazards of environment (see Figure 2.1). The dermis lies beneath the epidermis and contains the hair follicles, nerve endings, blood vessels, fat cells, and sweat and oil-producing sebaceous glands. As one ages, the sweat glands decrease in size, number, and function, thereby causing increased skin dryness, which is usually pronounced on the lower legs

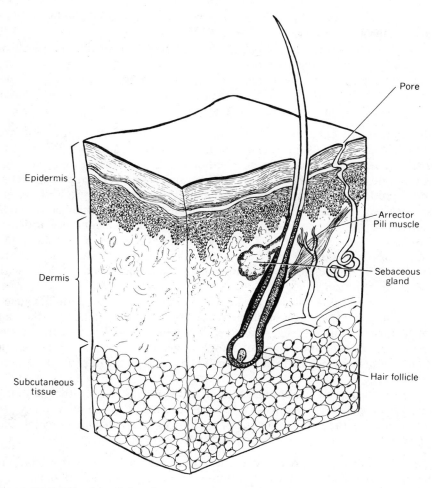

Figure 2.1 Epidermis and dermis.

and is aggravated by a low-humidity environment. Wrinkling normally occurs with use—that is, habitual frowning or smiling and various facial expressions tend to accent furrows. Loss of elastin fibers within skin collagen
and the cross-linkage process of the fibers themselves add to ''sagging'' and
inelasticity of old skin. Uneven pigmentation can be caused by internal or
external causes, such as diabetes, malnutrition, liver disease, vascular and
metabolic disorders, neurological diseases, and heredity. Often irregularities

in skin coloring can be linked to normal skin changes or to a combination of natural alterations and disease states.

The thinning of the skin is largely due to a reduction of subcutaneous fat (storage fat). This change is most marked in the extremities, and especially in men, in whom skinfold thickness averages 1.2 cm. from age 25 to 29; 1 cm. from age 65 to 79; and 0.9 cm. over 80 years. In women, the change is not as great, decreasing only from 1.5 cm. at ages 25 to 39 to 1.4 cm. over age 50.[30]

Hair. Age-related changes in hair color, density, and body distribution are diverse. While each of these characteristics is largely a matter of heredity, general patterns of change occur within the genetic framework of both sexes. For example, some hair loss and thinning is universal beginning in the middle and later years, and a progressive loss of hair appears in both sexes. Men lose more from the scalp than do women, and axillary hair often tends to disappear among females. Racial factors are also significant in hair distribution, color, and density. In Japanese women who are ten or more years postmenopausal, axillary hair has virtually disappeared.[31] Such changes are thought to be associated with diminished endocrine function along with genetic constitution.

Graying hair is a normal consequence of aging for most people, caused by the diminished function of pigment cells (melanin production) in the hair root within the hair follicle. Again, as with hair loss, graying of the hair is variable, contingent upon genetic factors, racial differences, and presence or absence of disease (which in certain instances hastens the decline of melanin production).

In Caucasian men, although scalp hair decreases, hair in the ears may increase. In some cases, male hormones produced by aging women are responsible for their development of facial hair. Such hair is cosmetically undesirable but can be safely removed under proper medical supervision.

Nails. The rate of nail growth decreases over the life span, with variations between males and females and differences among digits of the hand. In a study of thumbnail growth, an average decline was found from 0.83 mm/week among subjects in their 30s to 0.52 mm/week in the ninth decade—a 38 percent decrease.[32]

The rate of linear nail growth of males is greater than females up to about age 60, but thereafter growth is reversed. The nail of the middle finger grows faster than the thumbnail. External factors, such as environmental temperature (nails grow faster in November than in July), nail biting, and poor nutrition, and internal influences of hormonal efficiency and circulatory changes also can affect nail growth. The appearance of the nails, as well as growth rate, changes during advanced years. They become opaque and yellowish, ridged longitudinally, and likely to split. Decreased circulation, particularly in the toenails, may lead to thickening rather than thinning. Nail brittleness may occur, especially among persons with arthritic joints.

Aging Kidneys and Bladder. The primary function of the kidneys and bladder is to maintain a constant alkalinity and chemical composition of the blood by removing blood waste products and excesses in water and salt through the urine. The kidneys provide physiologic mechanisms for excreting most of the end products of bodily metabolism. The bladder serves as the receptacle for the accumulation of urine until it empties itself through the urethra by the detrussor muscles, triggered by the micturition reflex—whereby voluntary control is learned.

The length of the female urethra is 2 to 3 cm. (1 inch) long, in close relation with the front wall of the vagina, into the vestibule of which it opens.[33] The male urethra is considerably longer (see Figure 2.2). This anatomic difference accounts, in part, for immediate need in micturation among females, particularly older women with weakened detrussor and sphincter muscles (see the section in Chapter 6 on Kegel exercises).

Aging kidneys are characterized by anatomical changes and decreased function. In youth, each kidney contains about one million nephrons. These unit structures are reduced in number by one-half to two-thirds by 75 years of age.[34] Renal blood flow is slowed to approximately one-half its rate, from 1200 ml. per minute to 600 ml. per minute. Such changes signal a slowing down of the kidneys' ability to remove waste and regulate body water and salt, as well as filtering out and returning important nutrients to the bloodstream.

The kidney is also an endocrine organ and produces important hormones, one of which is renin—a blood pressure regulator. Other hormones produced by the renal organ are aldosterone and erythropoietin. These hormones are associated with regulation of salt balance and hemoglobin in the blood cells.

In addition to the normal losses of kidney mass and function that accompany aging, specific problems may further impair the ability of the kidneys to regulate waste removal or salt and water balance. Disorders frequently found in elders include hypertension, vascular disease, and diabetes.

Each of these conditions is described with considerable detail in Chapters 4 and 7. In brief, uncontrolled hypertension damages the kidney and impedes its ability to filter out body poisons and sustain salt/water equilibrium. Atherosclerosis and arteriosclerosis are two major types of vascular diseases that affect the oxygen-carrying vessels to the kidneys. Such sclerotic changes in blood vessels further decrease renal function and may result in body swelling, or edema, as well as an increase in blood pressure by

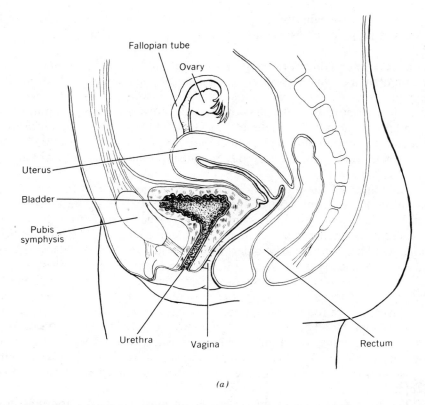

(a)

Figure 2.2 (a) Pelvic organs and relationship of urethra and bladder in the female; (b) Pelvic organs and relationship of urethra and bladder in the male.

the production of renin. Diabetes accelerates vascular disease, and when it affects the circulation of the kidneys, the results are essentially similar to hypertension and atherosclerotic changes in the blood vessels.

Notwithstanding the normal changes that slow kidney and bladder functions, adequate performance may continue well into old age with minimum discomfort (barring serious diseases) when prudent attention to proper nutrition, exercise, and lifestyle is pursued.

Gastrointestinal System Changes. Internal changes in the gastrointestinal system represent a major factor affecting the nutritional status of the senior adult. The discussion here focuses upon the principal changes in the mouth, esophagus, stomach, and alimentary tract that affect the absorption and assimilation of nutrients by the body.

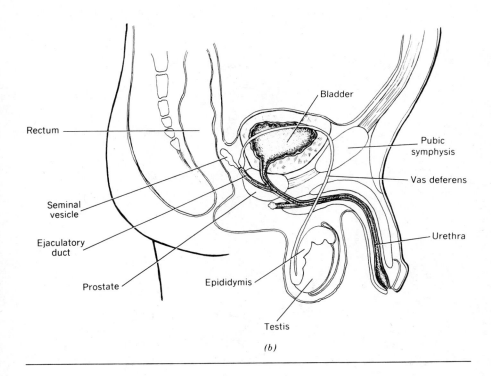

(b)

The gastrointestinal tract and process (see Figure 2.3) begins with the mouth, with chewing, swallowing, and dissolution of food through the esophagus, stomach, and small, and large intestines, and finally, excesses of nondigestible foodstuffs eliminated through the anal canal and rectum.

The number of taste buds declines with age, usually by 40 to 45 in women and 50 to 60 in men.[35] Sour and bitter are usually detected on the palate, whereas the tongue is more acute in detecting sweet and salt. Acuity of each taste sensation gradually declines, with pronounced decrements after 70.

Old persons wearing upper dentures have diminished taste sensitivity for sour or bitter, but greater perceptions for sweet and salt. Thus, they may increase their use of condiments and salt, which, in turn, may exacerbate general health by contributing to obesity and hypertension.

The sense of smell also becomes less keen with advanced age. Together with loss of taste acuity, reduction in saliva may occur, since this secretion is stimulated by flavor and taste perception. However, losses in taste and olfactory acuity vary significantly among seniors, and perceptions may remain stable in some individuals throughout the life span.

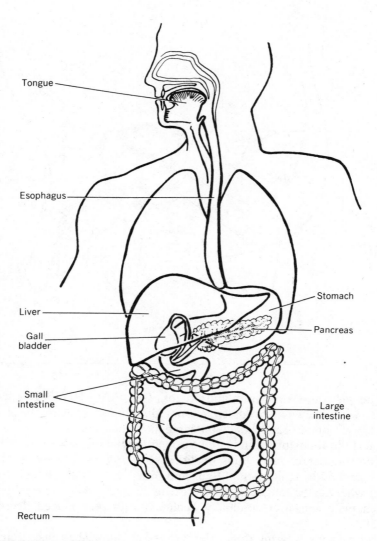

Figure 2.3 Gastrointestinal tract.

The teeth provide the important mechanical function of chewing, which is the first stage of digestion. As food is chewed, it is mixed with saliva, which contains the enzyme ptyalin necessary for starch digestion. More than 50 percent of persons at age 65 have no teeth.[36] Consequently, edentulous elderly are prone to chewing and swallowing difficulties. Dentures are used by many older persons, but their effectiveness is much less than that of natural teeth.

Motility of the gastrointestinal tract decreases with age. The action of swallowing (peristalsis) slows, with an increase in nonpropulsive contractions of the esophagus.[37] The stomach, too, declines in efficiency to some extent, failing to produce adequate hydrocholoric acid, which can result in decreased absorption of iron and vitamin B_{12}. Aging of the small intestine is reflected by reduction of gut mass and weakening of muscle fibers.

Secretion of the enzymes of the pancreas, trypsin and amylase, also declines and affects regular absorption of amino acids and monosaccharides. Calcium and lipids are less readily absorbed in the small intestine. These changes in salivary, stomach, and intestinal secretions often lead to gastritis; however, such abdominal inflammation may be caused by assorted pathologies and infections of the intestinal tract, not solely by the aging process.

The large intestine contains the colon, which extends from the cecum to the rectum and functions as a receptacle of the small intestinal contents. It absorbs water, sodium, and chloride and secretes potassium, bicarbonate, and mucus.[38]

Three common gastrointestinal conditions that frequently occur among senior adults—hiatal hernia, diverticulitis, and constipation—interfere with the normal functioning of the alimentary canal and cause considerable discomfort.

Hiatal Hernia. The occurrence of hiatal hernia increases with age. It often appears after age 50, and has been reported in 67 percent of persons over 60; it is more common in women.[39] Hiatal hernia is a protrusion of the stomach into the chest cavity through a hole in the diaphragm. Heartburn, difficulty in swallowing, flatulence, abdominal pain, and chest distress may accompany the disorder, which can be eased by relief of intraabdominal pressure of tight clothing, avoiding lifting and straining, and, in the case of obesity, weight reduction.

Diverticulitis. Colonic diverticulitis is characterized by an inflammation of small pouches protruding from the intestinal wall. These small pouches (diverticula) result after years of constipation, which weaken the bowel wall and form sacs. When the diverticula become inflamed, infected, or blocked, diverticulitis develops. Pain, bloating, and vomiting may occur; severe bleeding from the rectum and fever may appear in complicated cases. Medication and diet usually relieve episodal attacks. Maintaining adequate muscle tone of the abdominal muscles, particularly of the compressor muscle (transverse abdominis), helps to relieve constipation, and subsequently results in less strain upon the diverticula.

Constipation. The notion that the bowels must move every day is common among older persons. Subsequently, they often overuse laxatives, which may lead to adverse effects, including further sluggishness of the bowels. First and foremost, the idea that daily bowel action is not necessary should be emphasized among older adults. Bowel action every two or three days may be normal for certain persons, depending upon individual metabolic makeup and behavioral characteristics.

Adherence to proper food intake is also essential for the avoidance of constipation. The adequate intake of bran and fluids should be stressed. Fiber adds bulk to the diet. The increased bulk greatly speeds up transit through the digestive tract—in one study, transit time decreased from 48 to 12 hours when the subjects switched from a low- to a high-fiber diet.[40]

It also is important to educate the elderly about the decline of the thirst mechanism with aging, which may result in insufficient fluid intake. Adequate water in the system is important for the prevention of fecal impaction. Diet should include wheat bran, cereals, grains, vegetables, and fruits with edible skins, all rich sources of fiber. In general, one should ingest enough water each day to produce about one liter or more of urine per 24 hours.[41] Older persons under multiple medications are especially prone to dehydration and may require additional fluid intake.

Physical inactivity and loss of muscle tone affect the regularity of bowel movement. As indicated earlier, the transverse abdominis is primarily responsible for voluntary expiration and expulsive movement necessary for defecation. Exercises that increase the rate of respiration, such as brisk walking or jogging, activate the transversus by triggering the body's need for ventilation. Sit-up exercises, with deliberate expiration at the end of the effort, are excellent for improving the strength of this compression and expulsion muscle. Counting aloud at the end of the upward movement of the sit-up (concentric contraction) and at the end of the return to the supine starting posture (eccentric contraction) is an effective technique of tracking the contraction sensations while exercising. (See Chapter 5 for further details of the sit-up exercise.)

Aging and the Endocrine System. The endocrine system is a highly complex, interrelated network that produces secretions called *hormones*. These hormones are released into the blood stream and affect bodily functions including growth patterns, sexual characteristics, metabolism, water balance, immune responses, glucose tolerance, and neural reactions. The following discussion examines the general endocrine changes, with reference to exercise and fitness, in the mature years.

Contemporary research in the area of exercise has focused upon the body's response to the release of endorphins and its effect upon the psyche, and on the regulatory effect of exercise upon glucose tolerance. Appropriate exercise, along with diet and insulin protocols, is generally accepted as an important modality in the management of diabetes—a common disorder in the elderly. Although the data is not conclusive concerning the positive hormonal relationships of exercise, relaxation, and the pituitary gland, the phenomenon of the "runner's high" does indeed exist.

Two of the most conspicuous hormonal age changes involve the reduction of the production of *estrogen* in females and loss of *testosterone* in males. Estrogen declines with a reduction in ovary size, function, and loss of reproductive capacity after the fifth decade. Estrogen loss is associated with breast involution, adipose skin, bone changes, and menopause. Testosterone reduction in men is a slow and gradual process, less abrupt than estrogen loss in post-menopausal women.

Adrenal hormone studies show that the secretion rate of the steroid hormone *cortisol* is diminished; however, adrenals may continue to function adequately into later life. Cortisol promotes the formation of glucose by the breakdown of glycogen, plays a role in fat-water metabolism, and affects muscle tone. Such functions of cortisol continue effectively into advanced years in the healthy elderly.

Aldosterone is produced by the adrenals and is a principal electrolyte-regulating steroid. Aldosterone secretion is lower in elderly individuals. This hormone, together with the renin adrenal vasopressor mechanism, controls sodium, water, and potassium balance. The efficacy of these adrenal-regulating mechanisms may be further impaired in older hypertensive persons on diuretic and potassium medications.

The thyroid gland, lying in the neck just above the chest (see Figure 2.4), secretes the hormone *thyroxin*, which regulates the body's energy level, or metabolic rate. In the elderly, the thyroid gland decreases in size and mass. Such reductions may result in a low manufacture of thyroxin and a condition called hypothyroidism, which is characterized by lethargy, loss of alertness, intolerance to cold, dry skin, and mental and sensory dullness. The overactive thyroid, resulting in hyperthyroidism, produces greater quantities of hormones that cause an increased metabolic rate with weight loss, rapid pulse, and sleeplessness. An overactive gland may be enlarged or of normal size. However, research studies indicate that an enlarged thyroid gland with characteristics of protruding eyeballs is rarely seen in the elderly.[42]

Goiter, an enlargement of the thyroid sometimes accompanied by thyroid deficiency, may occur in older persons. Such swelling is visible to the casual observer, and if the gland is sufficiently enlarged it may cause some difficulty in breathing or swallowing. An overactive or underactive thyroid is usually responsive to medication, which includes thyroid extracts, synthetic hormones, or radioactive iodine (RAI) depending upon the specific syndrome.

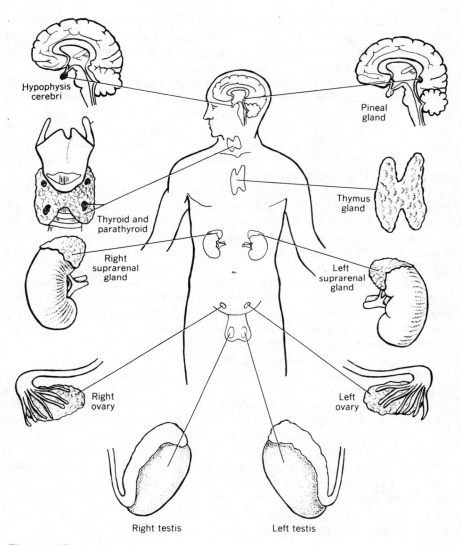

Figure 2.4 Endocrine system.

The nervous, respiratory, and cardiovascular systems also change in their anatomical structural and functional capacities. These changes are discussed in Chapters 3, 4, and 5.

Mental and Emotional Changes

The impression that intelligence, memory, and cognition decline with advanced age is widespread. Such a view may stem from observations of residents in nursing homes, where memory loss and intellectual misunderstandings are common events.

Intelligence and Aging. One problem that arises in relation to intelligence centers around its interpretation. The lexicologic meaning of intelligence refers to "faculty of understanding; capacity to know; intellect, reason, etc."[43] Such a connotation implies the acquisition of knowledge and information, but does not differentiate intelligence into specific components such as its verbal, social, creative and mathematical aspects—nor does the definition consider the *application of knowledge* to solve a particular problem at hand. Thus, when judging intelligence and recognition in an older person, specificity in terms of kinds of intelligence, and what he or she does with acquired information, become exceedingly important. For example, knowing the mathematical elements of the fulcrum, resistance, and force points in a third class lever when lifting a heavy load with a shovel is meaningless, unless the individual can apply the knowledge of gaining leverage by placing the forward hand close to the load, thereby easing the task.

Intelligence is multidimensional, and multiple causes contribute to its development. Some people rely more heavily on personality and social intelligence, others on cognitive and analytical skills to successfully function in everyday living.

Because of individual differences, people tend to become "more themselves" as they grow older, and general standardized intelligence tests designed for youth are inappropriate for persons past 60. A general test that adequately assesses intelligence of older persons has yet to be developed. The shift of our perception of intelligence from a unitary perspective to a multifactor concept adds complexity to its measurement.

An interesting classification of intelligence types was advanced by Cattell in the early sixties.[44] Cattell identified two types of intelligence: fluid and crystallized. Fluid intelligence is the ability to recognize and reorganize one's perceptions, and it is considered to reflect functioning of biological parameters, including neurological and vascular structures. This type of cognitive functioning is thought to increase until adolescent maturity and to decline thereafter. In contrast, crystallized intelligence is largely verbal, conceived in terms of cultural assimilation, and influenced by formal and informal education throughout life. Crystallized intelligence is considered to be more resistant to decline.

Elsayed et al. investigated the effects of a physical fitness program upon 70 university faculty members and businessmen from age 24 to 68 years.[45] The fitness program consisted of three 90-minute sessions each week for four months, involving warmups, jogging, progressive running, and self-selected recreational activities. The results of the study indicated that those who received high fitness scores at the end of a four-month period had a significantly higher total fluid intelligence score than the low-fit group. The investigation further revealed that neither physical condition nor age had any effect on crystallized intelligence. Powell and Pohndorf investigated the relationship between fluid intelligence and exercise, studying 71 adult males between the ages of 34 and 75.[46] they found that in general, better fitness measures accompanied higher fluid intelligence scores. These studies lend credence to the belief that physical fitness may be related to certain kinds of intelligence, particularly of the fluid type, which is based upon physiological structures and performance. The research also provides examples of the complex nature of mental ability. Certain types of intellectual achievement require physical performance and manipulation of objects; others involve verbal, creative, and social skills.

Some investigators believe that decline in intellectual functions may not be seen before ages of 50 or 60, and that even then, the reduction is small, which suggests that people who perform well when young will perform relatively well when old.[47]

The question arises; "Does intelligence decline with age?" A reasonable response would address the specificity notion: "It depends upon what *kind* of intelligence is being assessed." The following notions about aging and intellectual functioning support the specificity concept:

- Verbal and word fluency remain strong in healthy elderly persons.
- Cognitive tests that require speed of response obscure mental powers of older adults.
- Older persons perform better on tests that are meaningful and related to significant activities within their environment.
- Decline may be due not to age, but to cultural and social environment.[48]
- Physical fitness has a positive relationship between reorganization of one's perception (fluid intelligence) and aging.
- Decline with age of many intellectual functions may not be seen before ages 50 or 60, and even then the decline may be small.[49]

Memory and Aging. When a young person forgets the car keys, it is dismissed as a normal event; however, when the same behavior is demonstrated by a senior adult, opinions such as "He is getting old" or "She is senile'' are often expressed. Forgetting one's keys, wallet, or other common everyday items should not always be considered a result of aging. While poor memory is often described as one of the major symptoms of old age, research indicates that only certain aspects of the memory may actually decline with increasing age.[50]

Memory is the capacity of retaining and reviving impressions, or of recalling or recognizing previous experiences. Memory is usually classified into two broad categories: short-term and long-term. A further breakdown includes the following components:

1. *very short-term memory:* information is retained for a second or two.
2. *intermediate short-term memory:* information is retained and recalled for a period from a few seconds to several minutes.
3. *intermediate long-term memory:* information is retained and recalled after one-half hour or up to several days.
4. *old or remote memory:* information involves storage with recall after weeks or years.

Memory loss, excepting pathological brain dysfunctions, depends upon the material involved. For example, memory that requires very little mental processing of information, such as the ability to dial phone numbers or remember letters for a few seconds, seems to be retained well into advanced age. However, the ability to retain information for minutes, hours, or several days appears to lessen. Thus, older persons may find it difficult to remember what they read in yesterday's newspaper or what their recent purchase at the grocery store was, yet information from old or remote memory is usually well recalled. People tend to remember their childhood or specific events in their lives that have happened up to 30 or 40 years earlier. Such recollections of the past often have therapeutic value through the process of reminiscence and life review described by Butler and Lewis.[51] Remembering events of the past allows the older adult to reflect on previous life experiences and offers an opportunity for self-expression, placing daily living into an orderly perspective; it also aids in the task of coping with losses, which usually increase as the life cycle continues.

Other factors also appear to affect memory acuity. For example, people tend to remember what is really important to them, rather than items or events that are insignificant. Meaningful information is more likely to be retained than trivia; however, separating meaningful items and events from trivial things is an enigmatic process among persons of all ages. The following aids are useful in strengthening the memory process of older adults:

- Use visual images and auditory clues when presenting material that is to be retained and recalled.

- Apply sound principles of motivation: people remember what is important in their lives.
- Encourage older persons to talk about past experiences, and listen to them.
- Allow self-pacing and sufficient time for recall of events.
- Stress the importance of proper nutrition and physical fitness in developing memory efficiency.

Personality and Aging. As with younger people, great variability in personality exists among older adults. A single pattern of characteristics typical of the older adult simply does not exist. Aged persons are often branded as "rigid," "crabby," or "inflexible." When valid, such stereotypical descriptions reflect an extension of the person's temperament and personality demonstrated in youth and middle-age years and are not a consequence of aging. Essentially, the safest generalization is that personality remains relatively unchanged throughout the adult life span.[52]

An interesting study by Reichard, Livson, and Peterson classified personalities of older men into five major categories according to their character structure and adjustment to aging: (1) the mature, (2) the rocking-chair, (3) the armored, (4) the angry, and (5) the self-haters.[53] The mature type consists of those who are well integrated and maintain close personal relationships, accepting the strengths and weaknesses of their age. Rocking-chair personalities tend to disengage from the verve of society and are content to disregard most of life's activities. The armored types are those who strongly protect their independence with well-integrated defense mechanisms, and who continue to hold on to their work for as long as possible. The angry ones are those who are bitter about life in general and respond aggressively or suspiciously to other people. Finally, the self-haters turn their bitterness and hatred inward, with periodic bouts of all-engulfing depression. The mature, rocking-chair, and armored types in the study were seen as well adjusted within the characteristics of their personalities, whereas the angry and self-haters had adjusted poorly. Additionally, the majority of those adjusting poorly had a life-long history of personality problems.[54] It is unknown how well this typology would apply to women; however, it would seem that basic characteristics and adjustments may be similar. Neugarten contends that the element of introversion increases with age during the second half of life.[55] Most studies to date imply that one's basic personality extends itself, with some modification depending upon physical health, background, heredity, culture, religion, etc., into the senior years of life.

Sexuality and Aging

Sexuality, at any age, is a personal and private matter—and because the topic is less open for a number of reasons, including embarrassment, uncomfortableness, and myriad societal negative attitudes (which range from "sex is ridiculous after 60" to "sexual activity hastens wearing out"), a plethora of myths, misunderstandings, and untruths exist about human sexual activity. The development and nurturing of a healthy attitude toward sexuality must be based upon factual information about sexual expression in old age.

A substantial amount of data about sexual interests, biological and psychological changes, and societal attitudes of older persons has been gathered. Evidence supports the premise that sexual interest and expression continue for the majority of persons past 60, but society still holds negative attitudes about sexual activity among the elderly.[56] Yet sexual expression is each individual's personal concern—some are not interested in its pursuit, others desire to continue a lifestyle that includes intimate physical contact. Butler and Lewis cogently express this point of view:

> "[T]hose who have neither a desire for nor an interest in sex, or who have deliberately chosen a lifestyle in which sexuality plays little or no part, have a right to their decision. Each of us is entitled to live the life he or she finds most fulfilling. . . . On the other hand, those older people who enjoy sex deserve encouragement and support as well as necessary information and appropriate treatment if problems arise."[57]

The above view does not seek to impose or prescribe sexual conduct for individuals, but accents the individualistic nature of sexuality, and the individual prerogative of personal choice without social stigma.

The following section presents a summary of normal biological and behavioral sexual changes that occur in later years, and of the role of fitness in the preservation of sexual functioning.

Sexual Interests. Interest in sex does not disappear with age. Those individuals who were not interested in sex in youth most likely continue to show little interest in the matter during their senior years. On the other hand, men and women who enjoyed sexual activity in their youth tend to be sexually active when old.[58]

Studies reveal that frequency of sexual activity does decline in both sexes, more so among women than men. The factors explaining the decline stem from a number of causes. For both men and women, a central determinant of interest is physical health and fitness. Sexual interest and performance is relegated to low priority when acute or significant chronic illness dominates the everyday living environment of senior adults. Decline in sexual interest among women also has been attributed to the factor of widowhood, since males generally die earlier than females, and women are less likely to remarry than men. Also, sexual desire may wane because of hostility, depression, or simple boredom.

Normal Physiological Changes in Older Men. Sexual capacity in men reaches its peak in the late teens and early 20s, with a gradual decline in the 50s, 60s, and beyond. However, changes are slow and subtle without sharp or abrupt biological reversals.

As is true of other physiological parameters, considerable variability exists in sexual capacity among males. Aging men are generally slower to achieve a full erection than younger men, for whom psychological stimulation alone is usually sufficient to cause physical arousal.[59] The ejaculate is also less forceful and abundant past 60. Although slower erection and less ejaculatory power is evidenced in older men, their pleasure is not reduced; in fact, older men may maintain erection longer once achieved, without premature ejaculation, often a problem among younger males. This normal age change thus allows the advantage of longer love making.

Some men falsely believe that slowness of erection and ejaculation is a sign of impotence, but such changes do not mean either reduction in sexual capacity for intercourse or impotency. However, impotency may arise from psychogenic sources such as excessive use of alcohol; work-related or money problems; stress and tension; fatigue; or an unhappy sexual relationship. The solution of such problems through appropriate guidance and counseling will restore the sex drive.

Normal Physiological Changes in Older Women. Menopause signals a subsequent reduction in the production of estrogen. Such a decline may cause a thinning of the vaginal mucosa. Additionally, less lubrication in the vagina may occur, which can irritate the vaginal wall. These physiological changes vary among women, and need not diminish sexual capacity or ability. In fact, little change occurs in regard to a woman's capacity for orgasm into the 70s and 80s. Vaginal lubrication, which is the biological counterpart of male erection, takes longer as the woman ages. Dryness of the vaginal tissues may cause itching or painful intercourse and may trigger infections of the bladder. Vaginal lubricants often relieve dryness and lubrication problems.

Estrogen therapy, although widely used to relieve the symptoms of menopause, is still controversial because of its association with cancer of the uterus. Careful evaluation and prescription by a physician is essential when weighing the possible health risks of estrogen therapy. It should be noted that estrogen is not only produced by the ovaries, but also secreted by the adrenal glands. Thus, these hormones are continuously secreted, although in reduced quantities. There is some indication that regular sexual activity stimulates estrogen production.[60]

Common Illnesses and Sexual Problems. Several illnesses, acute and chronic, have particular effects upon the libido and sexual activities of older persons. As indicated earlier, illness can destroy sexual interest until physical health is at least partly restored.

Many people believe that sexual activity after a heart attack is life-threatening. It is true that a heart attack may temporarily interrupt sexual expression because of a depressive emotional reaction. However, once the heart damage is healed (in about 8 to 14 weeks), there is no physical reason why the cardiac patient should not return to sexual activity, unless the cardiovascular system has been seriously impaired. The energy cost of sexual intercourse is equivalent to that of climbing a flight of stairs; heart rate ranges from 90 to 150 beats per minute, with an average of 120 beats—about the level of light to moderate physical effort.[61] Thus, it is obvious that a basic threshold of physical fitness is required for successful sexual performance.

Diabetes mellitus may cause impotence in men. It is difficult to determine whether its effect on erection capacity is psychogenic, vascular, or neurologically based. Control of the disease through appropriate medication, diet, and exercise is essential for improving diabetes-induced impotency. The effects of diabetes on sexuality of women is not known at the present time.

Chronic prostatitis and prostatectomy also may produce impotence in some men. The prostate gland is a walnut-size structure that is vulnerable to inflammation and enlargement, particularly in men past 55. The incidence of prostatitis increases considerably past 60. Glandular enlargement or inflammation may interfere with nerve impulses that allow blood in and out of the penis, impairing organic erection. Prostatic inflammation usually responds positively to antibiotics; it also is lessened by reduced alcohol intake, ample intake of water, and avoidance of extended periods of sitting (such as long trips in the car).

Removal of the prostate gland may or may not cause impotency. After a prostatectomy, the semen is deposited in the bladder and not ejaculated. Loss of the feeling of masculinity may be experienced by some men, resulting in impotence. Sage pre- and postoperative counseling is effective in restoring sexual desire and capacity. Finkle and Finkle have shown that counseling and encouragement can help individuals recover sexual potency even in the presence of organic disease, including heart attack, diabetes, and prostatitis.[62]

Nor should hysterectomy or removal of the ovaries produce any loss of sexual desire or performance in women. Decline in libido, if any, stems from psychological sources. Some women experience severe emotional disruption after major surgery such as hysterectomy, mastectomy, colostomy, and other operations where body parts are lost. These individuals need reassurance that such procedures need not result in loss of femininity or libido. Emotional support from family, friends and the attending physician is vital in assisting men and women to regain their self-confidence after surgery.

Nonprescription and prescription drugs are frequently used by the elderly. Certain medications can significantly alter sexual desire and capacity.

For example, tranquilizers such as Mellaril may affect the ejaculatory mechanism. Librium, a minor tranquilizer, although used for anxiety reduction, may reduce libido among women. Certain antihypertensive drugs such as Aldomet and Reserpine, through their controlling effect upon the neural system, may decrease sexual interest and cause impotence.

Great variability in drug reactions exists among individuals. Although medications are important for the treatment of many medical problems, each drug user should be well-versed in probable side effects, including sexual consequences. Alcohol often disguises its sedative effect by making people friendly and more talkative. Such behavior may be falsely interpreted as the result of neural stimulation, when, in fact, alcohol lowers judgment and inhibitions by depressing the brain. Thus, while a person may feel initially stimulated, alcohol beyond a moderate amount produces drowsiness and interferes with sexual performance in males and females. Other side effects of alcohol are discussed in Chapter 7.

Fitness and Sexuality. We have indicated that sexual performance among older persons generally requires light to moderate levels of physical exertion. Poor physical fitness can act as an obstacle to sexual activity whenever the energy level is low.

Brisk walking, jogging, bicycling, or swimming are excellent activities for the maintenance of efficient cardiovascular functions for healthy sexual activity. Maintaining good muscle tone and control, especially of those muscle groups surrounding the back, abdominal, and pelvic areas, are particularly important for the improvement of sexual performance. Chapter 5 offers exercises and activities specifically targeted for the enhancement of the upper and lower trunk muscles.

Some older women may develop weakened pelvic muscles surrounding the circumvaginal musculature, particularly the pubococcygeus muscle, which supports the bladder, urethra, and the outer portion of the vagina. A specialized set of exercises, devised by Kegel for urinary stress incontinence, also increases orgasmic responsiveness.[63] Kegel asserts that the weaker a woman's pubococcygeal muscle ability, the higher her sexual dissatisfaction is likely to be. In a study involving anorgasmic females, Kegel found that 78 of the 123 women who completed his exercise program experienced orgasm for the first time.[64] These exercises, which consist of a series of isometric contractions of the pelvic floor muscles, are described in Chapter 6.

Hypochondriasis

The neurosis of hypochondriasis is a gross preoccupation with one's physical and emotional health, accompanied by complaints in the absence of any discernible cause. It is considerably more frequent among women than men and appears to become more frequent with age. The message expressed by a hypochondriacal person is that he or she is sick and needs medical care. Another characteristic of the syndrome involves the individual's resistance to accepting his or her complaints as a sign of emotional distress.

Essentially, chronic health complainers often use hypochondriasis as a method of relieving anxiety and to seek sympathy, forgiveness, or assistance from other people. Hypochondriasis may become an escape mechanism to avoid facing the realities of various losses including those of job significance, family relationships, deaths, or social status. The condition is difficult to treat. Careful attention and long-term counseling by an understanding physician, with sincere support and encouragement from relatives and friends, may help to unfold the individual's source of mental and emotional conflicts.

AGING AND HOMEOSTASIS

The tendency of the body systems, especially the physiological mechanisms, to maintain stability of the internal environment, or constancy, is termed *homeostasis*. As the human organism ages, a slow and variable rate of decline in circulatory, neural, and hormonal efficiency governing the adaptive adjustments or homeostatic capacity occurs.

The diminished ability of the body to respond and adapt is triggered by physical or emotional stress. For example, neural and hormonal control mechanisms that regulate blood sugar and body temperature become less efficient in advanced age. Thus, older people become more vulnerable to internal destabilization when exposed to extremes in temperatures. In the instance of glucose tolerance reduction, the probability of diabetes rises with excessive weight. It is well known that emotional stress, through its effect on the hormonal system, causes changes within the cellular environment of the body. In older persons, losses such as spousal death, job security, social status, change of residential surroundings, and family problems can further reduce the adaptive capacity of biological systems necessary for effective functioning. The impact of stress—whether physical or emotional—means homeostatic disruption is greater, and the recovery time is slower with advancing age.

SUCCESSFUL AGING: A QUALITY OF BODY AND MIND

The most important affair in life is "living." Longevity is desirable, but the quality of the individual's personal productivity and contributions to the well-being of humankind far outweighs any quantitative dimension of aging.

Each person's fulfillment is esoterically meshed with body and mind—

an inseparable wholeness that reflects each individual's image through his or her actions and behavior. Physical fitness is one of life's basic foundations upon which to maximize personal dreams, aspirations, and contributions to fellow beings. Movement is part of homo sapien's functional living and environment, and the quality of intellectual and physical performance inescapably depends upon one's level of organic and dynamic fitness. Perhaps one of our society's most conspicuous changes is the demographic phenomenon of increased life-span. Medical technology has already expanded the aging population, and will continue to do so. We have conquered hundreds of diseases and maladies, but people have only "scratched the surface" of improving their health and well-being through preventive systems.

Rather than viewing aging from an arbitrary chronological dateline, we might ponder the following epigram:

"Age is a quality of body and mind;
If you lift your own dreams and hopes for mankind,
If you possess the zest for life in peace or strife,
If your flames of movement and enthusiasm are alive—not dead;
Then you are not old, but young instead."

Summary

The aging process is irreversible. Organ and tissue changes occur gradually at different rates in and among people. Rates of biological and psychosocial change are set by interacting genetic and environmental forces. The six biological theories presented in this chapter attempt to explain age changes at the cellular and organism levels. Certain theories accent the role of genetics, others stress the effects of environment as central to prolonging length of life.

The free radical theory proposes that chemical substances are produced at the cellular level that alter the DNA structure within the cell nucleus.

The wear-and-tear theory is based upon the premise that the body ultimately wears out, with an inevitable slowing of the metabolic processes until the human machine ultimately stops from exhaustion.

The cross-linking (collagen) theory bases its premises upon a build-up of collagen, which becomes stiffer with age. Collagen appears to replace water in bones and also deposits itself in an altered form within numerous body structures, cross-linking with the DNA strands so that they no longer function normally.

The autoimmune theory assumes that aging results from a breakdown of the body's immune system. This theory postulates that age-connected diseases such as diabetes, arteritis, arthritis, and cancer result from deviate antibodies produced by aging cells.

According to the genetic mutation theory, body cells undergo form and quality changes that hasten the aging process. Cells are altered so that they are unable to manufacture essential enzymes necessary for maintaining life.

The cellular error theory suggests that errors occur in the formation of a protein or enzyme. Such errors produce faulty compounds, which presumably accumulate rapidly, and progressively lead to age changes and death.

The activity, disengagement, and continuity behavioral theories of aging involve a psychosocial and health-fitness perspective. Essentially, the activity theory asserts a positive relationship between successful aging and the individual's level of mental, physical, and social involvement. The disengagement theorists regard the gradual withdrawal from societal activities as normal biological and psychological behavior as one grows older. The continuity theory holds that behavior in old age is an extension of one's previous lifestyle; and one's early habits, preferences, and dispositions continue into senior maturity.

Age changes occur in the broad categories of anatomical/physiological and mental/emotional/cognitive areas. Biological age changes of the skin, hair, kidneys, bladder, gastrointestinal, and endocrine systems may stem from intrinsic or extrinsic sources.

Hormonal changes in the aging involve insulin, endorphins, estrogen, testosterone, renin, cortisol, aldosterone, and thyroxin.

The text then examined fluid and crystallized intelligence types. Fluid intelligence is thought to increase until adolescence, then decline thereafter; crystallized intelligence, dependent upon past experiences such as education and environmental influences, is considered more resistant to decline. Some evidence indicates that higher levels of physical fitness enhances fluid intelligence. Short-term and long-term memory were identified and discussed.

The several patterns of personality discussed illustrate both well-adjusted and integrated types and the disintegrated sort found among "self-haters."

The review of biological and behavioral sexuality changes indicated that not all persons are interested in sexual activity, and those who were not interested in sex during youth are most likely to show little interest during the senior years. Illness and disability do not necessarily produce loss of libido. Alcohol and other drugs, identified as significant depressors of the neural system, in fact may cause episodes of impotency. Poor physical fitness also is an obstacle to normal sexual functions.

The dynamics of hypochondriasis were reviewed next. The topic of homeostasis was then examined, emphasizing the fact that adaptation to stress is slower in the elderly than in young persons.

The chapter concluded with a discussion of the concept of body/mind symbiosis and the philosophical premise that physical fitness is an essential cornerstone of life enrichment.

REFERENCES

1. Nathan W. Shock, "Biological Theories of Aging," in J. E. Birren and K. W. Schaie, eds., *Psychology of Aging* (New York: Van Nostrand Reinhold, 1977), p. 103.
2. Ibid., p. 104.
3. Ewald W. Busse, "Dialogue on Aging: Some Conceptions and Misconceptions," *Geriatrics* (November 1973), p. 166; and Rao D. Sanadi, "Metabolic Changes and Their Significance in Aging," in C. E. Finch and L. Hayflick, eds., *The Biology of Aging* (New York: Van Nostrand Reinhold, 1977), pp. 92–93.
4. Alex Comfort, *The Biology of Senescence*, 3d ed. (New York: Elsevier, 1979), p. 178.
5. Shock, "Biological Theories," p. 106.
6. Daniel Hershey, *Lifespan and Factors Affecting It: Aging Theories in Gerontology* (Springfield, Ill.: Charles C Thomas, 1974), p. 98.
7. Ibid., p. 99.
8. George A. Sacher, "Life Table Modification and Life Prolongation," in C. E. Finch and L. Hayflick, eds., *The Biology of Aging* (New York: Van Nostrand Reinhold, 1977), p. 626.
9. Shock, "Biological Theories," p. 111.
10. John W. Rowe and Richard W. Besdine, *Health and Disease in Old Age* (Boston: Little, Brown, 1982), p. 327.
11. Hershey, *Lifespan,* p. 107.
12. Comfort, *Biology of Senescence,* p. 210.
13. Shock, "Biological Theories," p. 106.
14. L. E. Orgel, "The Maintenance of the Accuracy of Protein Synthesis and Its Relevance to Aging," *Biochemistry* 49(1963): 517–521.
15. Erdman Palmore and George L. Maddox, "Sociological Aspects of Aging," in E. W. Busse and E. Pfeiffer, eds., *Behavior and Adaptation in Later Life* (Boston: Little, Brown, 1977), p. 48.
16. Larry G. Peppers, "Patterns of Leisure and Adjustment to Retirement," *The Gerontologist* 16, no. 5 (1976): 441–446.
17. Erdman Palmore, "Predictors of Successful Aging," *The Gerontologist* 19, no. 5 (1979): 427–431.
18. Thomas J. Decarlo, Lawrence V. Castiglione, and Memet Cavusoglu, "Lifetime Leisure Patterns' Relation to Successful Aging" (Paper presented to the 54th Annual Convention of Eastern District Association, American Alliance for Health, Physical Education and Recreation, Mt. Pocono, Pa., 8 March 1976.
19. Walter M. Bortz, II, "Disuse and Aging," *Journal of American Medical Association,* 248: 10, 1203–1209, 1982.
20. Ibid.
21. G. L. Maddox, "Activity and Morale: A Longitudinal Study of Selected Elderly Subjects," *Social Forces,* 42, no. 2 (1963): 195–204; and B. Lemon, V. Bengston, and J. Peterson, "An Exploration of the Activity Theory of Aging: Activity Types and Life Satisfaction among In-movers to a Retirement Community," *Journal of Gerontology* 27 (1972): 511.

22. E. Cummings and W. Henry, *Growing Old: The Process of Disengagement* (New York: Basic Books, 1961).
23. Jaber F. Gubrium, *The Myth of the Golden Years* (Springfield: Charles C Thomas, 1973), pp. 20–21.
24. Suha Beller and Erdman Palmore, "Longevity in Turkey," *The Gerontologist* 14 (1974): 373–380.
25. Robert N. Butler and Myrna I. Lewis, *Aging and Mental Health,* 3rd ed. (St. Louis: C. V. Mosby, 1982), p. 35.
26. John Piscopo and James A. Baley, *Kinesiology: The Science of Movement* (New York: John Wiley & Sons, 1981), p. 508.
27. R. J. Havighurst, B. L. Neugarten, and S. S. Tobin, "Disengagement and Patterns of Aging," in B. L. Neugarten, ed., *Middle Age and Aging* (Chicago: University of Chicago Press, 1968).
28. Sharon L. Vander Zyle, "Psychosocial Theories of Aging," *Journal of Gerontological Nursing* 5, no. 3 (1979): 45–48.
29. Isadore Rossman, "Anatomic and Body Composition Changes with Aging," in C. E. Finch and L. Hayflick, eds., *The Biology of Aging* (New York: Van Nostrand Reinhold, 1977), pp. 214–215.
30. Ralph Goldman, "Decline in Organ Function with Aging," in E. Rossman, ed., *Clinical Geriatrics,* 2d ed. (Philadelphia: J. B. Lippincott, 1979), p. 45.
31. Rossman, "Anatomic and Body Composition Changes," p. 215.
32. Victor Selmanowitz, Ronald L. Rizer, and Norman Orentreich, "Aging of the Skin and Its Appendages," in Finch and Hayflick, *Aging,* p. 500.
33. John V. Basmajian, *Primary Anatomy,* 8th ed. (Baltimore: Williams & Wilkins, 1982), p. 243.
34. Anna M. Ticky and Lois J. Malasanos, "Physiological Parameters of Aging," *Journal of Gerontological Nursing* 5, no. 1 (1979): 42–45.
35. Gail R. Marsh, "Perceptual Changes in Aging," in E. W. Busse and D. G. Blazer, eds., *Handbook of Geriatric Psychiatry* (New York: Van Nostrand Reinhold, 1980), pp. 159–160.
36. Edward B. Elkowitz, *Geriatric Medicine for the Primary Care Practitioner* (New York: Springer Publishing, 1981), p. 98.
37. K. Soergal, F. Zboralsken, and J. Amberg, "Presbyesophagus: Esophageal Motility in Monagenarians," *Journal of Clinical Investigation* 43 (1964): 1472.
38. Kowit Bhanthumnavin and Marvin M. Schuster, "Aging and Gastrointestinal Function," in Finch and Hayflick, p. 714.
39. Bernard Strauss, "Disorders of the Digestive System," in I. Rossman, ed., *Clinical Geriatrics* (Philadelphia: J. B. Lippincott, 1979), p. 272.
40. Robert C. Cantu, *Sports Medicine in Primary Care* (Lexington, Mass.: Callamore Press, D. C. Heath, 1982), p. 30.
41. Elaine B. Feldman, *Nutrition in the Middle and Later Years* (Boston: John Wright PSG, 1983), p. 23.
42. Rowe and Besdine, *Health & Disease,* p. 143.
43. *Webster's Third New International Dictionary of the English Language, unabridged* (Springfield, Mass: G. & S. Merriam, 1971), p. 1174.

44. R. B. Cattell, "Theory of Fluid and Crystallized Intelligence: A Critical Experiment," *Journal of Educational Psychology* 54 (1963): 1–22.
45. M. Elsayed, A. H. Ismail, and R. J. Young, "Intellectual Differences of Adult Men Related to Age and Physical Fitness before and after Exercise Program," *Journal of Gerontology* 35, no. 3 (1980): 383–387.
46. R. R. Powell and R. H. Pohndorf, "Comparison of Adult Exercisers and Nonexercisers on Fluid Intelligence and Selected Physiological Variables," *Research Quarterly* 42, no. 1 (1971): 70–77.
47. Jack Botwinick, "Intellectual Abilities," in Birren and Schaie, *Psychology of Aging,* pp. 580–605.
48. Jack Botwinick, "Psychological Aspects of Aging" (Paper presented at the 5th Annual Conference of SAGE, Buffalo, N.Y., 7–8 October 1977).
49. Botwinick, "Intellectual Abilities," p. 603.
50. Martha Storandt, "Psychological Aspects of Aging," in Rossman, *Clinical Geriatrics,* p. 556.
51. Butler and Lewis, *Aging and Mental Health,* p. 193.
52. Storandt, "Psychological Aspects," pp. 556–557.
53. S. F. Reichard, F. Livson, and P. G. Peterson, *Aging and Personality* (New York: John Wiley and Sons, 1962), pp. 170–171.
54. Ibid.
55. Bernice L. Neugarten, "Personality and Aging," in Birren and Schaie, *Psychology of Aging,* p. 636.
56. Eric Pfeiffer, "Sexuality and Aging," in Rossman, *Clinical Geriatrics,* pp. 568–575.
57. Robert N. Butler and Myrna I. Lewis, *Sex after Sixty* (New York: Harper & Row, 1976), pp. 1–9.
58. Martin A. Berezin, "Normal Psychology of the Aging Process, Revisited—I, Sex and Old Age: A Further Review of the Literature" (Paper presented at the 15th Anniversary Annual Scientific Meeting of the Boston Society for Gerontologic Psychiatry, Boston, 1 November 1975).
59. Pfeiffer, "Sexuality and Aging," p. 570.
60. Butler and Lewis, *Sex after Sixty,* p. 18.
61. Butler and Lewis, *Aging and Mental Health,* p. 145.
62. Alex L. Finkle and Paul S. Finkle, "How Counseling May Solve Sexual Problems of Aging Men," *Geriatrics* (November 1977), pp. 84–89.
63. Fay E. Sultan and Dianne L. Chambles, Pubococcygeal Function and Orgasm in a Normal Population," in B. Graber, ed., *Circumvaginal Musculature and Sexual Function* (Basel: S. Karger, 1982), pp. 6–7.
64. Ibid., p. 7.

3

Anthropometric and Kinesiologic Aspects of Aging

INTRODUCTION

The human musculoskeletal form is unique. It reflects all shapes and sizes, depending to a large extent upon our ancestors. Long ago—before 400 B.C.—Hippocrates recognized extremes in body types, naming them *habitus apoplecticus* (the short thick type), and *habitus phthesicus* (the long thin type). Today, we still use the basic anthropometric concept of Hippocrates, although modified and refined to include: (1) endomorph (predominately soft, round, obese), (2) mesomorph (well-developed musculature, athletic form); and (3) ectomorph (thin, lean musculoskeletal profile). Even though 343 different body types are categorized, about 50 combinations of the basic *endo, meso, ecto* forms are most frequently reported by contemporary anthropologists.[1]

Some controversy does exist over whether body build changes from its genetic endowment. According to W. H. Sheldon, somatotype does not change, and everyone has a "biological identification tag" with a predisposition toward one or more combinations in each of the obese, thin, and muscular categories.[2] Sheldon further maintains that an individual's somatotype follows a trajectory or pathway through which the living organism will travel under standard conditions of nutrition and in the absence of serious disease. It is commonly observed that the descriptive gross endomorph will not become a tall, lean, fragile ectomorph with the passing of time, nor can the

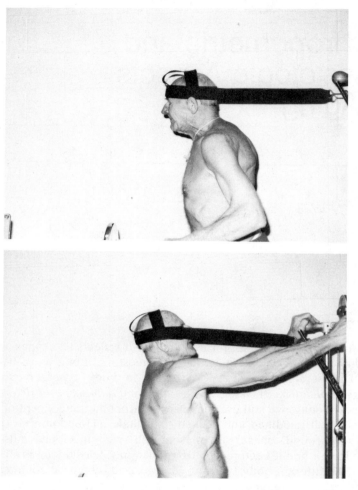

Figure 3.1 An 81-year-old mesomorph in action—strengthening neck muscles.

tall, lean ectomorph or "walking stick," possessing extreme linearity and fragility, become a short, full-bloomed obese endomorph.

If we accept the premise that body build does not basically change, then what does happen to the human form between the upright appearance of youth to the typically shorter and, in some cases, stooped physique of the older adult? The skeleton, including the bones of the vertebral column, head, face, chest, hips, and feet, indeed does change in composition, size, and shape. Muscles also change in morphology and mass, altering the posture of the long-living person.

It is reasonable to assume that each of us falls under a genetic body build label described by Sheldon. Our biological identity of physique, which is derived from the basic inherited embryonic tissues of endoderm, mesoderm, and ectoderm, gives us our own personal somatotype tag. Although we are given a genetic stamp, our bodily structure can and does change within the parameters of our own somatotype pattern. The maturing of the human organism brings about changes irrespective of our endowed body type. The element that is not constant is the degree of change itself. Some people change more rapidly than others depending upon a host of interacting components inside and outside the body. This chapter examines modifications that relate to the musculoskeletal system, and how those changes affect mobility and motor performance.

Certain anatomical alterations in bone composition, collagen deposits, and the spinal column normally occur with aging; however, the extent of change is astonishingly variable among individuals. Research studies continue to support the premise that changes in structural and functional characteristics occur more quickly among inactive, sedentary persons than those who maintain physical fitness. Body structure retains its basic genetic embryonic tissue makeup, but the physique does change within its personal genetic pattern depending upon the nutritional habits, activity level, lifestyle, and environmental milieu of the individual.

Debate continues over whether many alterations are caused by disease or result from normal aging. For example, spinal discs become thinner in older persons, yet the point at which spinal pain, herniation, and osteoarthrosis become more than from normal aging and pathology is often a fine distinction.

In some cases, musculoskeletal changes may be caused entirely by disease, and physical activities of any kind may not improve the condition. In such instances, active exercise is contraindicated. For example, rheumatoid arthritis is a systemic disease of unknown cause characterized by a chronic inflammation of the body's connective tissue and joints; in its acute stage, passive exercise, rest, and heat, rather than active movement, should be pursued. Vigorous exercise may lead to greater inflammation and debilitation when joint pain and swelling are present. Examples such as this point to the need of customizing activity programs according to the individual's medical status and dynamic physical fitness profile.

ANTHROPOMETRICAL AND SKELETAL CHANGES

Stature and Posture

Anthropologists generally agree that individuals at varying periods past maturity are shorter than youthful groups within any given population. Decreases in stature of one to three inches, and even more—especially in women—are reported as occurring over a lifetime.[3]

It is interesting to note that the reduction in height is not due to decreases in the appendicular skeleton (arms and legs), but rather to a shortening in the length of the axial skeleton (vertebral column). The appearance of long arms and legs upon a short torso may give the impression that legs and arms become longer with aging, but actually the vertebral column shrinks while arm and leg lengths remain constant. Some bowing of the legs may occur, however, due to the weight load carried by the legs over the years.

Changes in the spine, such as thinning due to compression stress on the intervertebral discs, reduction in its water-binding capacity, and increased bowing, or kyphosis (rounding of upper back), all contribute to shortness of stature. Although these spinal column changes occur in varying degrees, one positive benefit from a biomechanical view is the shortening of the lever arm from the hip joint to the upper trunk's center of gravity. A reduced height can be an advantage in moving the upper trunk in a sit-up action from supine to the upright posture. The strength demanded of the trunk and abdominal muscles for a sit-up is less because of the decreased length of the lever arm from its axis of rotation (see Figure 3.2).

The Spine

The spine is the body's central and most complex biomechanical structure. The spinal column is a collection of 33 bones: 7 cervical, 12 thoracic, 5 lumbar, 5 sacral (fused together to form the sacrum), and 4 vestigial vertebrae, called the coccyx or tail bone (see Figure 3.3). The coccyx is also fused into a single mass. The tail bone no longer has any useful purpose. In fact, among older persons this rudimentary vertebrae is vulnerable to contusions and bruises in exercises such as sit-ups since this part of the spine contains little fat pad protection.

Intervertebral Discs. The intervertebral discs, which are responsible for approximately one-fourth of the total length of the spinal column, act principally as shock absorbers, along with curvatures of the spine itself. The movement between adjacent vertebrae is extremely limited and restricted to gliding actions; however, the sum total is considerable with movements of flexion, and extension, rotation, and adduction/abduction typical in the normal column.

Stability of the spine is provided by both intrinsic and extrinsic structural arrangements. Ligaments and discs furnish intrinsic stability and muscles give extrinsic support to the column. (These support factors are discussed in later sections of this chapter.)

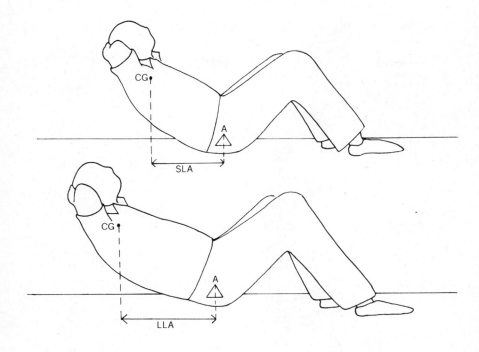

SLA = Short lever arm
LLA = Long lever arm
CG = Center of gravity
A = Axis of rotation

Figure 3.2 Short and long lever arms created by variance in stature.

The intervertebral discs are of primary mechanical and functional importance. These round plates are subject to constant stresses, including compression, tensile stress, and shear strains. Compression is caused by the weight of the body and other loads, which tend to flatten the disc. Tensile stress results when spinal movements or forces are directed away from the disc surface; e.g., when strain is placed on the posterior aspect of the lumbar discs in a forward flexion movement of the spine. Shear strain occurs when forces or loads act on the surface on a plane parallel to the applied weight or load. Figure 3.4 illustrates these three types of stresses.

Disc Changes. As mentioned earlier, intervertebral discs tend to "thin out" in older persons. The *nucleus pulposus,* or soft core, of the disc loses its water-binding ability, and as the disc becomes dryer, its elasticity decreases. Consequently, the disc is unable to distribute stress loadings without injury to the structure.

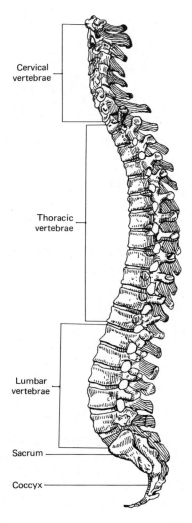

Cervical
vertebrae

Thoracic
vertebrae

Lumbar
vertebrae

Sacrum

Coccyx

Figure 3.3 Vertebral column. (From J. Piscopo and J. A. Baley, *Kinesiology: The Science of Movement* [New York: John Wiley & Sons, 1981], p. 34. Used with permission.)

In young adults (25 to 30) the nucleus of the disc has sufficient moisture and can act as gelatinous mass. Among older persons (over 60), however, deformation and herniation of the disc may occur with relatively light compression loads. Compression tests have shown that intervertebral discs behave normally, as an elastic body, up to a maximum pressure of 635 kg. (1398.77 lbs.) in specimens from young adults, but only up to 158.8 kg. (349.77 lbs.) in samples of older persons.[4] The differential of 1049 pounds represents a 75 percent loss in disc elasticity and resiliency of older adults.

The data clearly imply the avoidance of heavy weight lifting or exercise activities that place undue compression stress upon the spinal column.

Intrinsic and Extrinsic Support Factors. The main functions of the human spine are to protect the spinal cord and to transfer weights and stresses from the head and trunk to the hips. Stability and support of the column originates from two sources: Intrinsic stability is provided by the discs and surrounding ligaments. Extrinsic stability is furnished by the muscles of the trunk and back. The combined intrinsic and extrinsic support capabilities allow the spine to act as an elastic rod, with greater mobility in the cervical area graduated to lesser mobility ranges at the lumbar or low back spine.

Research studies show that disc height lessens with the aging process. As pointed out earlier, narrowing of the discs is due to loss of water content and the gelatinous mass of the nucleus pulposus.

Although biomechanical and morphological changes and osteoporosis are more pronounced in women than in men, movement limitations and stiffness of the spine is greater among males than females.[5] This mechanical characteristic indicates that the elastic properties of the disc, called visco-elastic behavior, affects spinal flexibility more than its flattening appearance from the aging discs. Although it is well known that spinal mobility losses are associated with aging in varying degrees among both sexes, we do not know whether these decrements are a result of spontaneous tissue alterations that cause stiffness or whether rigidity is a product of gross inactivity and absence of spinal column exercise.

The ligaments of the spine together with the discs provide important intrinsic support in all movements of the spinal column. The fibrous tissue bands serve to connect one vertebra to the next unit. Since ligamentous tissue contains tough inelastic fibers, the ligaments control excessive elongation and thus protect the spine from overstretching and undue tensile stress. While most spinal tissue is tough and fibrous, one set of ligaments, the *ligamenta flava,* contains considerable elastic properties and acts very much like rubber bands. These ligaments extend from the second cervical vertebra to the sacrum. In addition to providing spinal stability, this series of ligaments allows controlled flexion and extension of the spine, at the same time serving to protect the cord and vertebrae from overstretching. Orthopedic specialists consider the ligamentum flava to be the purest elastic tissue in the human body; however, it has been found that with aging, there is an increase in the amount of fibrous tissue.[6] The combination of the ligamentous fibers and the rubber-like properties of the ligamenta flava helps to protect the vertebral column from injury, also enhancing the smooth functioning of spinal movements with a minimum of resistance and energy expenditure.

The second source of spinal stability is provided by the extrinsic force

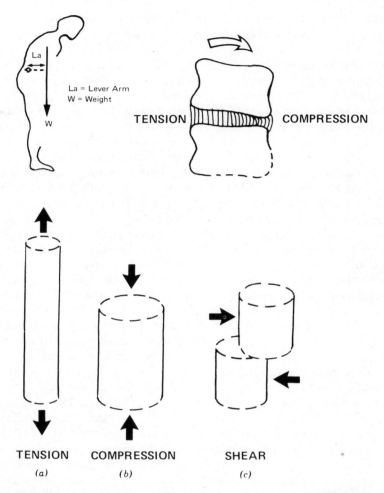

Figure 3.4 Stresses created by spinal column movements: (a) compression; (b) tensile; (c) shear. (From V. H. Frankel and M. Nordin, *Basic Biomechanics of the Skeletal System* [Philadelphia: Lea & Febiger, 1980], pp. 23, 269. Used with permission.)

actions of the trunk and back muscles. Numerous muscles surround the spine. Usually, back muscles are divided into three groups: upper limb, respiratory, and low back muscles surrounding the abdomen and trunk. Although upper limb (trapezius, latissimus dorsi, levators, rhomboids) and respiratory (posterior and inferior serratus) muscles also are involved, the discussion here focuses upon the third group, in the lower part of the spine (erector spinae, abdominals and iliopsoas), a common site of weakness and pain with the onset of aging.

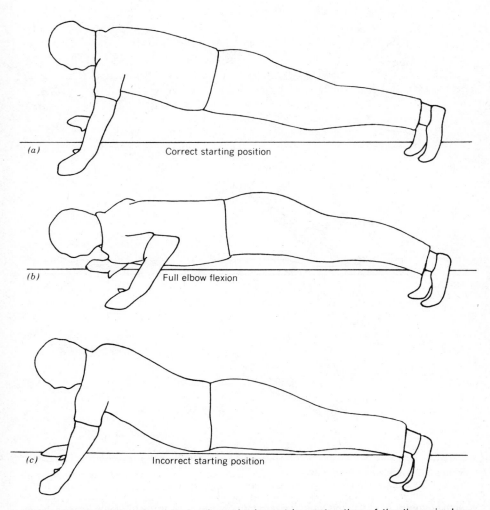

(a) Correct starting position

(b) Full elbow flexion

(c) Incorrect starting position

Figure 3.5 Stabilizing the spinal column by isometric contraction of the thoracic, low back, and trunk muscles in push-ups; note the sagging effect (c) when spinal muscles are relaxed.

The trunk and back muscles may reverse their extrinsic and force roles. In certain instances, spinal muscles act as a stabilizing unit. Other body actions require the spine to function as a prime mover. For example, the spine is a major mover in sit-ups, as the column flexes and extends; however, it becomes a stabilizing unit when an individual performs a push-up. The extrinsic muscles of back, thorax, trunk, and abdominals stabilize the spine, thereby allowing the push-up action without hyperextension of the spine or sagging in the middle, as shown in Figure 3.5.

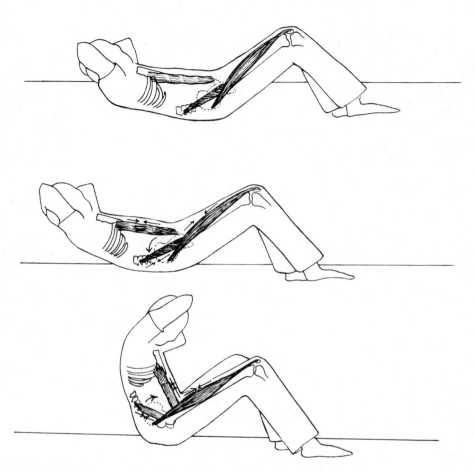

Figure 3.6 Spine as a prime mover in sit-ups; although the spine moves from the supine to the upright posture, the abdominal muscles (e.g., rectus abdominus, etc.) stabilize the pelvic girdle by producing backward tilting, while the trunk muscles (e.g., iliopsoas and rectus femoris, etc.) flex the hips (forward tilting), lifting the trunk to the upright position.

Figure 3.6 shows the spine as a prime mover in performing a sit-up. The extrinsic muscular support can provide protection to the spine as the column moves dynamically in the sit-up motion or holds isometrically as demonstrated by the push-up exercise.

Postural sway in the upright standing position tends to increase in the aging individual, particularly the anterior-posterior (front to back) sway.[7] This causes a shift in the body's center of gravity, resulting in the need for counterbalancing muscle forces to maintain balance and equilibrium. White

Table 3.1 Average Ranges of Spinal Joint Motion*

Joint	Averages (Degrees)
SPINE—	
Cervical	
Flexion	38
Extension	38
Lateral Bending	43
Rotation	45
Thoracic and Lumbar	
Flexion	85
Extension	30
Lateral Bending	28
Rotation	38

*All motions of a joint are from zero starting position. Thus the degrees of motion are added in the direction the joint moves from zero starting position.

Source: C. V. Heck, I. E.Hendryson, and C. R. Rowe, *Joint Motion: Method of Measuring and Recording* (Chicago: American Academy of Orthopaedic Surgeons, 1965), p. 86. Used with permission.

and Panjabi point out that such shifts in the center of gravity of the trunk require and activate the back, abdominal, and psoas (hip flexors) muscles respectively.[8]

Biomechanics of the Spine. Although the spine has 33 vertebrae, 24 articulate with each movement of flexion, extension, abduction, adduction, rotation, and the cone-like motion called circumduction. The intrinsic and extrinsic support factors discussed earlier supply the stability and force demands of the spinal column whether the individual is stationary or dynamically moving.

Table 3.1 shows the average ranges of spinal joint motion. These averages are merely guidelines. Considerable variations in range of motion exist among those of all ages, young and old, depending upon the organic and dynamic conditions of body joints and muscular tissue. Further details on the topic of flexibility are provided in the next chapter.

Effect of Changing Positions and Loads on the Spine. The changing anatomical and mechanical elements of the aging spine justify greater attention to posi-

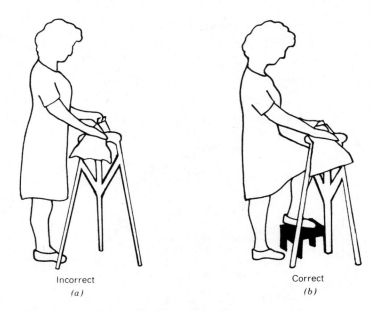

Incorrect   Correct
(a)   (b)

Figure 3.7 Reducing tension of low back by hip flexion.

tions and load stresses placed upon the back to avoid undue stress on the discs and the vertebral column. Standing, sitting, walking, and bending forward or backward all place some stress on the spine. Compression, tensile, and shear stresses can be held to a minimum by performing body movements correctly and maintaining adequate strength of extrinsic muscles surrounding the spine.

For example, Figure 3.7 illustrates correct and incorrect methods of doing a necessary household task. Most persons use position (a) when ironing clothes. This postural stance places greater stress on the lumbar disc because tension of the major hip flexor (iliopsoas), which is attached to the lower spine and upper thigh (femur), is increased. This muscle is elongated or stretched, fostering an exaggerated inward curvature of the lumbar spine (lordosis) as well as intensifying load stress on low back discs.

As we move, bend and twist in the dozens of positions required in daily living or participating in sports and exercise, stress is continuously placed on our backs. Nachemson studied the relative loads on the third lumbar disc for various body positions and, surprisingly, found that sitting exerts greater stress on the low back than does standing.[9]

Effects of Lifting Loads on the Spine. As aging proceeds, we find that the spine cannot tolerate compression loads that are no problem for younger persons.

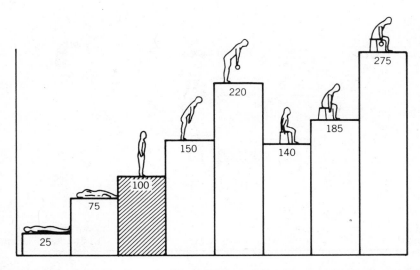

Figure 3.8 The relative loads on the third lumbar disc for various body positions in living subject are compared, with the load during upright standing depicted at 100%. (From A. White and M. Panjabi, *Clinical Biomechanics of the Spine* [Philadelphia: J. P. Lippincott, 1978], p. 334. Used with permission.)

Load tolerance depends largely upon the extent of disc and vertebral bone change. An understanding of the basic lever arrangement found within the musculoskeletal system provides a logical rationale for maintaining strong spinal muscles and avoidance of excessive obesity.

The forces that affect the spine, in addition to diverse body movements, also are produced by the lever action of the trunk and limbs. These forces can be increased or decreased depending upon the position and lever type involved in a specific movement. Internal and external lever types affect the amount of load exerted on the spinal column.

Figure 3.9(a) illustrates a first-class lever arrangement within the musculoskeletal system of the low back area. The axis or fulcrum is placed at the disc, with the load in front of the body (forward bending movement), and the force counterbalancing the load situated behind the axis. This sequence classifies the internal arrangement as a first-class lever. Anatomically, the anterior portion (distance from axis to the load of the lever arm) is much longer than the posterior lever arm (distance from axis to the force point).

Figure 3.9(b) illustrates an external third-class lever arrangement in a shoveling task, with axis located at rear hand, force point situated at the forward hand, and the load at the end of the shovel. In this case, the external arrangement can be changed to reduce the load upon the spinal discs. Less force is required when the lifter places the forward hand close to the loaded

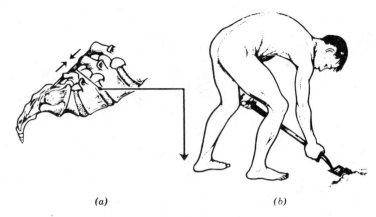

(a)   (b)

Figure 3.9 Effect of leverage upon the spinal column in ordinary movements. (From J. R. Armstrong and W. E. Tucker, eds., *Injury in Sport* [Springfield, Ill.: Charles C Thomas, 1964], p. 569. Courtesy of Granada Publishing Limited, St. Albans, England.)

end, because the law of levers states that the longer the force arm (distance from axis to force point), the less force necessary to lift a load.

Assuming that the person is lifting a load of 50 pounds, as shown in Figure 3.9(b), it must be balanced by a contraction of the extensor muscles of the spine (erector spinae group) acting much closer to the internal fulcrum of the joint (intervertebral discs). The relationship between the long and short posterior levers has been computed as 15 to 1; and 50 pounds must, therefore, be balanced by a muscle contraction of 750 pounds shown by the lifting motion. When considering the total throwing force, in addition to counterbalance contraction, as in this example, 1500 pounds of force is exerted on the intervertebral joint. Older persons, particularly those with weakened or degenerated discs, should follow the basic rules of correct mechanics when lifting or carrying loads. The following basic guidelines are recommended:

1. Hold loads close to the body instead of away from it to decrease the anterior internal lever length in the musculoskeletal system arrangement.
2. Increase the length of the force arm when lifting an object or load, as in shoveling, by placing the forward hand close to the lifting end of the shovel.
3. Use the larger muscles of the legs by flexing the knees and keeping the load close to the body.

Obesity and Spinal Stress Loads. The weight of the body adds a considerable load on the discs. The weight and shape of the physique can increase or

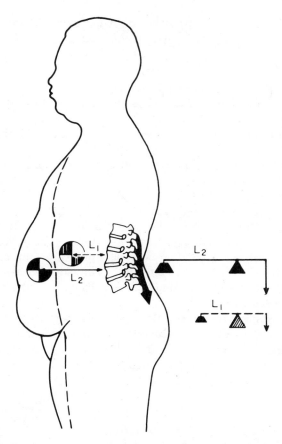

Figure 3.10 Lever effect of excessive weight and protuberance of the abdominal area. (From White and Panjabi, *Clinical Biomechanics*, p. 336. Used with permission.)

decrease disc stress. For example, Figure 3.10 shows the lever affect of excessive obesity on the disc center of rotation.

The mechanics involved in applying external weight causing undue stress on the disc in lifting activities are similar, except that the excessive weight and increased distance from the lumbar disc creates compression on the anterior disc portion and tensile stress (overstretching) on the posterior aspect of the disc. Consequently, avoiding excessive adiposity, which tends to increase around the abdominal area with aging, can relieve mechanical pressures and potential lumbar back discomfort and pain.

Activity and Exercise Hints for the Spinal Column. The vertebral column does undergo normal structural and functional changes that affect its movement efficiency. Given these changes, the following exercise and activity hints with respect to avoiding back pain and maximizing spine and trunk mobility are recommended:

1. Avoid specific exercises that induce pain.
2. Accent exercises and activities that enhance flexibility of the back and trunk muscles.
3. Perform exercises that strengthen back, chest, abdominal, and trunk muscles.
4. Avoid sudden jerks and twists in movements of the spinal column.
5. Avoid conditions such as excessive obesity that create overloading stress pressures on the discs.
6. Avoid excessively high-heeled shoes.
7. Avoid sit-up exercises when back pain is present; note that performing a sit-up with legs bent, which limits the action of the psoas (trunk muscle), creates greater disc pressure than exercising with legs straight. A simple "curl-up" exercise whereby the shoulders are slightly raised, clearing the floor from a supine position, is preferable. (See Figure 3.11.)
8. Avoid staying in one position over long periods of time—e.g., sitting at a desk or chair. Move from sitting or standing postures and comfortably stretch or bend.
9. Use a firm rather than soft bed.

OTHER ANTHROPOMETRICAL CHANGES

Other structural changes, in addition to shortened stature, also occur with aging and have relevance to movement efficiency. Figure 3.12 illustrates ten anthropometrical variables reported in a study by Damon, comparing specific structural differences from 2 to 79 years of age.[10]

Although Figure 3.12 depicts certain patterns, the reader should keep in mind that considerable variability does exist among older adults depending upon their genetic background, nutrition, lifestyle, and absence or presence of pathological conditions. However, clues to body shape and form are provided for a particular population segment.

Normal age changes of nose breadth, ear length, and head circumference have insignificant effect on bodily movements; however, weight, chest depth, skinfold, and abdominal depth can alter the caliber of mobility and motor performance depending upon the degree of physical change in bodily proportions.

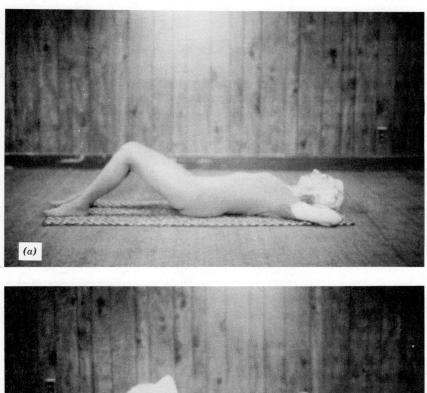

Figure 3.11 Curl-up exercise.

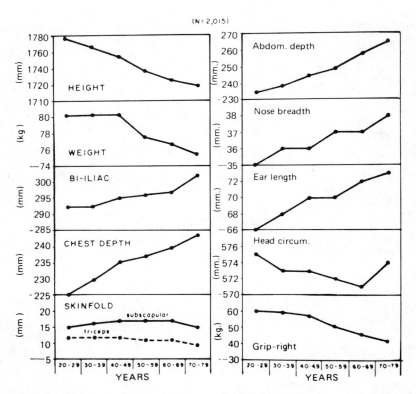

Figure 3.12 Physique and age-selected variables—white veterans' morna normative aging study. (From A. Damon et al., "Age and Physique of Healthy White Veterans," *Journal of Gerontology* 27 (1972): 205. Used with permission.)

Weight

Continued weight gain is typical after age 20 and throughout the 50s. These gains are followed by a modest decrease past 70; however, such weight loss is primarily due to a decline in lean body mass (muscle and bone). Extra adipose tissue may continue to develop within the organs, e.g., intestinal and kidney areas, with some gain as well in the subcutaneous abdominal site. Males and females differ in weight patterns. Men gain in weight to about age 55 whereas women continue to climb up to 20 years longer, and the decline among females is generally less.[11]

Weight gain or loss can present confusing information about physique and fatness. The central issue really stems from body composition changes rather than lightness or heaviness. Weight changes can be caused by alterations in muscle mass, bone composition losses, and alterations in adipose tissue deposits.

Research studies show that basal metabolism (minimum amount of energy necessary to maintain the cellular activity when the body is at complete rest) declines at the rate of 3 percent per decade from age 3 to over 80, or an average decrement of about 15 percent over this age span.[12] Therefore, calorie intake must be adjusted downward, or the older person must at least maintain (and in some cases increase) his or her physical activity level to compensate for the normal decrease in cellular energy requirements.

It is well known that when individuals expend high levels of physical energy, accompanied by restricted food intake, weight gain does not occur. Body weight, especially in the form of adipose tissue, serves as a structural restraint to the efficiency of human movement. Fat tissue is inert; it cannot generate muscular contraction, and, when present in excess, can change the human form so as to impede motion. An increase in adipose tissue coupled with the decrease in muscle strength creates a real loss in one's ability to move and handle the body efficiently, in addition to increasing the risk of physical injury.

The deterioration in physique can be a result of gross inactivity. It is possible for persons to remain the same weight, yet gain in fat tissue. Jokl reports on the condition of an international wrestler at 28 years of age, and at 63, when he had not trained for more than 30 years.[13] Figure 3.13 shows the dramatic change in the man's shape without any weight change. The ratio between the chest and abdominal circumference is reversed. Specific gravity declined by 5 percent, implying a reduction in muscle tissue and an increase in surplus fat.

Collagenous Tissue

The effectiveness of moving the body depends not only upon the weight and shape of the body, but also on the transference capabilities of various movement forces through bone, tendons, ligaments, and joints. The mechanical response pattern and reaction to various stresses placed upon these musculoskeletal systems by various and multiple body movements significantly depends upon the composition of the principal substance called collagen.

Collagenous tissues consist of a protein substance that helps provide density to bone and the essential tensile strength qualities required of the tendons and ligaments surrounding the joints. The tensile strength of a tendon is four times the isometric strength of muscle.[14]

Collagenous tissues contain three types of fibers: collagen fibers, elastic fibers, and reticulin (net framework) fibers. The collagen fibers provide strength and stiffness to the tissue, the elastic fibers furnish extensibility, and the reticulin fibers supply bulk. Although each type of fiber remains in the bones, tendons, and ligamentous tissues as one ages, the nature and distribution of collagen appears to change in composition and amount. For

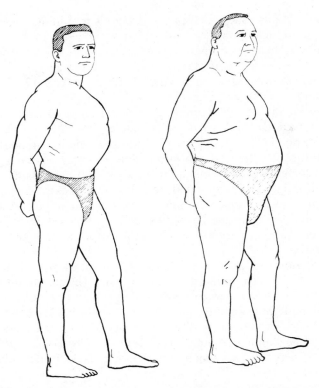

Figure 3.13 Physique at 28 and again at 63. (From E. Jokl, M.D., *Physiology of Exercise,* 1964. Courtesy of Charles C. Thomas, Publishers, Springfield, Ill.)

example, the increase in bone porosity and loss of bone mass in old age is well known. Along with mineral loss of calcium phosphate, collagen and reticulin fibers are also reduced and contribute to a weakening of the matrix of the bone itself. Extreme resorption of bone accompanies the condition known as osteoporosis. The topic of fitness and osteoporosis is further discussed in Chapter 6.

The primary functions of a ligament are to stabilize a joint during motion and to prevent injury from excessive movement. Most ligaments in the body contain collagen fibers, and they serve these functions very well in youth because of their excellent strength qualities in tolerating the stress loads placed on joints in the array of daily dynamic body movements.

Aging tends to produce changes in the ligaments similar to alterations found in immobilized joints. A significant reduction in the strength and stiffness of the ligaments occurs with advanced age.[15] It is yet to be determined whether changes in collagenous tissues within the ligamentous and surrounding structures are due to disuse, poor nutrition, or pathological conditions resulting from disease.

Tendons attach muscles to bone or fascia tissue sheaths under the skin. Tendons are abundantly supplied with collagenous fibers and provide tough anchor strength to muscle-bone attachments. During aging, muscles lose their strength and contractile qualities. These losses are attributable to some degree to cross-linkage of collagen fibers from tendon to muscle.[16] Since collagen fibers are considerably less elastic than muscle fibers, increased rigidity of joints may well be caused by collagen build-up in tendons and all the cellular elements surrounding connected bones.

Joints

Three types of joints are found in the body: fibrous, cartilaginous, and synovial. Fibrous joints, those sutures located in the skull, do not move. Cartilaginous joints represent those articulations found in the vertebral column, and synovial joints are free-moving articulations typical of those connections found in hands, feet, arms, and legs. Cartilage is found in intervertebral discs, ligaments, and tendons of the synovial joints along with synovial sacs containing lubricating fluid. These structures change in composition with aging. Elastic tissues decline within the cartilage network of the vertebral discs, thereby reducing its shock-absorbing qualities. The molecular structure of the cells actually changes, showing greater deposits of nonelastic fibrous connective tissue.[17]

In early life, the vertebral disc contains sufficient moisture to act like a gelatinous mass with considerable resiliency, allowing it to resume its normal form after compression. Notable variance exists in the degree of disc change; however, it is important to remember that activities, that exert great compression stress on discs, such as dead lift type exercises found in weight lifting, can injure the spine. Such exertions should be avoided because of the structural disc changes that occur with normal aging.

A similar declining resiliency occurs in the synovial joints of the arms and legs. The composition of the cartilage changes from a translucent quality to an opaqueness, with a correspondent loss of elasticity. Calcification of the cartilage may also develop in the surrounding structures including the tendons and ligaments. This hardening deposit adds to the loss of rebounding qualities of the cartilage and prevents its return to a natural shape when exposed to compression and stretching stresses.

Bone Changes

Some bone loss and change is a universal concomitant of the aging process.[18] As with all other anatomical changes, variability in bone changes exists

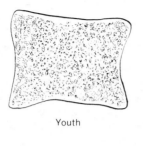

Youth

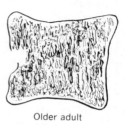

Older adult

Figure 3.14 Bone changes—from youth to osteoporotic older adult.

among older adults. For example, blacks appear to manifest less loss of bone density than do whites, and women tend to have more bone loss than men, particularly after 40.[19] Smith reports that some women lose 30 percent of their bone mineral mass by age 70. This condition, which is identified by a soft bone structure and enlarged spongy cavities, is called osteoporosis.[20]

Figure 3.14 illustrates the bone changes from a youth of 20 to a person of 70. Understanding of the cause of normal bone loss and of decrements resulting from pathological conditions remains uncertain. Research studies increasingly point to poor nutrition and lack of exercise as central to the cause of bone loss and a subsequent decline in bone strength.

At the present time, several important concepts, based upon scientific evidence, have been determined:

1. Rate of bone loss is about 1 percent per year for women after 30, and slightly less for men after 50.
2. Bone loss is a universal age-related phenomenon with differences in degree among individuals.
3. Bone loss may be associated with estrogen and testosterone production changes.
4. Role of diet is linked with bone loss (i.e., deficiency in calcium and Vitamin D).
5. Long periods of bed rest and physical inactivity result in bone loss at any age.
6. Bone growth can result from regular exercise by applying Wolff's Law (forces and stresses on bone causes structural changes).

7. Reduction in loss of bone mass may reduce the older person's vulnerability to hip, spine, and shoulder fractures.[21]

Specific methods for the prevention and reduction of osteoporotic bone through alterations in nutrition and physical activity patterns are discussed in Chapter 6.

Muscles and Muscular Changes

Approximately 40 percent of the body is composed of skeletal muscle, and an additional 5 to 10 percent is made up of smooth or involuntary cardiac muscle. This section focuses upon the nature and characteristics of skeletal (voluntary) muscles, with particular attention to persons past 50. In order to place muscle characteristics and changes within the context of older adults, a brief review of the role and functions of muscle is presented.

Role and Functions. Six hundred skeletal muscles of various sizes and shapes are found in the body. Muscles, together with the skeleton, provide shape to the human form and protect the soft structures within from injury. Muscles further provide the source of energy to move, change direction of motion, and hold an object in position against the pull of gravity or some other external force. In the human body, force is created by the contraction of muscles, and the speed of muscular contraction, which together make up power.

Motion cannot take place unless the force from muscular contraction is present, and as such, it is a vital fitness component in producing and maintaining mobility. Muscles have multiple roles and may serve as prime mover, antagonist, stabilizer, or neutralizer depending upon the task at hand. Muscles also may reverse their normal roles. For example, the bicep is a prime flexor of the elbow joint; however, it becomes an opposite or antagonist muscle when the elbow is deliberately extended.

Muscles act as stabilizers when they contract isometrically to hold a segment or bone in place. For example, the abdominals assist in stabilizing the pelvis to prevent the back from bowing when one is performing push-ups (see Figure 3.5). Muscles that cause body parts to move within a desired pathway are called neutralizers. For example, the right abdominal external oblique muscle, when contracting alone, will flex the trunk to the right and rotate it to the left, while the left external oblique muscle will flex the trunk to the left and rotate it to the right. When they contract together, they flex the trunk forward, neutralizing one another's role as lateral flexors and rotators to produce forward flexion of the trunk on the hip.

Reciprocal Innervation. Another important role of the skeletal muscles, in concert with the neural system, involves the neuromuscular mechanism called *reciprocal innervation*. Simply stated, muscles function in pairs—when one muscle is contracting (agonist), the opposite muscle is relaxing (antagonist). High-level motor skills such as racquetball, badminton, and handball, as well as efficient swimming and jogging, require free reciprocal innervation muscle interplay between flexors and extensors. This mechanism implies that when a prime mover is stimulated, inhibitory action of the opposing muscle (antagonist) results. Figure 3.15 illustrates the paired rhythmic contraction and extension in jogging.

Reciprocal innervation is also identified with *reciprocal inhibition*. Actually, both terms are part of the same concept. For example, during the pull-up action, flexion of the biceps brachii (agonist) automatically triggers inhibitory neural impulses to the triceps brachii (antagonists), and a free-flow movement of the elbow joint results.

The principle of reciprocal innervation, broadly conceived, is that it coordinates paired muscle interplay; that is, when one muscle is excited, the corresponding antagonist is inhibited. Functional levels, and in some cases, superior qualities of reciprocal interplay between muscle groups can be sustained well into old age when these neuromuscular mechanisms are stimulated through continued sports participation and regular physical exercise. Such sports as racquetball and handball enhance the agonistic and antagonistic muscles interplay by their demands for free-flowing motion requirements in striking the ball or moving the body in controlled patterns during competitive play. Free-flowing motions, also called ballistic movements, are characteristic of walking, jogging, turning, and other everyday body ambulation maneuvers. All these mobility patterns include reaction and movement time responses that are part of the reciprocal innervation mechanism.

Spirduso compared persons between 20 to 70 years of age who participated in racquet sports and handball with a control group of inactive individuals. She found that reaction and movement time decrements due to age were 22.5 percent in nonactive men but only 8 percent in a physically active group.[22] These data certainly emphasize the importance of maintaining reasonable levels of physical activity to prevent atrophy and involution of neuromuscular mechanisms, which too often tend to decline rapidly, unless muscle, nerve, and other body regulatory metabolic functions are stimulated and used regularly.

Muscle Composition. Skeletal muscle (the type attached to the skeleton) is composed of contractile fibers. These fibers form clusters called *fasciculi* or *bundles*. Skeletal or voluntary muscles are striped and covered with a thin layer of connective tissue called *epimysium,* from which a partition or wall designated as the *perimysium* passes, dividing the muscle into fasciculi. Each fasciculus contains a number of parallel fibers separated by a sheath

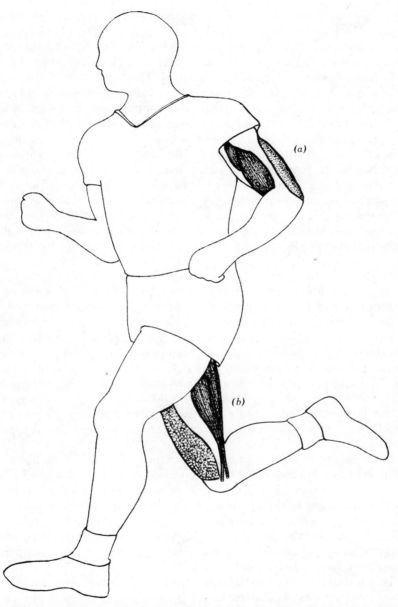

Figure 3.15 Reciprocal innervation of flexors and extensors: upper body—biceps flexing while triceps are extending; lower body—hamstrings flexing, quadriceps extending.

called the *endomysium*. Each fiber consists of *sarcoplasm* (within the muscle cell), which is striped and composed of alternate light and dark portions. Embedded in this structure are *myofibrils* enclosed by a membrane called the *sarcolemma*. The sarcolemma has remarkable electrical properties used for the transmission of contraction impulses. The sarcoplasm contains soluble proteins, glycogen, fat, phosphate compounds, and ions. Also suspended in the red viscous fluid are nuclei, mitochondria (small particles of living substances, which carry on the metabolism of the muscle), phosphocreatine (PC), and adenosine triphosphate (ATP).

Myofibrils, which are found in the sarcoplasm, are composed of filaments called *actin* and *myosin*. These filaments are arranged into geometric units called *sarcomeres*. Although actin or myosin cannot contract separately, together they form a complex protein called *actomyosin* and are responsible for the contractile properties of muscle that result from a breakdown of chemical substances called *adenosine triphosphate* (ATP) and *phosphate creatine* (PC). Figure 3.16 shows the structure of a skeletal muscle.

Skeletal Muscle Fiber Types. Human skeletal muscle is composed of two principal types of fibers: Type I—slow contracting, termed *slow twitch* or *red fibers;* and Type II—fast contracting, termed *fast twitch* or *white fibers*. The red fibers, because of their chemical characteristics, are well adapted for endurance. They contain greater amounts of *myoglobin* (red color of muscle) and are able to perform long periods of *aerobic* ("with oxygen") work. These fibers are used when the individual is performing slow or moderate exercise. The white fibers are quite different. They are designed for fast movements and immediate energy release, and they fatigue easily. These fibers are used for sprinting, running, or performing an exercise at a fast rate.

Each person is born with a certain ratio of fast and slow fibers, and current evidence indicates that this proportion cannot be changed by training or nutritional regimens. It follows that persons with a larger proportion of white fibers are faster by their genetic make-up than individuals with predominantly red fibers. Although fibers do not increase in number, it is possible to increase the size and metabolism of white and red fibers through various training and conditioning procedures by applying the specificity of training principle discussed in Chapter 4.

This brief review of the basic structure and function of muscles raises curious questions about muscles during the aging process. Does muscle morphology change? What happens to muscle metabolism? Can muscular form and efficiency be maintained? The following discussion focuses upon these and related topics.

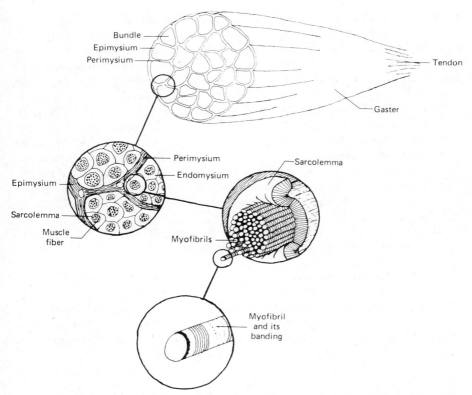

Figure 3.16 Skeletal muscle and fibers. (From J. Piscopo and J. A. Baley, *Kinesiology: The Science of Movement* [New York: John Wiley & Sons, 1981], p. 28. Used with permission.)

Form and Structure Changes. Morphological muscle change does not become noticeable until very late in life, and disuse is considered one important factor affecting the structure and function of muscular tissue.[23] Muscle weight and density decline with aging. The number and size of the fibers also decrease. Typically, collagen and fat adipose tissue increase in and around muscle and bone, particularly near body joints. Research on animals has shown that collagen content amounts to almost double that in young adults.[24] This increase in nonelastic substance may well account for some of the muscle dysfunction apparent in old age. The decrease in senile muscle mass is associated with a decline in protein concentration, and together with the increase of lighter connective tissue and fat accounts for some of the shrinkage in body form.

Marked losses in fiber numbers, as well as reduced volume, are found in the elderly. Some research suggests that greater losses occur in the fast Type

II fibers than in the slow Type I fibers.[25] The law of differential aging applies to muscle tissue as well as to other organs and systems of the body. For example, the diaphram shows late atrophy (shrinkage) and the slow soleus muscle of the lower leg shows early atrophy.[26] This raises the question as to whether constant use of a muscle slows its degeneration rate, since the diaphram is continuously exercised by automatic neural mechanisms.

Other studies indicate that fast-twitch fibers (white) decrease in both number and size, while slow-twitch fibers (red) decrease in number.[27] Larsson studied morphological changes of 51 males between the ages of 22 and 65 and found a decreased number of Type II fast-twitch fibers in the quadriceps femoris muscle (large muscle in front of the thigh) compared to Type I slow-twitch fibers.[28] His research provides some evidence that the distribution and composition of muscle structure at the cellular level does change in older skeletal muscle. The implications of such changes in designing specific conditioning exercises and activities for the maintenance of static and dynamic strength are explained in the next chapter.

Muscle Metabolism Changes. As a general rule, basal metabolism generally slows down at the rate of 3 percent per decade from age 3 to over 80.[29] However, it is possible for some 80-year-old persons to have metabolic rates as high as that of a 40-year-old.[30] Nevertheless, the typical older person does experience a slowdown in the production and transformation of energy substances needed for hundreds of uses required by the body.

The ability of a muscle to generate force is dependent upon the contractile elements found in the myofibrils that contain actomyosin. The union of these filaments is shown in the following equation:

$$\text{Actin} + \text{Myosin (AM)} + \text{Energy (E)} = \text{Actomyosin (AM)} = \text{Muscle Shortening}$$

The evidence is not clear whether the metabolic sequence is caused by aging or by inactive and sedentary living patterns. However, the following characteristics affecting metabolism are identified with aging skeletal muscles:

1. Reduced levels of muscle protein and nitrogen.
2. Decrease in water content and potassium.
3. Loss of distinct differences in composition of fast and slow muscle fibers.
4. Reduced capacity of processing the chemical substances adenosine triphosphate (ATP), phosphate creatine (PC), and glycogen.
5. Increase in collagen and fat in and around the muscle itself.

The energy transport and transfer system of muscular work involves the above chemical components in an orderly and sequential series. This physical and chemical process (metabolism), whereby catabolism (foods are broken down and ATP formed) occurs and anabolism (build-up of cells for the maintenance of muscle tone and function changes) takes place, generally becomes impaired or reduced in aging. However, significant metabolic changes do not occur until very old age.

Effects of Exercise and Disuse

Atrophy, or wasting away, of muscle tissue takes place rapidly when muscles are not used, in younger persons as well as older individuals. Although slowness of muscle contraction speed is common among older adults because of some loss of fast-twitch fibers, muscle tone, hypertrophy, and functional capacity can be maintained through participation in regular exercise activity.

Orlander et al. studied age-related changes in human skeletal muscle metabolism of sedentary men aged 22 to 68 and in older men 66 to 76 years who were more physically active.[31] Muscle biopsies were taken from the vastus lateralis (upper thigh muscle) and cellular tissue structure, and the investigators found that physically active men in their 60s and 70s maintained as great a metabolic flow in muscle cells as did the young men. It can be said with confidence that appropriate exercise activity will retard the decline of muscle senescence, and every individual (barring pathological conditions) thus can maintain satisfactory metabolic response necessary to sustain sufficient muscle strength and endurance well into old age. The positive effects of conditioning upon muscles are similar for all persons whether the individual is young or old, male or female.

AGING AND MOTOR PERFORMANCE

The variability in motor performance among persons over 55 is astonishing. Certain older adults are capable of running 26-mile marathons, while others do not even possess sufficient ambulatory skills for everyday walking, turning, and bending tasks. Although motor skill and performance are a result of integrated anatomical and physiological mechanisms, an examination of neuromuscular elements as they relate to human movement is presented in the next section.

Central Nervous System Changes

It is generally accepted that there is a loss of brain cells with advancing age. It has been calculated that adults lose 100,000 neurons per day.[32] Although this seems like a massive amount, we still have cells to spare, with about 20,000 million neurons found in the cerebrum (main portion of the brain, consisting of right and left hemispheres). Gradually, brain cells change in composition to varying degrees, reflecting greater accumulation of *lipofuscin* (fatty substance) and *glial* (glue-like tissue) elements, which impair sensory perception and motor responses. These structural changes are shown by slower reaction time and loss in ability to coordinate gross (involving big muscle) and fine (involving precision movements) neuromuscular tasks. However, the degree and type of neuromuscular losses are by no means uniform between and among long-living persons. As pointed out earlier, older adults who maintain a physically active lifestyle generally react and move faster than their sedentary peers.

Normal brain function requires threshold levels of oxygen to its cells supplied by the blood vessels. Too often, the vessels become arteriosclerotic (hardened) and atherosclerotic (narrowed), hampering the oxygen flow to the cerebrum. Subsequently, depressed cerebral blood supply contributes to the individual's inability to make quick mental decisions required in many everyday motor actions. Sports such as racquetball, handball, volleyball, tennis, and badminton tend to stimulate sensory and motor neurons, and at the same time, when played with sufficient intensity, condition the cardiovascular system, lessening or postponing decrements in neuromuscular functions.

Motor Learning and Aging

The ability to learn motor skills depends to a great extent upon the individual's level of physical fitness, rather than age. Motor performance involves integrated levels of muscular, nervous, and cardiovascular functions, all of which together affect the neuromuscular system. Muscles give the energy for generating force; cardiovascular actions serve the oxygen transport system by carrying nourishment to the cells; and the nervous system provides the electro-chemical means of exciting neuromuscular connections between nerve and muscle. As is the case with other body systems, striking differences exist here among older persons.

As pointed out earlier, Spirduso's research provides evidence that reaction time, which involves transmission of neural impulses from nerves to muscles, does not need to slow when threshold levels of physical fitness are maintained through such sports as racquetball and handball. The ability to perform motor tasks is intricately intertwined with the speed with which the nerve impulse moves through the neurons that ultimately stimulate a particular group of muscle fibers to contract. Some slowing in the rate of speed in nerve conduction does develop, but such change is relatively small—about

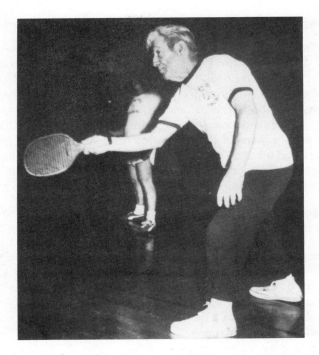

Figure 3.17 Maintaining reaction time and neuromuscular efficiency through wall tennis. (From J. Piscopo and C. A. Lewis, "Preparing Geriatric Fitness and Recreation Specialists," *Journal of Physical Education and Recreation* 48, no. 8 (1977): 24–29. Used with permission.)

10 percent.[33] Therefore, the physical-chemical processes of neural transmission of impulses, which affect the quality of a motor skill, can be enhanced through participation in physical activities that stimulate and excite the neurons of the brain, spinal cord, and synaptic (nerve-muscle) junctions.

Older adults probably need more time in learning new motor skills due to the general decline in vision, hearing, and other sensors such as kinesthesia (body sense), which involves balance and equilibrium. Both nerve and muscle cells are *post-mitotic*; that is, once these cells are lost, they do not regenerate. Thus, it seems logical to follow a course of action that allows us to maximize the functional use of our remaining cells.

Although exercise cannot guarantee life-span extension, overwhelming evidence indicates that functional capacity of the neuromuscular system is higher among physically active people than unfit sedentary people, irrespective of age.

Balance and Equilibrium Changes

Understanding balance and equilibrium changes of older adults is important because of their connection with the high rate of falls within this special population. Persons over 65 account for 25 percent of all accidental deaths, and in seven of ten fatalities from falls, the victim is elderly.[34] Balance control stems from both internal and external sources. Internal sources are vision, ears, and sensory receptors of proprioceptors and kinesthesia. External sources are mechanical elements such as position and placement of the line of gravity and location of the gravity center and its supporting base. The following discussion focuses upon several important structural and functional changes that accompany aging.

Internal changes. The internal structural changes involved in balance and equilibrium involve eyes, ears, proprioception, and kinesthesia.

Eye and Ear Changes Affecting Balance. Research shows that a vast difference exists when a balance skill is performed with eyes open or closed. This reality can be quickly demonstrated by walking a low balance beam with eyes open, then with eyes closed: it is much easier to walk the beam with eyes open. Vision provides a point of reference and, therefore, is important for the maintenance of balance.

Visual impairments are common among older adults. For example, for some persons, color discrimination, especially between blues and greens, tends to fade. The power of accommodation or adjusting the eyes to focus at various distances is diminished after the age of 40, especially in relation to the ability of the lens and ciliary muscles to focus on a chosen object (presbyopia). Some older persons lose acuteness in determining depth perception, a problem, for example, in walking up or down stairs. Glare is also a problem for older persons, because the pupil does not open and close as quickly to allow the correct amount of illumination. Visual acuity also declines, especially in darkness and in viewing for moving objects (see Table 6.5).

Each of these visual changes can affect the balancing ability of the older adult when walking, bending, or turning the body. Since aging eyes lose some acuity and discriminating ability as to light and dark, their contribution as a visual fixation or point of reference in dynamic and static balance movements is lessened. Maintaining balance and equilibrium through the development of other sensory mechanisms, and the place of visual losses, are discussed in Chapter 6.

The ear not only serves as a receiver of sound, but also acts as part of the sensory balance control mechanism. The ear is divided into three major segments: external, middle, and internal or inner. The external and middle ear deals primarily with the conduction of vibrations via the eardrum and three ossicles: *malleus* (hammer), *incus* (anvil), and *stapes* (stirrup). The internal ear, or labyrinth, contains the structures and fluids that affect balance and equilibrium.

The power of coordinating the movements of the body and maintaining balance rests in the cerebellum of the brain; however, this power of coordination, which involves equilibrium, is shared with the vestibular apparatus of the inner ear. The vestibular apparatus is the sensory organ that detects sensations of equilibrium, particularly head orientation. Whenever these detectors signal a head position other than that associated with upright normal posture, control centers initiate movements of the head to correct its position with the line of gravity force, triggering the well-known axiom, "the body follows the head."

Although conductive hearing losses (through mechanical defects of ear bones) have little relationship to balance, impairments to the internal structures that disturb the ear fluid often affect balance. Various changes in head movements causing posture adjustments introduce neural signals to the brain, which tend to move the body in the direction initiated by the head. The vestibular mechanism has particular implications for older persons. Sudden and quick head motion changes can cause the individual to lose balance. In certain older persons, vertigo or dizziness may be caused by Ménière's disease. In such cases head movements and balance exercises should be avoided.

Proprioception. An integral component of balance and equilibrium involves sensory nerve terminals in the muscles, tendons, and joints called *proprioceptors*. These receptors, often referred to as "muscle sense," together with inner ear vestibular mechanisms, are important elements in skilled movements requiring balancing competence, such as daily tasks of walking, standing and changing body position in bending, twisting, and sitting.

Sensitive nerve endings called *Ruffini's corpuscles* and *Pacinian corpuscles* are principal proprioceptive receivers found in muscular tissue. Pacinian nerve endings are found in connective tissue, especially in the palm of the hand, sole of the foot, and about the joints. Muscular contraction stimulates these nerve endings in the connecting tissues, tendons, and joints, sending messages to the cerebellum about the actual state of contraction. This information and communication from the brain's cortex (or gray matter) is integrated by the cerebellum, resulting in an adjustment of the rate and force of muscular contraction necessary for the balancing task at hand.

The acuity of these sensory receivers and the processing network via their neural pathway declines as we grow older. This phenomenon is proba-

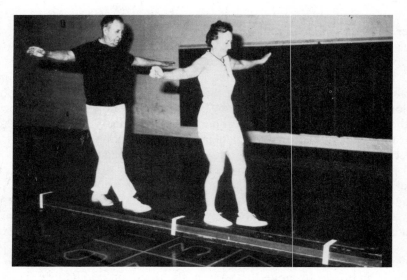

Figure 3.18 Enhancing upright dynamic balance skills through beam walking.

bly due to the loss of brain cells, particularly in the cerebellum, and the lack of body movement activities that innervate and stimulate the function of the sensory receivers.

Such activities as those shown in Figure 3.18 help to sustain propriocep-tive sensitivity in the feet as the individual walks down the beam. Active body movements used in dance, bowling, shuffleboard, horseshoes, fitness exercises, and swimming also are excellent ways to cultivate proprioceptive impressions and neural efficiency for the improvement of safety balance skills. The development of the sensors depends significantly upon their stim-ulation and use.

While strength has little, if any, relationship with the attainment of a balance position, this fitness component does have value in correcting bal-ance errors. The greater force made available by increased strength can alter errors in joint angles, which are important in maintaining the correct align-ment of the gravity line over its supporting base. For example, tripping over an obstacle (a common cause of falls among young and old), requires im-mediate restoration of balance. Muscles that manifest sufficient strength have the advantage of providing the necessary energy transfer for a person to resume a balance position more quickly, and with less likelihood of injury from a fall. An expanded discussion of proprioception and its relevance to efficient movement is presented in Chapter 5.

Kinesthesia.* Kinesthesia or kinesthesis is the neuromuscular mechanism by which one is aware of position and movements of body segments, or the whole body as a unit. Often this awareness is identified as "position sense." Balancing ability is a part of kinesthesia. In fact, visual clues, ears (vestibular mechanism), and proprioception are intricately related to the ability of the individual to initiate and maintain balance at all ages. Figure 3.19 illustrates postures and motions of body segments that are perceived by the kinesthetic sense.

A person's position sense is dependent upon the neuromuscular system operating as an integrated unit. This involves sensations that arise from the sensory receptors of the muscles and joints (proprioceptors) which are funneled to the brain for movement modulation and adjustments.

Kinesthesia is part of the body's internal sensory feedback system. The "feel" or kinesthetic sense is used more extensively when other balance sensors are reduced or eliminated. For example, walking on a low beam as shown in Figure 3.18 uses eyesight to transmit visual information about balance and the body position to the brain in the walking pattern. If the performers close their eyes, kinesthetic sensations take over, and the maintenance of correct form and balance largely depends upon the acuteness of the individual's kinesthetic sensitivity. Actually, one's optimum position sense results from the coordinated role and function of such components as balance, flexibility, muscle tone, and, indirectly, the five sensory organs. Inputs from other sensory modalities shape the physiological response we call kinesthesia. The "position sense" is a remarkable body control mechanism that receives input from other sensory organs to fulfill its role of indicating "where" and "how" we are postured in the realm of human movement.

At what point can kinesthetic clues best be used in motor performance? Does kinesthesia improve with training? Is this sense mechanism a general quality or specific to a particular motor skill? Does this quality diminish with age? The blueprint of constitutional individual differences provides the mold for the development of skeletal muscular position sense. Certain persons by virtue of their neuromuscular makeup appear to possess inherent qualities that allow this sense to be developed more quickly and to a greater extent than others. However, several general conclusions based upon research studies can be advanced about the nature of kinesthesia:

1. Athletes, musicians, mechanics, and other individuals who engage in activities where skilled motor performance is part of the task generally have high levels of kinesthesia.

---

*The terms *kinesthesia* and *kinesthesis* connote similar meanings and are used interchangeably in this discussion.

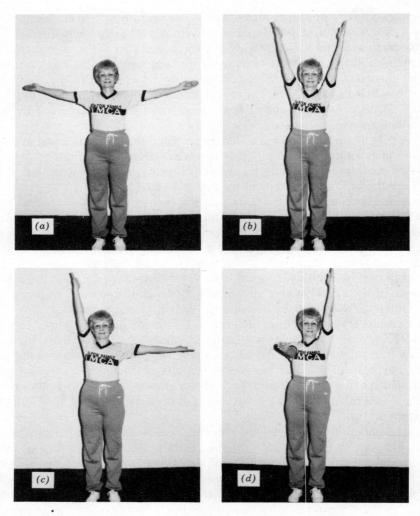

Figure 3.19 Changes in body segment positions perceived by the kinesthetic sense.

2. Kinesthesia largely involves the acuity of the skeletal muscle receptors for its detection, and the central nervous system centers for its control, with the muscles themselves serving as movers.
3. Kinesthetic ability can be improved with practice of motor skills.
4. Kinesthetic ability becomes more important as the motor skill level increases.
5. Balance is an important element of kinesthesia. When balance ability improves, kinesthesia perception also tends to get better.

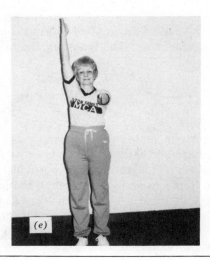

6. Kinesthesia appears to be a specific quality, not a general trait; however, skilled motor performers score higher marks than do unskilled individuals in kinesthetic tests.
7. Kinesthetic acuity exists with astonishing variability among aging adults, depending upon the absence of disease, and stimulation and frequency in using the muscle receptors.

One message is clear about kinesthetic perception—unless muscle receivers, which contain our sense organs, are stimulated and used regularly, their "feedback" functions are lost. Activities such as dancing, racquetball, balancing tasks, swimming, golf, and bowling are only a few of the hundreds of physical activities and sports that help the older adult sustain high levels of kinesthetic ability.

OTHER CHANGES IN PHYSICAL CHARACTERISTICS

A striking difference between budding maturity and aging in terms of structural change is its rate. Young people change rapidly, and changes can be readily observed over a period of only months. However, later changes in size and shape of the head, face, height, chest, hips, and feet occur over many years and are hardly discernible to the older adult.

Head

The shape and size of the head changes slightly as one ages. Figure 3.12 shows a slight increase in head circumference from 35 to 39, followed by a decline to 65, with more shrinkage after 65. These changes are probably due to expansion and shrinkage of the sutures (fibrous joints) of the skull and alterations in cranium thickness. The length of the head tends to increase after 50.

Face

Several changes that occur modify the appearance of the face. The overall face height increases through 30 to 34, which gives some individuals a long and fine look; thereafter, its length declines, particularly at the lower part, due to the wearing out and some loss of teeth. The chin and nose become closer together, especially if most of the teeth are missing, and a thinning of the lips occurs. The nose becomes progressively longer, with an increase in width from ages 55 to 59. Thus, for most long-living persons, the facial features become more pronounced.

Height

Hebbelinck points out that full height is reached by the late teens or early 20s.[35] Stature remains constant from 30 to 40 years, after which a decrease starts, beginning slowly, but subsequently becoming progressively faster. As noted earlier, decreases of up to three inches occur by the age of 80, males and females have lost an average of 6 cm. or 2.4 inches, with most of the loss occurring in the spine.[36]

Although some height loss occurs in most persons, differences exist between racial groups. A study conducted in the southeastern United States involving over 700 whites and blacks between the ages of 50 and 104 years showed that black males lose about 4.2 cm. (1.88 inches) in height every 20 years compared to the 1.2 cm. (0.48 inches) of the white population.[37] The implications of this research are that care should be observed when generalizing about specific stature decrements among all people. Height and weight are factors frequently used to determine drug dosages, metabolism, nutritional requirements, and exercise heart rate specifications; therefore, racial variability should be considered when developing corrective health standards for long-living persons.

Decreased sitting height (of the spine) is caused in part among some elderly who habitually carry themselves in a postural slump with exaggerated flexion of the knees and hips. Conditioning and toning posterior muscles of the upper back, hips, and legs can counter the forward "slouch" posture.

Chest

It is clear that the chest increases in size with aging. Figure 3.12 shows a continuous increase in chest depth from 225 mm. (9.0 inches) to 265 mm. (10.6 inches) over a 59-year age span (20 to 79). The chest also tends to become rounder. These changes are probably due to increased connective and fatty tissue surrounding the chest.

Hips

Most studies show a widening of the pelvis, as contrasted with a narrowing of the shoulders.[38] The patterns are similar among men and women. Abdominal girth also enlarges, with a greater percentage increase in women. Shepherd reports a 6 to 16 percent increase in men and a 25 to 35 percent increase in women.[39] It is curious to note that even though men generally manifest fewer adipose deposits than women, especially around the abdominal and hip areas, longevity records continue to favor females over males. Yet we know that the caloric cost of movement increases with obesity, and the level of efficiency is also reduced. A puzzling question arises: Does this adipose differential provide some degree of longevity protection for females? This enigma is worthy of further investigation and research.

Feet

The foot is a complex body part that can become quite rigid when necessary for standing, or very flexible for such activities as walking or picking up pebbles with the toes operating as a prehensile tool. Feet tend to widen with age. Common problems of the feet after 60 include bunions, corns, and callouses. Muscles, ligaments, and tendons surrounding the foot weaken, particularly the ligaments supporting the big toe.

This muscular weakness coupled with wearing stylish shoes that cram the toes together creates a drifting of the first metatarsal bone of the foot, often causing a bunion as shown in Figure 3.20. The pressure from the shoe forces the big toe sideward. The result is a drifting of the first metatarsal (first of the five long bones connected to the toes) toward the center, increasing its angulation. When this happens, the tendons, which normally flex and adduct (draw toward the middle of the foot), begin to rotate or turn, subsequently forcing the head of the first metatarsal to turn more to the middle of the foot (see Figure 3.20b). Bone growth actually occurs, with a bunion developing. Surgical correction is usually necessary once the bones become organically set.

The worst offenders of the feet are tight-fitting shoes that cramp the big

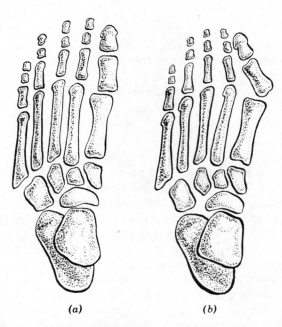

(a)   **(b)**

Figure 3.20 Bunion formation: (a) bones of normal foot; (b) bunion of the large toe.

toe. Ill-fitting shoes are also a major cause of corns and callouses. Usually, changing to footwear with appropriate heel height and width can prevent the build-up of these conditions and promote walking without pain or discomfort.

Summary

The human physique reflects a wide variety of sizes and shapes. Although somatotype characteristics are genetically determined, anthropometrical changes in structure do happen with the passage of time. This chapter has examined the specific changes that occur in the spine and the way those alterations shorten the stature of the older adult.

The intervertebral discs, ligaments, and muscles function as prime movers, neutralizers, and intrinsic and extrinsic support mechanisms of the back. The biomechanics of the spine reveal that the vertebral column is quite flexible and capable of acting as a supple steel rod with considerable flexion, extension, lateral, and rotary movements. However, improper mechanics of lifting and excess obesity can exert undue stress upon the musculoskeletal support structures of the discs and back.

Weight gain and loss trends appear throughout the lifespan in both sexes. Men tend to gain weight to about age 55, whereas women generally continue to climb up to 20 years longer; and the eventual decline among females is usually less.

Changes in collagenous tissue also occur with aging. Certain types of collagen accumulate in the joints and contribute to inflexibility patterns of body movements.

Bone changes are inevitable, although the degree of change between individuals is highly variable. Bone mass usually decreases, but white females lose more bone matter than black women, and males show less loss than females. Research also reveals that proper nutrition and sensible standards of exercise participation play a significant role in retaining bone mass and strength.

Skeletal muscles provide the source of force through their ability to contract and relax. The concept of reciprocal innervation means that muscle groups work in pairs. Evidence shows that fast reaction time can be sustained for some older persons who participate in physical activity.

Aging brings about structural changes in muscle tissue, changes that develop in the cells themselves. Muscle weight and density decline more rapidly among physically inactive people. Muscle metabolism steadily slows from age 3 to 80, yet some older persons are known to have metabolic rates as high as that of a 40-year-old. Exercise plays a significant role in maintaining the integrity of muscle metabolism throughout life; however, the specific operative way in which this phenomenon occurs has not been clearly determined.

Although the brain loses thousands of cells each day, this organ functions remarkably well into old age depending largely upon the quality of oxygen and nourishment cells receive from the cardiovascular system. Physically fit individuals generally experience less brain function loss that inactive persons. Older adults can learn new motor skills; the principal differences between them and the young are related to the speed and method of presentation.

Balance and equilibrium skills are important safety concerns of the elderly, since these are associated with accidental falls. Balance proficiency stems from eyes, ears, kinesthesia, and proprioceptors. These sensory structures change with aging and subsequently affect the balance ability of older adults. Conductive hearing losses seldom affect balance control; however, disturbances of the internal chambers of the ear can cause dizziness and vertigo. Maintaining muscle strength, however, can be important in correcting balance errors. And, as one's balance and kinesthetic sense are intertwined, such activities as dancing, bowling, golf, racquetball, and swimming stimulate and invigorate the body's kinesthetic receivers and subsequently improve balance and body position orientation.

Finally, the other physique changes discussed, in the dimensions of the head, face, height, chest, hips, and feet, also support the conclusion that the physique does change with age. However, structural modifications occur over many years and are hardly discernible to the older individual.

REFERENCES

1. John Piscopo and James A. Baley, *Kinesiology: The Science of Movement* (New York: Jonn Wiley & Sons, 1981), p. 94.
2. W. H. Sheldon, *Atlas of Men: A Guide for Somatotyping the Adult Male at All Ages* (Darien, Conn.: Hafner Publishing, 1970), p. 25.
3. Isadore Rossman, "Anatomic and Body Composition Changes with Aging," in C. E. Finch and L. Hayflick, eds., *The Biology of Aging* (New York: Van Nostrand Reinhold, 1977), p. 189.
4. James M. Morris, "Biomechanics of the Spine," *Archives of Surgery* 107 (September 1973): 421.
5. Augustus A. White and Manohar M. Panjabi, *Clinical Biomechanics of the Spine* (Philadelphia: J. B. Lippincott, 1978), p. 42.
6. Ibid., p. 18.
7. F. J. Imms and O. G. Edholm, "Studies of Gait and Mobility in the Elderly," *Age and Ageing* 10 (1981): 147–156; and Betty R. Hasselkus and Georgia M. Shambes, "Aging and Postural Sway in Women," *Journal of Gerontology* 30 no. 6 (1975): 661–667.
8. White and Panjabi, *Biomechanics of the Spine*, p. 49.
9. A. Nachemson, "Towards a Better Understanding of Back Pain: A Review of the Mechanics of the Lumbar Disc," *Rheumatology and Rehabilitation* 14 (1975): 129–143.
10. A. Damon et al., "Age and Physique in Healthy White Veterans in Boston," *Journal of Gerontology* 27 (1972): 202–208.
11. Rossman, "Changes with Aging," p. 194.
12. Nathan Shock, "Systems Integration," in Finch and Hayflick, *Biology of Aging*, pp. 642–643.
13. Ernest Jokl, *Physiology of Exercise* (Springfield, Ill.: Charles C Thomas, 1964), pp. 34–35.
14. Roy J. Shephard, *Physiology and Biochemistry of Exercise* (New York: Praeger Publishers, 1982), p. 130.
15. Victor H. Frankel and Margareta Nordin, *Basic Biomechanics of the Skeletal System* (Philadelphia: Lea & Febiger, 1980), p. 101.
16. David A. Hall, *The Ageing of Connective Tissue* (London: Academic Press, 1976), p. 82.
17. Ibid., p. 60.
18. E. L. Smith, T. S. Christopher, and R. W. Purvis, "Bone Mass and Strength Decline with Age," in E. L. Smith and R. C. Serfass, eds., *Exercise and Aging: The Scientific Basis* (Hillside, N.J.: Enslow Publishers, 1981), p. 61.
19. Rossman, "Changes with Aging," p. 194.
20. Everett L. Smith, "Exercise for Prevention of Osteoporosis: A Review," *The Physician and Sports Medicine* 10, no. 3 (1982): 72–73.

21. Smith and Purvis, "Bone Mass and Strength," pp. 59–87; and John L. Aloia, "Exercise and Skeletal Health," *Journal of the American Geriatric Society* 29, no. 3 (1981): 104–107.
22. Waneen Wyrick Spirduso, "Reaction and Movement Time as a Function of Age and Physical Activity Level," *Journal of Gerontology* 30 (1975): 435–440; and Spirduso and Clifford Phillip, "Replication of Age and Physical Activity Effects on Reaction and Movement Time," *Journal of Gerontology* 33 (1978): 26–30.
23. E. Gutman, "Muscle," in Finch and Hayflick, *Biology of Aging,* pp. 448–449.
24. Hall, *Ageing of Connective Tissue,* p. 62.
25. Robert H. Fitts, "Aging and Skeletal Muscle," in Smith and Serfass, *Exercise and Aging,* pp. 31–41.
26. Gutman, "Muscle," p. 463.
27. Toshio Moritani, "Training Adaptations in Muscles of Older Men," in Smith and Serfass, *Exercise and Aging,* pp. 149–166.
28. Lars Larsson, Gunnar Grimby, and Jan Karlsson, "Muscle Strength and Speed of Movement in Relation to Age and Muscle Morphology," *Journal of Applied Physiology* 46 (1979): 451–455.
29. Shock, "Systems Integration," p. 642.
30. Ibid.
31. J. Orlander et al., "Skeletal Muscle Metabolism and Ultrastructure in Relation to Age in Sedentary Men," *Acta Physiologica Scandinavica* 104 (1978): 249–261.
32. D. M. Bowen and A. N. Davison, "Neurochemistry of Aging and Senile Dementia," in G. Barbagallo-Sangiorgi and A. N. Exton-Smith, eds., *The Aging Brain* (New York: Plenum Press, 1980), p. 25.
33. Spirduso, "Reaction and Movement Time," p. 439; and E. Gutman and V. Hanzlikova, *Age Changes in the Neuromuscular System* (Baltimore: Williams & Wilkins, 1972), p. 98.
34. Metropolitan Life Insurance Co., "Accident Mortality at Older Ages," *Statistical Bulletin* 55 (June 1974): 5–8.
35. Marcel Hebbelinck, "Kinanthropometry and Aging: Morphological, Structural, Body Mechanics, and Motor Fitness Aspects of Aging," in F. Landry and W. A. R. Orban, eds., *Physical Activity and Human Well-being* (Miami: Symposia Specialists, 1978), p. 97.
36. Ibid.
37. J. R. McPherson, D. R. Lancaster, and J. C. Carroll, "Stature Change with Aging in Black Americans," *Journal of Gerontology* 33 (1978): 20–25.
38. Rossman, "Changes with Aging," p. 189.
39. Roy J. Shephard, *Physical Activity and Aging* (Chicago: Croom Helm, 1978), p. 60.

4

Fitness and the Aging Process: Implications for the Prevention of Illness

DEFINITIONS AND INTERPRETATIONS

Fitness means diverse conditions of health to different individuals. Interpretations of fitness range from a simple state state of freedom from disease to the Greek philosophy embracing the body beautiful, with the notion that a superb physique signifies good health. Fitness and health also assume different meanings at various stages in human growth and development. For example, to those in the prime of young adulthood, fitness may denote qualities of muscular strength and physical prowess in motor and athletic skills; on the other hand, for persons in their 70s and 80s, well beyond maturity, fitness takes on other meanings, such as absence of physical pain and discomfort, freedom from disease, sufficient mobility for independent living, freedom from stress, or merely coping with problems of everyday living. It is obvious that fitness and health definitions and interpretations depend upon the philosophical orientation and knowledge of the individual.

Three important characteristics about fitness and health emerge.* First, fitness is a dynamic, not a static, quality; second, fitness is a *personal* matter; and third, fitness is multi-dimensional, not only embracing physical well-being, but also involving mental, social, emotional, and spiritual factors—all interacting upon each other, resulting in "poor," "good," and other grada-

*The words *Fitness* and *Health* are used interchangeably throughout this text.

tions of fitness. Whether health is poor or good depends upon three factors: (1) genetic or inherited characteristics, (2) environmental circumstances, and (3) personal lifestyle. Hoyman defines health as personal fitness for survival and self-fulfillment and delineates four interrelated components: physical fitness, mental health, social well-being, and spiritual faith.[1]

Figure 4.1 demonstrates the concept that the health-disease spectrum is a continuum, ranging from zero health to optimum health. The model is based upon the premise that favorable ecologic factors tend to push one up into the zones of wellness and health, and unfavorable elements tend to thrust one down into the zones of disease.[2]

Dynamic Fitness

Levels of fitness are not static. Change is the rule, rather than the exception, according to the effect of the interacting variables shown in figure 4.1. The genetic factor is irreversible; that is, we cannot change our inherited blueprint with regard to basic body framework, those somatotype characteristics that give us our own individuality. However, such health aspects as dynamic fitness, functional capabilities, freedom from disease, stress, and social and emotional well-being are reversible and often slide up and down the ecological scale depending upon the type of lifestyle and environmental circumstances we have created. Each individual's genotype is predetermined, but living that fosters a positive set of interacting personal and environmental influences can enhance the fitness level of everyone.

As the years go on, a constant change in base-line functioning occurs. Metabolism, muscular strength, endurance, and joint mobility generally decline; however, these functional changes are often slow and hardly recognizable, particularly by people who see each other every day.

The rate of decline is (by far) more rapid among inactive sedate persons. A well-conditioned person will be able to perform greater physical work with less fatigue product build-up in the body and will be able to maintain higher levels of personal locomotion. A fit person also shows better neuromuscular coordination, more agility, and altered body composition of increased muscle mass and decreased adipose tissue.

The energy requirements for a given task are less for individuals who are physically conditioned. In short, the person who manifests higher levels of muscular strength, endurance, and flexibility and who avoids extreme obesity can not only do more work or play with less fatigue but also possesses greater energy reserve to maintain physical, mental, and psychological coping mechanisms. Physical fitness for the older person is defined as the ability of the individual to function efficiently and safely in everyday work and play activities without undue fatigue and with enough reserve energy to

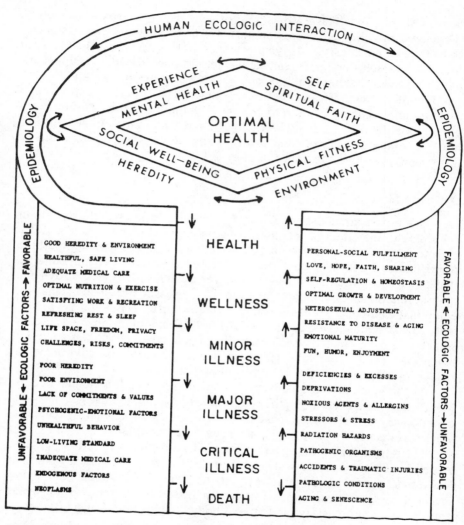

Figure 4.1 An ecological model of health and disease. (From H. S. Hoyman, *Journal of School Health*, SLV, no. 9 (1975): 514. Used with permission.)

meet unexpected physical demands. For example, performance of such tasks as walking, bending, turning, twisting, lifting packages, standing, sitting, climbing stairs, and moving in and out of a car all demonstrate functional efficiency requirements for normal activities. A sudden and unexpected shift in body weight to avert a fall, or a quickening in walking pace while carrying a loaded suitcase to catch a plane or bus are examples of unforeseen physical situations that require reserve energy to react successfully.

Unexpected physical demands on energy reserves also are involved in the enjoyment of leisure opportunities by older persons. For example, among the most popular leisure preferences of retirees are travel and sightseeing tours to those distant places described in attractive brochures, but precluded in early adulthood by lack of time. Now their greater discretionary time options, coupled with modern technology and rapid transportation, mean domestic and foreign travel is available to older people of most socioeconomic levels—but a stroll through the Gardens of Tivoli necessitates the physical stamina of leg strength and joint mobility to walk up the hundreds of steps found in this famous tourist attraction. Thus, it is clear that higher levels of physical fitness enhance the quantity and quality of leisure enjoyment which can enrich the mental, emotional, and social components of good health.

FITNESS PARAMETERS AND MOTOR PERFORMANCE

Although fitness benefits or impairments affect the whole person, the discussion here focuses upon the biological and kinesiological changes that accompany the aging process and their implications for the improvement of mobility and vigor. The central theme throughout this book is that the need to maintain physical fitness is basic for the enhancement of human effectiveness. A sedentary existence, in its extreme manifestation, ultimately leads to physical, emotional, and, finally, mental degeneration. As Dr. Raymond Harris poignantly reported in his testimony to a Senate subcommittee on fitness for older persons:

> Impaired mobility in middle age and older people, often the result of poor physical fitness, leads to social isolation, personality, and emotional deterioration and poor mental health.
> Muscular degeneration and physiological changes resulting from restriction of physical exercise lead to greater clumsiness, and increased fear of physical activity. Physical exercise programs that encourage older persons to be more active, independent, and mobile provide economic benefits by reducing medical problems and hospital costs.[3]

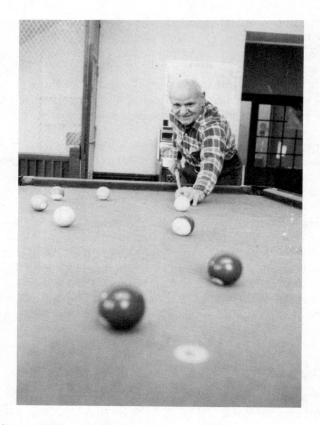

Figure 4.2 Leisure activities require reserve fitness energy.

His statement points out the dire consequences to the individual and society of deconditioning and poor physical fitness.

Muscular Strength and Endurance

Muscle composition, shape, and metabolism do change with advancing age. As pointed out in Chapter 3, the principal role of skeletal muscle is to give shape to the human form, provide protection to the soft internal organs, and supply the source of force, through its contractile nature. Essentially, two types of muscular contractions are used to perform motor tasks: dynamic (isotonic), and static (isometric). Dynamic contractions occur when a muscle is contracted and moves through a range of motion. External work (positive work) is performed. Tension is developed by shortening the muscle, which is physiologically called a *concentric-isotonic* movement. Tension and external work (negative work) may also be developed by lengthening the muscle. This, physiologically referred to as an *eccentric-isotonic* movement, is also a form of external work. Lifting a cup of tea from the table to the lips exemplifies a concentric-isotonic movement of the flexors of the elbow joint. Lowering the cup with control to the table, after sipping, is an example of an eccentric-isotonic movement. In both cases, flexor muscles of the elbow are contracting and under tension, even though opposite motions are performed. Daily motor tasks of older persons include dozens of such types of movements. It is important to know that muscular strength can be improved by concentric and eccentric isotonic exercises.

Isometric contraction occurs when tension of a muscle is created by pushing or pulling against an immovable object. Internal work is produced by the biochemical action of muscle metabolism, but changes in muscle length and movement do not take place.

Figure 4.4 illustrates an isometric contraction that places tension upon the pectoral (chest) muscles without movement. In other words, the chest muscles are not significantly lengthening or shortening. Research studies by Hettinger and Miller in the early 1950s showed that strength can be improved when a static exercise is held for a six-second position.[4]

Isotonic and isometric exercises are two contrasting methods that both improve strength. Isometric training offers the advantages of economy of time, cost, and storage space for equipment; however, this form of exercise does not promote joint flexibility and poses a potential hazard of creating the *Valsalva effect*. Also called the Valsalva maneuver, this involves breath holding during the exhalation effort of an exercise with the windpipe closed, producing increased pressure. During the hard muscular contraction used in isometric exercises, increased pressure on the chest is formed, which may be great enough to slow or inhibit the blood flow from the veins to the heart, resulting in an increase of blood pressure. When contraction has been completed and the pressure on the blood vessels is decreased, the dammed-up blood rushes into the heart and blood pressure rises. Older persons and frail people with weak vascular walls have been known to suffer ruptured blood vessels as a result of performing an isometric contraction—straining at the stool, for example.[5]

Historically, the medical profession has frowned upon all isometric exercises for older persons because of the potential inordinate rise in blood pressure. However, recent research has provided evidence that both dynamic movements and static contractions result in increased systemic arterial blood pressure, and the measure of rise depends upon the degree of tension exerted on the muscle, along with various other factors, such as using the big muscles of the legs and trunk rather than doing arm exercises.[6]

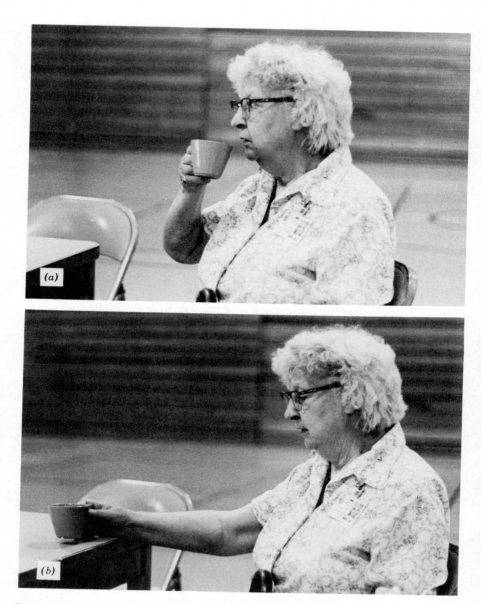

Figure 4.3 Concentric and eccentric movements: (a) lifting a cup (concentric); (b) lowering a cup (eccentric).

The Valsalva effect can be avoided provided free breathing is done during exercise, without breath holding. This procedure keeps the glottis (windpipe) open and counteracts the increased intrathoracic pressure. Consequently, potential danger to the cardiovascular system is lessened.

Furthermore, isometric work exists in everyday living. Lifting, holding, or moving an arm or leg involves some muscle contraction with a static movement. For example, the older adult carrying a bag of groceries and unlocking a house door with the opposite hand is performing an isometric contraction of hand, arm, and chest while holding the grocery bag. Many leisure and occupational tasks require lifting and holding assorted weights. Light weight lifting and low-level isometric exercises can condition and improve strength so that the senior adult can mow the lawn, hold a package, or steady a body position, when necessary, with less stress and strain.

Heavy weights and isometric exercises that require maximum muscular tension, however, should not be allowed. Persons with coronary or arterial disease should generally avoid resistive-type exercises and isometric work depending upon the pathology of their condition.

Incorporating rhythmic breathing, while exercising, is extremely important, particularly during low-level isometric work. Robert Spackman, a physical therapist at the University of Southern Illinois, devised a system of breathing in conjunction with isometric exercises. His technique consists of counting aloud while exercising, forcing the exerciser to inhale and exhale, thereby reducing pressure build-up in the cardiovascular system.[7]

The following protocol, developed by Spackman, has been used for over 30 years with senior adults into their 90s without any problems or injuries.

SPACKMAN METHOD FOR ISOMETRIC EXERCISE
Never Hold Your Breath—Breathe Normally!

1. Slowly ease the contraction. Slowly begin to push or pull as hard as you can without pain, holding for 6 seconds.
2. As you ease the contraction on, begin counting aloud: 1000-and-one, 1000-and-two, for 6 seconds.
3. Ease the contraction off slowly at the end of 6 seconds.
4. Relax for 6 seconds.
5. Repeat the exercise three times holding for 6 seconds each. *Breathe normally!*
6. Always count aloud during each exercise.
7. Should you have any pain, ease the contraction off and only push as hard as you can without pain.
8. As your strength increases, all pain should disappear.
9. If pain persists, stop the exercise and see your physician.[8]

A series of isometric exercises is shown in the Appendix A. Isometric training can improve muscular strength, and for some individuals free of cardiovascular impairments it provides a useful way of exercising. The primary focus is to improve the functional strength capabilities of the individual for better performance of everyday living chores, with conservation of some energy for recreational activities requiring muscular force. In any case, when deciding to use resistive or isometric exercises, the older adult should seek medical clearance before embarking on a program of this type.

Variations of Isotonic (Dynamic) Exercises. The surge of physical fitness interest, at all ages, has generated a variety of strength training modalities. Three types of resistive training systems have evolved: (1) free weights and weight machines (i.e., Universal Gym Apparatus), (2) Nautilus System, and (3) isokinetic system. These modes are popular with younger persons, especially for supplemental athletic training and rehabilitation purposes. However, each method can be employed by older persons, provided light-resistive loads are used. All these procedures are effective for improving muscular strength and body posture—two significant goals, irrespective of age.

Free weights, Universal Gyms, and Nautilus Systems are quite common, with the first two generally found in local Ys and the latter featured at private fitness centers in metropolitan city areas. Isokinetic instruments are costly items and generally found in university research centers and hospital settings.

Free Weights. Free weights refer to the lifting of dumbbells or use of a standard cross-bar with assorted weight sizes, usually from five to several hundred pounds. This mode is probably the least expensive and is easily adaptable to progress in increasing loads; however, changing weight loads does pose the risk of injury.

The Universal Gym system uses discs or stacked weights that allow the participant to move through a range motion. A fixed weight is predetermined and the resistance is greatest at extreme joint ranges because the length of the resistance arm (distance from center of gravity to the point of rotation) is farthest away from the axis of rotation. For example, less force is required to flex the elbow joint with or without a load when the joint angle is less than 45 degrees, rather than at an angle more than 90 degrees.

The Universal Gym is a form of weight training, and when used in a sequential and progressive way with correct rhythmic breathing, it can restore muscle mass to deconditioned individuals. This type of conditioning also has merit in the amelioration of osteoporosis (bone weakness) since it falls into the category of "weight bearing" activities which tend to stimulate bone accretion.

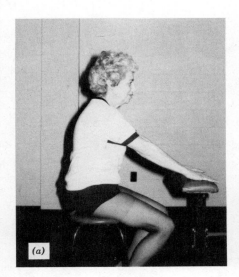
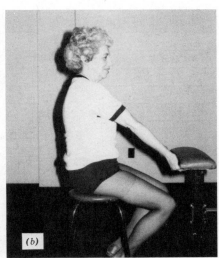
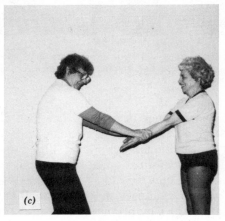

Figure 4.4 Improving chest strength through light isometrics: (a) downward pressing movement of the hand (arm extension); (b) upward pressing movement of the hand (arm flexion); (c) arm flexion (partner offering resistance).

Nautilus System. Nautilus training is another form of weight training using up to 20 separate machines, each designed to exercise specific muscle groups of the neck, shoulders, arms, hips, back, and legs. Nautilus equipment uses the principle of resistance exercise whereby different amounts of loads are applied during the course of an isotonic movement. A cam system is used to regulate the resistance, which changes to match the ability of the joint to

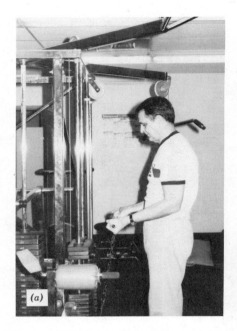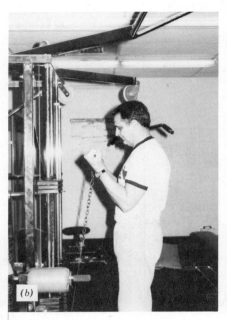

Figure 4.5 Strength development: (a) joint angle more than 90 degrees (greater resistance); (b) joint angle less than 45 degrees (less resistance).

produce force through its range of motion. The load changes of the resistance arm on the machine are preset to coincide with the average strength curves for specific joint motions. (See Figure 4.6.)

For example, in a typical situation, at the start of a movement, available force is at its lowest level; thus the radius of the cam is small and resistance is low. However, as the exerciser moves to another position, force increases, so the radius of the cam becomes proportionally larger. The radius of the cam automatically increases and decreases in exact proportion to the changing demands of the turning lever arm of the body part exercised. This instrument allows the individual to perform an exercise with full range of motion.[9]

Isokinetic System. Another name for this type of isotonic exercise is *accommodating resistance exercise.* This form of training, done with a special machine called a *Cybex,* allows the joint to move through a full range of motion with the speed of movement held constant. An automatic governor controls the resistance and speed, which is preset before the exercise is started. (See Figure 4.7.)

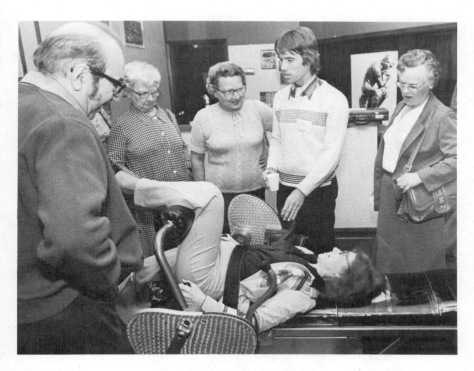

Figure 4.6 Nautilus System—hip and back machine. (Courtesy of Nautilus Fitness Center, Williamsville, N.Y., and Robert L. Smith, Photography.)

Several studies show that this type of exercise procedure is better than standard forms of weight training (lifting free weight) relative to strength and body composition.[10] However, the Cybex is expensive, and perhaps has a greater value in hospitals where therapeutic and rehabilitation modes requiring careful quantitative measurement techniques are necessary.

Each of these exercise instruments provides effective gains in muscular strength development, and anyone at any age can increase strength, provided correct principles of exercise progression and execution are applied. Table 4.1 summarizes the pros and cons of four available conditioning modalities.

In assessing strength development, consideration should be given to the differentiation between muscular strength and muscular endurance. Muscular strength is the ability to exert force during a single maximal effort. Muscular endurance is the ability to exert force during a series of repeated efforts. Each of these qualities merits attention since so many human move-

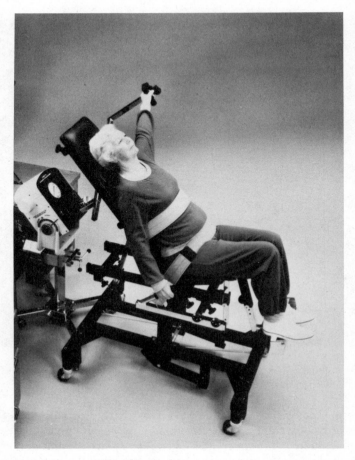

Figure 4.7 Isokinetic system—shoulder abductor/adduction exercise. (Courtesy of Cybex, a Division of Lumex Inc., Ronkonkoma, N.Y.)

ments require single strength exertion while other tasks involve sustained muscular work. For example, the maximum number of steps a person can climb is a test of muscular endurance, whereas the maximum grip strength determined by a hand dynamometer is a muscular strength measurement.

The principal difference between the two types of strength is that the endurance event must be supported by the circulation, and the energy requirements are very different from those of a single effort.[11] The question thus arises, What kind of strength and how much muscular force does an older person need? Of course, the law of individual differences prevails

Table 4.1 Exercise Modes for Muscular Strength Development

Type	Equipment	Pros	Cons
Isotonic	Free weights, e.g., dumbbells, barbells, Universal Gym, and other types of weight machines	Generally available at most Ys; least expensive, easy to use, less boring psychologically than isometrics	May take extra time to change weights; potential risk of injury with bars when using free weights
Isometric	A variety of commercial and home devices	Little or no equipment necessary; requires less time	May become boring because progress is difficult to observe; potential risk of creating Valsalva effect; does not contribute to flexibility development; not recommended for persons with hypertension or cardiac problems
Variable Resistance System	Nautilus equipment with cam device	Instrument allows variable resistant loads to match the joint ability to produce force throughout a full range of motion; applies appropriate biomechanical principles of lever arms and force production—uses positive and negative work to develop strength	Highly specialized equipment generally available only through private fitness centers; large space area needed to accommodate various machines
Isokinetic	Cybex instrument	Allows maximum resistance at a constant speed throughout range of motion	Expensive; essentially a rehabilitation, testing, and research instrument

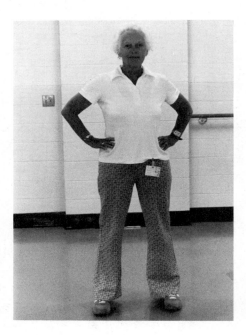

Figure 4.8 Muscular strength and endurance are essential fitness factors
for good posture and independent ambulation.

when setting muscular fitness goals, depending on the medical fitness lifestyle, needs, and interests of each individual. Essentially, strength development and maintenance serve two basic purposes that have specific relevance
to the average person over 50: (1) to provide myogenic tone (muscle firmness
through exercise) for the maintenance of good posture; and (2) to provide the
energetic source of power and force needed for independent ambulation in
work and play. The high levels of strength development, which accompany
heavy weight training regimens, are not recommended for most older persons because of the potential danger to the cardiovascular system.

Principles of Muscular Strength and Endurance Development. Muscle development and hypertrophy will occur at any age, male or female, young or old,
able-bodied or disabled, provided the individual is free of serious physiological dysfunctions or pathological disease. Studies have shown significant
improvement in muscle composition and strength through a variety of isotonic, isokinetic, and isometric modes.[12] Two principles that affect the development of muscular strength and endurance are the overload principle
and the specificity of training principle.

Overload Principle. The overload principle is a basic concept in fitness physiology for strength improvement. It refers to subjecting the various muscle

groups to greater resistive loads than normally encountered in everyday activities. The older person should remember that *overloading* is a relative term. Excessive resistance training for the younger or elite athlete is quite different from the overload regimen designed for the senior adult seeking good ambulatory proficiency.

Older adults should not exercise to the point of maximum loading. Overloading can be applied to the muscle by three methods: (1) increasing the magnitude of load (weight); (2) increasing the number of repetitions of the exercise; and (3) changing body position, favoring or not favoring the mechanical leverage positions of the movement performed. The first two methods should be obvious, with greater work generated. The third method involves some kinesiologic principles. For example, when performing a simple sit-up, it is more difficult to execute the movement with hands laced behind the head than placed along the thighs. Mechanically, the center of gravity is higher in the chest area with arms and hands in the head region than when placed parallel to the floor beside the thighs. By changing the gravity center, the lever arm is lengthened from its axis of rotation (hip joint) and consequently more strength is required to raise the trunk off the floor. Figure 4.9 illustrates three different positions of the arms that increase the length of the resistance arm and the force necessary to perform a sit-up.

Using this mechanical principle of levers, exercises can be designed to meet individual tolerance levels without undue fatigue or pain. Gains in strength will occur with any of the three methods described—provided greater tension is induced in the muscle fibers. A typical daily training routine includes several sets of contractions, each involving two to ten repetitions of an overloaded lifting effort.[13] A load of 50 to 60 percent of maximum effort is usually tolerated. However, the older person should *always* train at submaximal levels with each load individually prescribed by a physician or qualified professional physical educator.

Specificity of Exercise Principle. Strength training programs should be specific in terms of (1) muscle groups being strengthened, and (2) purpose of the exercise performed. That is, exercises to strengthen various muscle regions should be designed to directly activate the involved muscles. For example, if one wishes to strengthen the quadriceps (front) and biceps femoris (hamstring) of the upper thigh, he or she must apply resistive loads to knee flexion and extension so that the activity will specifically involve that region of the body. Arm and chest exercises contribute little, if anything, to the improvement of the leg muscles. Likewise, toe-touching exercises from a standing position do not strengthen the abdominal muscles; instead, they serve to stretch the hamstrings of the upper leg.

The purpose of the activity should also invoke the specificity of training

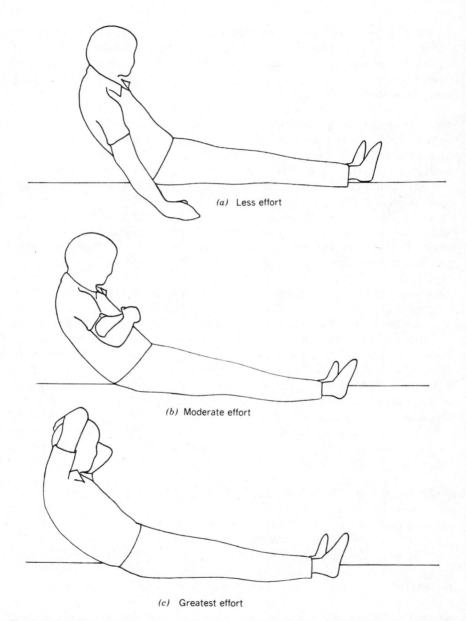

(a) Less effort

(b) Moderate effort

(c) Greatest effort

Figure 4.9 Applying the overload principle by changing the position of the arms in performing a sit-up: (a) less effort; (b) moderate effort; (c) greatest effort.

principle. For example, if one is aiming for greater strength increments throughout a particular joint range of motion, isometric conditioning will not contribute to this objective. Applying the specificity principle of resistive loading at each point through a full range of joint motion develops dynamic strength as opposed to static or isometric strength. Instruments such as the Nautilus equipment and the isokinetic machine (Cybex) use the overload and specificity principles

The overload and specificity principles of exercise apply to all ages. The fundamental difference in using the principles with older persons is that adaptations in intensity and duration are required. Because of biological age changes, stress loads and length of exercise periods should be less, and adapted to declining strength, flexibility, and neuromuscular coordination characteristic of persons past maturity. Although faster gains in muscular strength will result by using heavy weights with fewer repetitions, older persons should use lighter weights with more repetitions, which will pose less potential danger of injury to the musculoskeletal and cardiovascular systems.

Stronger muscles translate into quicker walking, turning, bending, striking a ball, or using a racket in badminton with greater command. Improving muscle quality and quantity is beneficial at any age; it becomes more important with advancing years. Joints are better protected with good muscle tone and tensile strength. Isotonic, isometric, and isokinetic exercise modes, although specific in their contribution to strength development, all serve to stave off muscle atrophy, help to preserve the integrity of the skeletal form, and protect the body's soft organs and bones which tend to become more fragile with advancing age. Research professor Dr. Harrison Clarke points out the importance of muscular strength, which too often is forgotten in our automated and computer-oriented society:

> Man's existence and effectiveness depend upon his muscles. Volitional movements of the body or any of its parts are impossible without action by skeletal muscles. Thus, obviously, one cannot stand, walk, run, jump, climb, or swim without the contraction of many muscles throughout the body. Smaller muscles perform intricate functions, including writing manuscripts, playing musical instruments, singing, using hand tools, catching and throwing balls, and the like. Muscles perform vital functions of the body. The heart is a muscle; death occurs instantly when it ceases to contract. Breathing, digestion, and elimination would be impossible without muscular contractions. . . . The good condition of muscles, their strength and endurance is essential to man.[14]

Most people would be hard-pressed to dispute Clarke's statement. Well-conditioned muscles are vital in many ways to the enhancement of human effectiveness.

Flexibility

The term *flexibility* is defined as the range of joint motion or of a series of joints. Flexibility may be passive or active. Passive flexibility is considered a slow, sustained stretch; that is, lengthening a muscle to an extended position and holding for several seconds, typically 6 to 10 (see Figure 4.10a). Active flexibility, known as dynamic or ballistic stretching, is the ability to move a joint through its range while performing a normal activity or changing body posture from one position to another (see Figure 4.10b). Dynamic flexibility really represents "body movement freedom," and its quality and quantity are most relevant to dynamic movement in walking, bending, turning, and twisting motions of common activities.

Nature and Functional Aspects of Flexibility. The articulating biomechanical structures of the human being are made up of bone, tendon, ligament, fascia, and cartilage. Bone provides the rigid physical support for joint articulation. Tendons serve as attachments to muscles, bones, other tendons, ligaments, or fascia and have the function of conveying the pull from one bone to another segment. Ligaments contain bundles of fibers richly supplied with the collagen that gives joints tensile strength and limits the extent of separation, thereby assisting in preventing injury. Ligaments are strong, pliable, inextensible (incapable of being stretched) yet tough fibers that hold joints together. Fascia is composed of superficial and deep fibrous connective tissues of varying thickness and density. Its thickness and density depends upon the functional demands for elasticity. Articular cartilage is a gristle-like connective tissue that lies in bony cavities and serves as a protective cushion for articulating surfaces. Each of these structures contains different amounts of collagen. It has been suggested that increased rigidity of connective tissues surrounding joints and musculature is due, in part, to greater masses of collagenous substances, particularly among the elderly.[15]

Muscular extensibility or amplitude also determines one's degree of flexibility. Dynamic-type activities that allow joints to proceed through a full range of motion enhance the extensibility of muscular tissue. Heavy resistance-type and isometric exercises tend to shorten fibers and thus restrict flexibility.

The contractile qualities of muscular tissue may be extended indefinitely with proper nutrition and physical activity, barring pathological conditions. Morphological changes in muscle with old age do not become noticeable until a very late state, and secondary changes are due primarily to disease and nutritional deficiency.[16] Such activities as swimming and stretching-type calisthenics are highly recommended for maintenance of muscular contractility and flexibility.

General agreement exists among authorities that flexibility is a highly

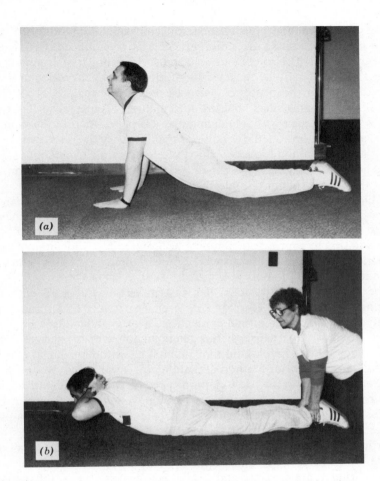

Figure 4.10 Flexibility movements of the upper trunk: (a) passive: (b) active.

specific factor rather than a general component, and flexibility shown in one joint does not reflect the range of movement in other joints.[17] That is, the range of motion of the elbow joint does not ensure a similar flexibility range of the knee joint.

Aging and Flexibility. Joint range of motion or flexibility is usually subordinated and often excluded in physical fitness test batteries. Although one may argue the significance of flexibility in the ranking of fitness components among youth, this factor takes precedence over other fitness elements in older persons because it is an indispensable prerequisite of mobility.

The anatomical and physiological musculoskeletal conditions of youth and the elderly of course are different. Several pronounced dissimilarities are: (1) greater calcification of cartilage and surrounding tissues among older people; (2) a tendency for muscles to shorten with age, particularly those groups located on the posterior surfaces and lower regions of the body, including trunk, hamstrings, and leg musculature; (3) increased "stiffness" of males over females with advancing age; (4) prevalence in the elderly of arthritic and other orthopedic conditions that intensify the restriction of joint motion; (5) tension and anxiety, which often strike older persons and may impede body flexibility; and (6) much less elasticity and compression tolerance of the spinal column in older persons.

A closer look at human flexibility and aging reveals the influence of genetics and environment. Tissue changes, such as lessened resiliency and cartilage calcification, are progressive. Sufficient levels of calcium in the diet, in addition to appropriate amounts of protein, iron, and vitamins and in conjunction with regularly performed slow-stretching exercises, can retard the stiffening of body joints.

The shortening of the muscular system can be retarded with slow-stretching type exercises. Hormonal differences between males and females may offer clues to the empirical evidence of greater flexibility among older women. However, the cause of this phenomenon remains unclear. Exponents of yoga (slow-stretch-hold movements) exalt the beneficial effects of this activity as a superior method of maintaining suppleness. Notwithstanding the merits of low-gear, slow-motion types of stretching exercises, their limited benefits to the cardiorespiratory system should be recognized. Other activities that stimulate the heart/lung mechanisms should also be a part of the exercise regimen.

Arthritic and other orthopedic-type conditions are common ailments of the elderly. Joint mobility can be fostered with activities that relieve the weight-bearing joints of stress and strain and possible further inflammation. swimming is excellent for orthopedically limited persons who possess a minimum level of stroke skills. A bicycle ergometer (stationary bicycle) is another exercise option that can be used to enhance flexibility while relieving body weight stress on the lower limbs. Specific exercises for the improvement of flexibility are presented in the next chapter.

Cardiovascular-Respiratory Efficiency

Cardiovascular disorders are the most common causes of death among the elderly. Such conditions as congestive heart failure and heart rhythm disruptions (arrhythmias) are quite common in aging hearts. *Arteriosclerosis* (hardening of blood vessels) is the most common type of heart disease and the usual cause of heart failure of the elderly.[18] *Atherosclerosis* (narrowing of blood vessels) is also a common vascular disease of the elderly; however, this condition can and does occur at any age. Atherosclerosis, a companion to arteriosclerosis, is a frequent cause of *ischemic heart disease* (deficiency in the blood supply to the heart muscle due to a constriction of the coronary arteries). *Hypertension* (high blood pressure) accelerates the potential for acute heart and vascular diseases.

All of these conditions also decrease pulmonary (lung) blood flow since oxygen transportation is dependent upon adequate cardiac output (amount of blood expelled per unit of time). Thus, a central task of the cardiovascular-respiratory system is to provide oxygen to the cells of the body. The heart, lungs, and blood vessels together are responsible for this objective.

The following discussion focuses upon physical fitness with respect to its effect on the cardiorespiratory and vascular systems.

Circulorespiratory Relationships and Limitations. Decreased circulorespiratory function occurs with age. The ability of the heart and lungs to utilize oxygen decreases with age, and so the resultant complaint of fatigue is frequently heard from the elderly. The thoracic cage and chest wall decrease in pliability and elasticity, directly reducing the respiration efficiency of the lungs (inspiration and expiration capacity). The internal structure of the lungs tends to become rigid with cell loss and increases in collagen substances. The net result is manifested in decreased ventilation and muscular force of the chest.

Deep breathing and coughing can be a problem for certain older persons. Weakened intercostal muscles, which are used to lift and lower the rib cage for breathing, often fail to maintain an adequate capacity. The transversus muscle of the abdominal group plays an important part in the expiratory phase of breathing. The diaphragm assumes a prominent role in quiet breathing, particularly during the inspiration phase.

Older persons need good breathing and coughing efficiency to rid the respiratory system of congestive mucus, which may serve as a breeding ground for pathological organisms. Activities and exercises of an aerobic nature that stimulate the diaphragm, intercostals, and transversus muscles should be an integral part of a training and conditioning regime for older persons. Brisk walking, jogging, swimming, and diaphragmatic breathing exercises help to maintain chest wall elasticity.

The "cold hands and feet syndrome" is a common disorder of the elderly. This condition is partially explained by the lack of adequate blood circulation to the skin, which results in lower skin temperatures. Dynamic exercise improves circulatory efficiency by increasing the pumping action of the heart, which results in delivery of more blood to the extremities. The

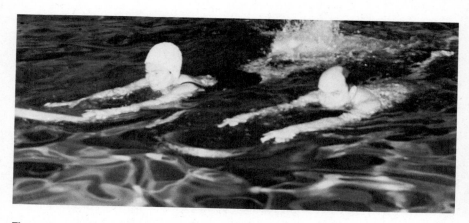

Figure 4.11 Improving peripheral vascular circulation of the legs using a kickboard. (From J. Piscopo and C. A. Lewis, "Preparing Geriatric Fitness and Recreation Specialists," *Journal of Physical Education and Recreation* 48, no. 8 (1977): 29. Used with permission.)

combined and integrative effect of exercise upon the cardiovascular and respiratory systems helps to bring more blood to the surface and thus serves as a body-temperature regulatory mechanism.

Activities that focus upon improving peripheral vascular circulation by using the big muscles of the legs as in walking, jogging, swimming, and dancing are natural ways to improve blood circulation. Heavy resistive exercises, on the other hand, create higher blood pressure and may constrict circulatory flow to the periphery of the arms and legs. Swimming is especially appropriate for individuals with joint and other orthopedic restrictions since the buoyancy of the water provides a cushion and minimizes load strain upon weakened joints.

Figure 4.11 illustrates an excellent exercise activity for individuals who are affected with vascular problems of the legs. Specific exercise programs designed for heart-lung-circulatory fitness are presented in Chapter 5.

Exercise and Heart Efficiency. Heart action and efficiency vary greatly at all ages, and individuals who are unconditioned for a variety of reasons can be at risk with increased exercise. For example, for physically inactive persons with coronary heart disease (CHD) whereby higher metabolic rates result from exercise, indiscriminate physical activity may be harmful. When exercise is prescribed, programs should be conducted under careful supervision. Any exercise programmer must consider: (1) type (what kind); (2) intensity (how hard); (3) duration (how long); (4) frequency (how often); and (5) progression (orderly sequence from low to high work-out levels).

Two important factors in determining the degree of exercise prescription are age and medical health of the participant. The American College of Sports Medicine has set forth a listing of medical conditions that require consideration before testing and physical activity. These are shown in Table 4.2.

The participant is well advised to discuss any of the above conditions with his or her physician and to seek explicit approval for physical activity participation before engaging in any type of exercise regimen. The discussion here applies principally to the asymptomatic (without symptoms of disease) persons, with normal cardiac changes and responses to physical activity.

Aerobic Efficiency. The term **aerobics** is a familiar one in the vocabulary of fitness and training personnel. Such phrases as "jazzercizes," "aerobic dancing," and "aerobics in motion," all refer to a basic physiological principle of work which literally means transforming energy of the body through the metabolic process in the presence of oxygen.

Aerobic capacity or power is generally considered a measure of cardiorespiratory endurance. This measure refers to the amount of oxygen used (liters or milliliters per kilogram of body weight) per unit of time (usually for one minute); it also is called maximal oxygen uptake (VO_2 max). As pointed out in Chapter 3, the metabolic process slows down with age; consequently, a loss of up to 50 percent of aerobic capacity is found among 60-year-old persons.[19] However, levels of VO_2 max in older persons can be surprisingly high. For example, Harold Chapman, a 71-year-old competitive Masters middle-distance runner set a record among men over 70 for running a mile in 6.05 minutes.[20] Chapman showed the following cardiovascular-respiratory measurements:

	Standing Position
Heart rate (beats · min^{-1}) at rest	57
Systolic blood pressure (mm Hg) at rest	123
Diastolic blood pressure (mm Hg) at rest	79
Maximal oxygen uptake (ml. kg^{-1} min^{-1})	57.3*

*Respiratory response to maximal uphill treadmill running (weight-adjusted)

Chapman's physical characteristics reflected extreme leanness (height 165 cm.), weight (54.8 kg.), and body fat (5.8 percent). The aerobic capacity values of this septuagenarian are similar to responses found in young athletes, with a much greater cardiac output than older nonathletes. His VO_2 max of 57.3 ml. $kg.^{1}$ min^{-1} was 74 percent higher than what is predicted for

Table 4.2   Contraindications for Exercise and Exercise Testing (Out-of-Hospital Setting)

A. *Contraindications*
   1. Acute myocardial infarction
   2. Unstable or at-rest angina pectoris
   3. Dangerous arrhythmias (ventricular tachycardia or any rhythm significantly compromising cardiac function)
   4. History suggesting excessive medication effects (digitalis, diuretics, psychotropic agents)
   5. Manifest circulatory insufficiency (congestive heart failure)
   6. Severe aortic stenosis
   7. Severe left ventricular outflow tract obstructive disease (IHSS)
   8. Suspected or known dissecting aneurysm
   9. Active or suspected myocarditis or cardiomyopathy (within the past year)
  10. Thrombophlebitis—known or suspected
  11. Recent embolism, systemic or pulmonary
  12. Recent or active infectious episodes (including upper respiratory infections)
  13. High dose of phenothiazine agents
B. *Relative Contraindications*[a]
   1. Uncontrolled or high-rate supraventricular arrhythmias
   2. Repetitive or frequent ventricular ectopic activity
   3. Untreated severe systemic or pulmonary hypertension
   4. Ventricular aneurysm
   5. Moderate aortic stenosis
   6. Severe myocardial obstructive syndromes (subvalvular, muscular, or membranous obstructions)
   7. Marked cardiac enlargement
   8. Uncontrolled metabolic disease (diabetes, thyrotoxicosis, myxedema)
   9. Toxemia
C. *Condition Requiring Consideration and/or Precautions*
   1. Conduction disturbances
        a. Complete atrioventricular block
        b. Left bundle branch block
        c. Wolff-Parkinson-White anomaly or syndrome
        d. Lown-Ganong-Levine syndrome
        e. Bifascicular block (with or without 1st block)
   2. Controlled arrhythmias
   3. Fixed-rate pacemaker
   4. Mitral valve prolapse (click-murmur) syndrome
   5. Angina pectoris and other manifestations of coronary insufficiency
   6. Certain medications
        a. Digitalis, diuretics, psychotropic drugs
        b. Beta-blocking and drugs of related action

Table 4.2 *Continued*

---

    c. Nitrates
    d. Antihypertensive drugs
  7. Electrolyte disturbance
  8. Clinically severe hypertension (diastolic above 110, grade III retinopathy)
  9. Cyanotic heart disease
10. Intermittent or fixed right-to-left shunt
11. Severe anemia (hemoglobin below 10 gm/dl)
12. Marked obesity (20% above optimal body weight)
13. Renal, hepatic, and other metabolic insufficiency
14. Overt psychoneurotic disturbances requiring therapy
15. Neuromuscular musculoskeletal, orthopedic, or arthritic disorders which would prevent activity
16. Moderate to severe pulmonary disease
17. Intermittent claudication
18. Diabetes

---

[a] In the practice of medicine, the benefits of evaluation often exceed the risks for patients with these relative contraindications.
Source: American College of Sports Medicine, *Guidelines for Graded Testing and Exercise Prescriptions* (Philadelphia: Lea & Febiger, 1980), pp. 12-14. Reprinted by permission.

his age and percent body fat. It is recognized that genetic endowment is a determining factor related to Chapman's superior cardiovascular functions, but these high values in aerobic performance certainly also come from the conditioning effects, which result from vigorous physical activity. His example provides some evidence that heart and lungs can function at high levels well into old age.

The measurement of aerobic capacity (VO_2 max), oxygen uptake, can be determined by laboratory tests using a treadmill and analyzing oxygen and carbon dioxide before and after exercise. This procedure is reserved for research purposes, and has little value for the activity practitioner. Field tests for measurement and evaluation using run-walk and heart rate threshold procedures provide a more practical method of assessing aerobic and cardiorespiratory fitness. Chapter 9 deals specifically with this topic.

Anaerobic Efficiency. Energy for muscular work is also provided by another aspect of the cellular metabolism process, called *anaerobic capacity*; it is used as a backup mechanism supplying the stored fuel reserves (adenosine triphosphate, or ATP) when the oxygen supply is inadequate for a given task. Muscle cells have the ability to make ATP from glucose (sugar) without oxygen through a biochemical process called *glycolysis*. This leads to the development of a fatigue substance in the blood known as *blood lactate*.

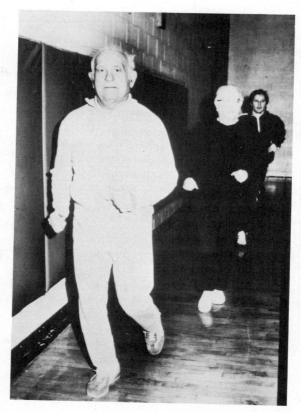

Figure 4.12 Maintaining high levels of aerobic capacity through jogging.

This mechanism is operative in activities that last from two minutes to at least ten minutes or longer.[21] Lactate accumulates in greater amounts at a faster rate and is removed more slowly in unconditioned individuals.

Building anaerobic power probably has less significance for older persons since most of the endurance activities of this group do not entail sprint work requirements. The majority of activities are performed using aerobic metabolism (with oxygen). However, it should be noted that the capacity of processing lactate is lessened in the elderly, and thus the onset of fatigue begins earlier particularly among unfit older persons.[22] Nevertheless, occasions may develop when the older person must call on extra reserve capacity to sustain an endurance task that will require this exercise metabolic phenomenon.

Although research is not conclusive, some evidence indicates that training improves anaerobic and aerobic capacity simultaneously. The practical implication of these metabolic phenomena clearly show that stamina involving cardiovascular, pulmonary, and muscular actions can only be attained by engaging in fitness activities that demand physical exercise and movement. Exercise gadgets that massage or passively stimulate the cardiovascular-respiratory and muscular systems represent futile attempts in seeking improved qualities of this endurance component.

Heart Rate and Aging. The heart rate is the number of beats per minute, and the pulse rate is the frequency of throbs (expansion and contraction of an artery) which may be felt with the finger, ranging from 50 to 100 beats per minute. Normally, the two values are identical. The resting heart rate can be taken at the *radial, carotid,* or *temporal arteries.* The intensity of exercise is usually determined by the rate of the heartbeat. Counting heart rate before and after exercise is important for the prescription of exercise intensity (see Chapter 5). A slight rise in resting heart rate occurs in adult life, but it varies from person to person at any age and from one situation to another. DeVries reports that it is almost meaningless to speak of a normal heart rate.[23] Average rates may be 78 beats per minute for one person and 40 for a highly trained endurance athlete. It is more important to note the heart rate changes for one individual, rather than to compare that person with a set of norms.

Even though resting heart rate changes only slightly, maximum heart rate (highest attainable heart rate capability of individual—MHR) progressively declines with age. The increase in MHR is in direct proportion to work required. However, this increase is only up to a point. That point of exhaustion is referred to as *maximal heart rate.* Maximal heart rates of 180 to 200 beats per minute have been observed in average young people with some values higher than 220 beats per minute reported.[24] The decline in MHR usually begins at 25, decreasing to a maximum rate for a 65-year-old of about 165-170 beats per minute. A basic formula of 220 minus age in years to establish exercise heart rate levels can be used in cardiovascular fitness programs. (Specific details of applying this formula are described in Chapter 5).

Cardiac Output. This indicates the total volume of blood expelled by the heart per unit of time (usually per minute). It is equal to the stroke volume (blood ejected at each heart beat) multiplied by the number of beats per time unit:

$$\text{Cardiac output} = \text{heart rate} \times \text{stroke volume}$$

Generally, cardiac output at rest declines about one percent per year from ages 19 to 86.[25] Again, as with other cardiac functions, wide variances exist

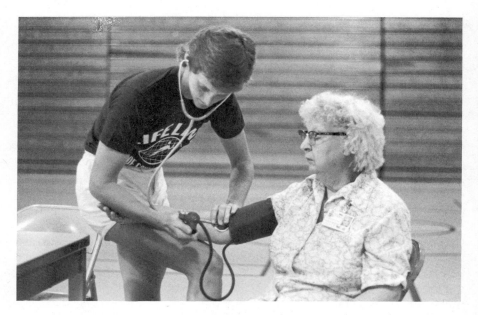

Figure 4.13 Measuring blood pressure using a sphygmomanometer.

depending upon the absence or presence of disease, overall fitness status, and genetic endowment. Some loss of heart muscle tissue, diminishing contractile power and elasticity, stiffening of heart valves, and fatty increments all tend to reduce cardiac output. These changes are accelerated with illness and gross physical inactivity.

Blood Pressure. The measure of force by which blood moves through the circulatory system is referred to as blood pressure and is defined as the pressure of the blood on the walls of arteries created by the action of the heart, elasticity of the walls of the arteries, and volume and thickness of the blood. The common method of measuring blood pressure is by use of a device called a *sphygmomanometer*, shown in Figure 4.13. This is an *indirect* method of taking blood pressure. Catheters measure direct pressure and are used in laboratory and research settings. The pressure is recorded in two numbers: the higher number is called *systolic pressure* (blood ejected from the heart—maximum pressure), and the lower number is called *diastolic pressure* (pressure between heart beats—minimum pressure). Thus a blood pressure reading of $^{140}/_{90}$ indicates a systolic pressure of 140 and a diastolic pressure of 90.

Basic blood pressure is the pressure during quiet rest. Generally, blood pressure increases with age; however, wide differences among populations exist. Genetics, culture, diet, and level of activity participation have considerable influence upon this circulatory component. Physiologically, blood pressure in the aging person greatly depends upon the loss of elasticity in the walls of the larger arteries—which tends to raise systolic and depress diastolic pressures—and at the same time, the increased role of the nervous system, which tends to stimulate contraction of the arteries and causes a rise in both. Therefore, systolic pressure typically rises with advancing years, while the diastolic may rise or fall.[26]

An interesting study by Fischer, investigating physically active males, demonstrated that active individuals in their seventh decade had lower systolic and diastolic pressure than inactive males.[27] He further discovered that arterial distensibility (stretching ability) was greater in the active group. This research suggests that physical activity helps to maintain higher transport capability of the blood (better circulation) by improving the elasticity of the blood vessels and simultaneously lowering blood pressure against the arterial walls.

Hypertension, a major contributing cause of deaths among the elderly, refers to a persistently high arterial blood pressure. Although such conditions as increasing stiffness of arteries, higher peripheral resistance to blood flow, and decreased kidney blood flow are associated with high blood pressure, this condition does not exist in all older persons. Other factors such as obesity, salt intake, and stress also contribute to hypertension. It appears that this disease has multiple etiologies and cannot be attributed to any one single cause. Nevertheless, it is generally accepted that regular and prudent physical activity tends to lower blood pressure.[28]

A note of caution must be interjected about the blood pressure effect of regular exercise and elderly individuals. Although some evidence has shown that exercise does tend to lower arterial blood pressure, more research is needed before conclusive proof is established. However, based upon the current evidence, we can state that engagement in regular exercise, together with reduction in gross obesity and high stress levels, can decrease the risk of hypertension and associated cardiovascular diseases.

Effect of Arm and Leg Exercises on Circulation. The heart-circulatory response to exercise varies with the type and intensity of its work requirements. In addition, the cardiovascular system also reacts differently to the part of the body and muscle groups involved. For example, when an individual is performing exercises using arm cranking devices, heart rate and blood pressure tend to rise more quickly than when using the large muscles of the legs on a bicycle. Clarke indicates that values for blood pressure are higher when work is performed with arms rather than with legs at a given level of submaximal oxygen consumption, and suggests that the smaller vascular beds in the miniature muscles offer greater resistance to blood flow.[29] Consequently, such tasks as shoveling snow and digging can present potential hazards for individuals with hypertensive conditions.

Wahren and Bygdeman investigated the circulatory adaptation to arm and leg exercises of subjects ranging from 25 to 65 years with a history of angina pectoris.[30] Their research showed that heart rate rose more steeply in relation to work intensity during arm exercise (arm pedaling) than during leg exercise (leg pedaling). Systolic blood pressure also showed steeper rises during arm exercise than in leg work. In addition to higher blood pressure and heart rates, greater lactate (by-product of fatigue) levels were found in the bloodstream with arm exercise than with leg work in a study conducted at the State University of New York at Buffalo.[31] Thus, arm exercises induce greater heart work loads and develop fatigue faster than do leg exercises.

Rhythmic exercises such as walking, cycling, and dancing are better activities for individuals with cardiovascular conditions. Arm exercises for this particular group should be viewed with caution. It is not suggested that arm exercises be eliminated from a conditioning program since many everyday tasks require hand and arm motions. However, overemphasis on such movements as arm flings, push-ups, overhead exercises, etc., with less attention to the big muscles of the trunk, hips, and legs is inadvisable.

Balance and Equilibrium Efficiency

A common notion about balance is that this fitness component is a general condition or state. Actually, balance is a specific skill related to a particular type of dynamic harmonious movement or to holding a particular stationary stance with stability and equilibrium under control. For example, balance required in walking is quite different from the equilibrium management in standing on a stepstool and reaching for an object. Normal walking patterns illustrate upright dynamic balance control. Standing on tiptoes represents another type of balance, called upright stationary balance. As pointed out in Chapter 3, balance stems from internal and external sources. Adapting the normal changes that occur internally (vision, ears, kinesthesia, and proprioception) and changing the surrounding external environment to allow for easier maintenance of such mechanical elements of the gravity center over its supporting base are key concepts in controlling balance and equilibrium.

Definitions and Classifications. Before prescribing activities that can improve balance skills, balance concepts must be defined and classified. Two broad types of balance are classified as stationary and dynamic balance. A subordinate category is further subdivided into upright and inverted balance.

Stationary balance, sometimes referred to as static balance, is defined as a hold position of the body in any given posture. Figure 4.14 illustrates upright and inverted stationary balance positions.

Dynamic balance is identified as the ability of the individual to maintain balance during a body movement. Figure 4.15 shows an upright dynamic balance movement.

Walking is an example of shifting the body's center of gravity—from one foot to another as the support base provided by each foot moves in a sequential and forward progression. Stability of the body, along with rhythm coordination and lower limb strength, is essential for efficient walking patterns. In a sense, the body loses its balance, then catches balance control again as each step is taken (see Figure 4.15).

Inverted dynamic balance applies when the body is moving in an upsidedown position in such skills as walking on one's hands or turning a somersault. Inverted dynamic balance skills are rarely used or necessary for older (and many younger) persons. They have specific relevance for athletes engaged in various sports where the body is moving continually in assorted inverted positions.

External Elements of Equilibrium. The acuteness of internal sources of balance control described in Chapter 3 changes from youth to maturity. Their keenness of function declines due to the normal alterations in the tissues that accompany the aging process. External sources of balance do not change and are constant. Such elements as gravitational constant (32.2 ft/sec^2), mass or weight of an object, center of gravity, line of gravity, and base of support are external factors that affect balance.

Mass or Weight and Center of Gravity. If mass or weight were the only factors affecting human balance, the heavier the object, the more stable the object would be. This factor is obvious in inanimate items such as bricks. Theoretically, the density and the center of a brick is also its center of gravity. The heavier the brick, the greater its stability. More weight evenly distributed over its supporting base tends to give the object stability. However, this concept applies to weight that is symmetrically distributed. The human body is asymmetrical, and its geometric center varies according to body build, age, and sex. The center of the body mass or center of gravity also changes when a person assumes different positions and postures such as sitting, standing, or leaning (see Figure 4.16).

Weight in older persons usually rises up to the middle and late 50s and then declines. Anthropometrical dimensions also change; i.e., increased chest size and abdominal girths further alter the location of the body's center of gravity. These varying weights and shifts in gravity centers of limb segments and the total body can create instability and loss of balance control in

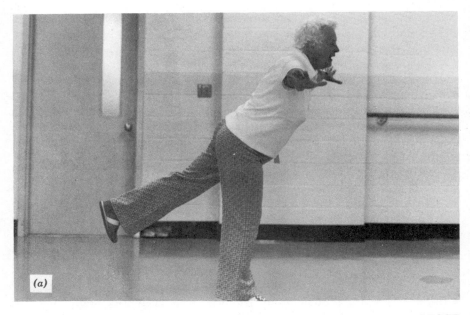

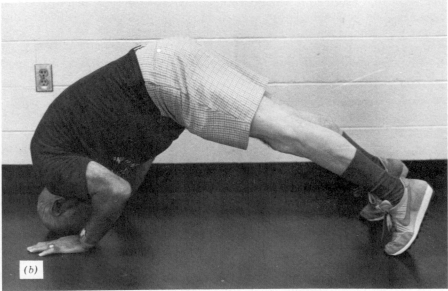

Figure 4.14 (a) Upright stationary balance; (b) Inverted stationary balance.

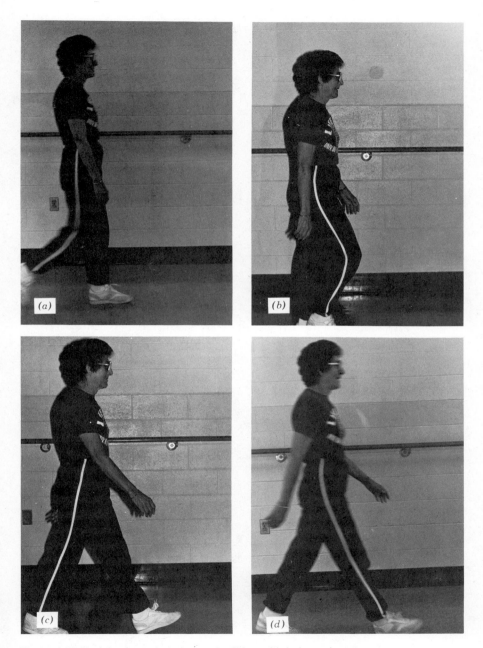

Figure 4.15 Upright dynamic balance—walking with balanced posture.

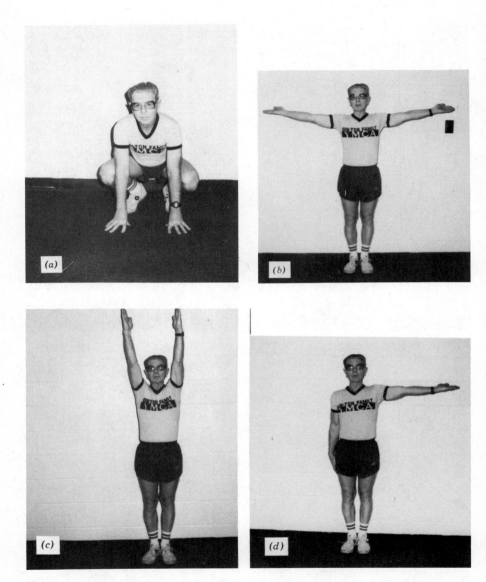

Figure 4.16 Center of gravity in various positions: (a) low CG; (b) higher CG; (c) highest CG; (d) shifting CG to one side of the body.

walking, turning, bending, and other assorted body movements used in work and play. Maintaining a reasonable level of muscular strength, particularly of the trunk and legs, which affect pelvic movements (where body center of gravity is located), helps to control the weight of the body by keeping the weight center within its supporting base (over the feet) in various standing postural movements. This factor is particularly important in falls caused by tripping. Individuals with strong hip, trunk, and leg muscles can regain their balance more quickly than those with weak musculature.

The center of gravity in the normal standing position of the adult male, arms hanging at the sides, is at a point at approximately 56 to 57 percent of the height. In women, it is at approximately 55 percent.[32] This weight center varies according to body build. Usually, older men are "top heavy," with larger chests and abdomens and thinner legs, and similar patterns are found among older women. However, exceptions to these body forms are not unusual. Orthopedic and skeletal deviations can affect the location of the center of gravity. For example, the gravity center of a person with hemiplegia (paralysis of one side of the body) as a result of a stroke will move to one side, near the heaviest part of the body. Individuals manifesting paraplegia (paralysis of the legs and lower part of the body) will possess a higher center of gravity than the person without disability. These shifts in gravity centers contribute to instability and can create balance problems within this special population group.

Line of Gravity and Base of Support. The pull of gravity is toward the center of earth. This fact establishes the direction and line of action or force called the *line of gravity.* An object or person maintains balance provided the line of gravity falls within its base of support. Figure 4.17 shows shifting centers of gravity in various positions. The line of gravity may be in front of or behind the gravity center; however, in each case, balance is maintained because the line of gravity falls near the center of the support. When one is carrying objects in front of the body, it is necessary to angle the trunk backward to maintain the line of gravity between the points of support. When carrying objects on one side of the body, it becomes necessary to angle the body sideward and raise the arm opposite to the side of the weight. This places the line of gravity between the points of support.

Calisthenic exercises that create changes in line of gravity, and activities such as walking on a zig-zag beam, as shown in Figure 4.18, allow the older person to practice maintaining the correct line of gravity over its supporting base principle, consequently sharpening acuity of maintaining upright dynamic balance.

The wider the base of support of an object, the greater its stability. Older persons can make use of this principle by placing feet shoulder width

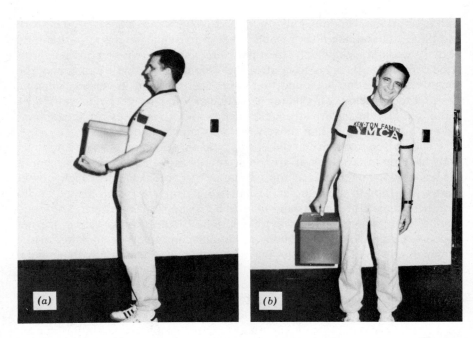

Figure 4.17 (a) Trunk angled backward to counterbalance weight; (b) Trunk inclined sideward to keep line of gravity over its supporting base (feet).

apart for better control in a standing position. Keeping the feet together narrows the support base and adds to instability.

Balance in Water. The application of basic laws of motion is quite different when individuals are swimming or exercising in water. In contrast to the normal gravity constant of 32 ft. per sec.^{2} pulling the individual toward the earth, water acts as a supporting medium. The body is 22 times lighter in the water than on land, and exercises can be done with less effort. This buoyancy advantage allows those individuals with arthritic and other joint problems to receive the benefits of physical activity without placing undue stress on their joints.

Older persons usually find it easier to float than younger individuals because of their body composition advantage. Specific gravity is much lower in older people, and consequently their ability to stay afloat requires less effort. The body rotates around its center of buoyancy, which is usually in the chest area. The hips and legs are heavier and less buoyant than the thorax, and accordingly create a downward force causing the body to assume a vertical float position, as shown in Figure 4.19a.

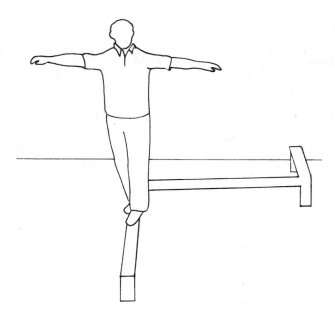

Figure 4.18 Zig-zag beam walking.

In addition to their lower specific gravity, older persons usually have their adipose tissue more uniformly distributed than younger individuals. Less downward force is generated by the legs, which in effect brings the center of buoyancy and the center of gravity closer together in the same vertical line, when one is floating in a horizontal position (see Figure 4.19c. This mechanical advantage in the water allows the older person to relax while he or she is floating—an excellent way to relieve stress and tension.

Balance Principles. Maintaining balance and equilibrium follows basic laws of motion. Following are several principles with particular relevance to improving balance efficiency for older persons:

1. *Maintain an adequate base of support;* e.g., keep feet slightly apart when standing.
2. *Lower the center of gravity when greater stability is needed;* e.g., attempt to crouch when it seems that a fall is imminent.
3. *Keep the line of gravity within the base of support;* stand and sit with proper body alignment so that line of gravity falls near or on its base of support.
4. *Widen the base of support in the direction of the force or movement;* e.g., lean into the wind with feet apart and one foot forward.

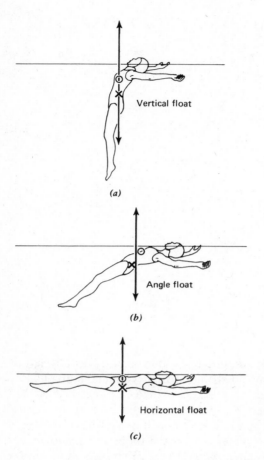

Figure 4.19 Various floating positions (O = center of buoyancy, X = center of gravity). (From J. Piscopo and J. A. Baley, *Kinesiology: The Science of Movement* [New York: John Wiley & Sons, 1981], p. 305. Used with permission.)

5. *Increase friction between the body and supporting surface for better stability;* e.g., wear rubber soles and appropriate footwear to increase gripping action of the shoe.
6. *Maintain adequate strength to provide the force necessary to regain balance after an unexpected loss;* e.g., develop strength of legs to counter the effects of tripping or falling.
7. *Focus vision on a stationary object rather than a moving item;* e.g., when walking a narrow path or plank, focus eyes on a fixed point in the distance.

SPORTS AND ATHLETICS IN AGING

The variation in athletic skill among persons over 60 is astonishing. Older people have attained phenomenal performances in athletics. Some notable feats include those of men in their 60s who throw a discus well over 100 feet; an 85-year-old female who completes a 1500-meter run in less than 14 minutes; men and women in their 70s and 80s who still compete in tennis, bowling, archery, swimming, marathons, baseball, and golf.[33] A new class of elders is appearing called "the super old." This group is composed of individuals between 60 and 80 who compete in regional and national report competition in a variety of events, from the mild exercise of shuffleboard to the intense physiologic effort required in the 100-yard dash. The Super Senior Tennis Organization together with the U.S. Tennis Association actively involves 1200 older players in competition. Tournament play is an important part of its members' lives. These senior athletes compete on grass, clay, and hard court surfaces in almost every state in the U.S.A.

Another example, which indicates that more older people are pursuing vigorous training, is the Master's Age-Specific Athletic Program. This organization sponsors world-class tournaments. Generally, Master's athletes show less accumulation of storage fat, lower blood pressure, and greater aerobic power than their contempories in the general population.[34]

It is clear that this class of elite seniors possesses superior qualities of functional performance, which inescapably enhance their quality and quantity of body mobility and locomotion. In addition, their social and physical sport involvement helps to build buffers against loneliness, depression, and dependence upon others. However, while it is certain that the quality of living can be richly rewarding for those who choose to participate and that these organizations help to motivate older adults to stay physically active, at this time, we do not have conclusive evidence that participation in athletics will directly prolong life span. The mysteries of such factors as genetics, gender, personality, nutrition, and lifestyle are intricately interwoven variables that affect longevity. Nevertheless, those who engage in athletic competition exhibit physical characteristics similar to those of youth, and evidence does exist that the biological decrements that accompany aging occur at a slower rate when the athlete continues participation in his or her selected sport. Several fitness characteristics related to athletic competition are discussed in the next section.

Body Composition and Build of Senior Athletes

Body build tends to conform to the nature of the individual's sport irrespective of age; for example, older distance runners tend to be lean and lighter in weight. Gymnasts and weight lifters retain muscular physiques. Barnard and his associates studied the fitness characteristics of sprint and endurance Master's runners of age range from 41 to 78 years.[35] They found that sprinters were younger and heavier than the distance runners, but that both groups had lower percentages in body fat than comparable categories of sedentary elders. Similar results, reflecting a predominance of lean body mass over fat tissue, were found in older U.S. champion track athletes and older marathon runners in Canada.[36] In each case, athletes had continued their training regimens for 25 or more years, which points out the importance of sustained participation in maintaining high levels of physique and body composition.

Muscular Strength

As indicated in Chapter 3, the steady decline in muscular strength becomes more rapid after age 50. Usually, maximum strength is reached at about age 25 or 30. Thereafter, the speed and power of contraction, as well as the capacity for sustained contraction, declines. Research is sparse on strength testing of individuals past 60, and this variable is usually assessed only by measuring isometric grip strength with hand dynamometers.

An interesting study of former Danish physical education students followed up their physiological functions after 40 years. Handgrip strength showed a steady decline in 18 of the 25 subjects examined (and the right hand remained stronger).[37] It was also found that the personal level of activity of all participants had decreased, with the exception of two individuals who continued systematic and hard training.

It is reasonable to infer that muscular strength can be retained or lost depending upon *use*, and that *disuse* results in greater muscle senescence, whether the participant engaged in past athletic competition or recreational vigorous activity in youth. The trainability of muscular strength increases quickly up to about age 30 and then drops steadily. For example, as shown in Figure 4.20, a typical sedentary man's maximum muscular trainability is below the level of a youth of 12 years.[38] Within limits, strength training can improve muscle capacity by fostering more efficient metabolic oxidation at the cellular level, thereby avoiding or delaying many of the mobility disabilities that result from muscle atrophy.

Cardiovascular Functions and Athletics

Past and recent research reinforces the premise that athletes who continue their training have less decrement in heart and circulation functions than sedentary individuals. This is particularly true of track athletes who continue to run or jog into their 60s and 70s. For example, Clarence DeMar, the famous marathon runner, made it a habit to run 12 miles every day, a level of training he maintained throughout his lifetime. He was still competing in 26-mile marathons at age 65, and he ran his last 15-kilometer race at 68, two years before his death from cancer. An autopsy showed that his heart was

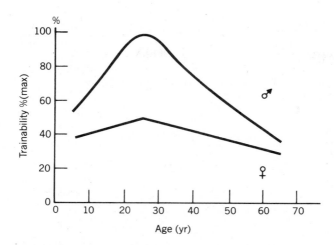

Figure 4.20 Trainability of strength at different age levels. (From M. Hebbelinck, "Kinanthropometry and Motor Fitness," in F. Landry and W. A. R. Orban, eds., *Physical Activity and Human Well-Being, Book 1* [Miami: Symposia Specialists, Inc., 1978], p. 106. Used with permission.)

well developed and the coronary arteries were approximately two to three times the normal size.[39]

However, it should be noted that college athletes often may not continue their participation in physical activity. In fact, Montoye et al. studied 628 former lettermen and 563 nonlettermen who attended Michigan State University at the same time.[40] His research showed that up to about age 45, a greater percentage of the former athletes engaged in some sport regularly. However, after that age the percentage of participation was significantly less than that of former nonathletes (see Figure 4.21).

Montoye's study was done in the mid-Fifties; since that time, the fitness awareness boom has grown, and millions of people are now engaged in some form of activity, with an increase from 24 percent in 1960 to 45 percent in 1981. It is estimated that half the adult U.S. population, a record of 70 million, practices some form of physical activity.[41] Most of the active individuals are young and middle-aged adults between 30 and 45 years of age; however, the activity level after 55 is also growing at a significant rate.[42]

More research is needed to verify or reject the findings of earlier studies. Nevertheless, the evidence is clear about the following positive cardiovascular benefits for those athletes who continue physical activity:

1. Lower blood pressures than sedentary peers.
2. Greater capacity for physiological work (improved oxygen transport and metabolism).

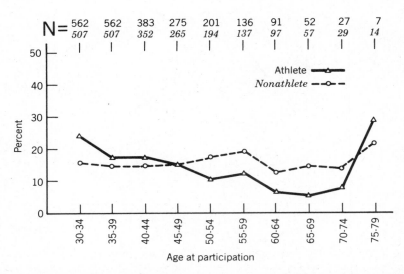

Figure 4.21 Changes of habitual activity with age. (From H. J. Montoye, V. Van Huss, and M. Zuidema, "Sports Activities of Athletes and Non-Athletes in Later Life," *The Physical Educator* 16, no. 2 (May 1959): 49. Used with permission.)

3. Reduced resting heart rate.
4. Greater vital capacity (improved breathing capacity).
5. Better electrocardiogram response.
6. Slower declining rate in circulorespiratory efficiency.

Opportunities for senior athletes to participate in a variety of sports are emerging. Organizations such as the National Senior Sports Association promote and publish newsletters about tournament play in golf, tennis, bowling, marathon running, skiing, bike racing, handball, swimming, track and field, and other athletic events. (See Appendix B for an annotated listing of organizations that provide programs and athletic competition for senior adults.)

EXERCISE AND RELAXATION

Relaxation is identified with ease, the lessening of tension, and comfort—the opposite of rigid, taut, stiff, or inflexible. Such terms as these can be applied to a state of mind ("he is too uptight and tense") or to muscle suppleness, flexibility, or ease of movement. Are these mental and muscular conditions related? Can exercise induce psychological relaxation? If these conditions are related, what kinds of activity contribute to relaxation?

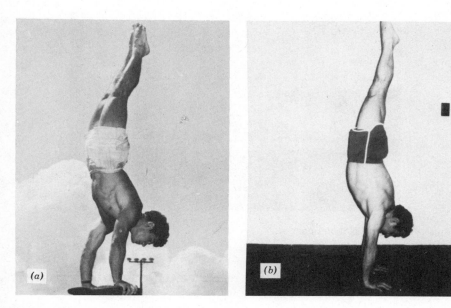

Figure 4.22 The author at 20 and at 61—motor skills can be retained with practice.

Resting muscle tone is affected by anxiety, which influences the flexibility and elastic properties of the muscle itself. Skeletal muscles must be in a relaxed state to achieve maximum motion mobility. In addition to somatotype, structural, and training modalities, a basic relationship exists between tension, anxiety, and one's flexibility pattern. Rathbone has drawn attention to the anxiety/flexibility relationship:

> Almost without exception, tense individuals have restrictions in joint flexibility. In the early states, this flexibility may be due solely to the inability of muscles to relax sufficiently to make possible full range of movement. In later states, the joint structures may become so tightened that flexibility cannot be regained.[43]

Some research has explored the relationship between anxiety and motor tasks, which is related to joint mobility. Muscular spasticity and rigidity increase during a period of stress.[44] One investigator found that subjects with low levels of anxiety required less time to perform certain motor skills than did high-anxiety persons, and that the former group was able to perform better than its high-anxiety counterparts.[45] The study also showed that the differences became more pronounced as the complexity of the skill increased. These findings support the premise that psychic factors have an

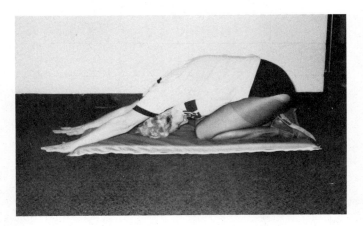

Figure 4.23 "Z" relaxation pose.

important influence in muscle tone regulation, which affects the range of joint motion. Tense individuals may well possess "stiff joints."

Exercise Types and Tension

A well-known activity that is highly related to flexibility and relaxation is hatha yoga. Stretching is basic to applying yoga techniques, as shown in Figure 4.23. This activity is a form of slow-motion exercise that involves moving from a muscle contraction to a stretched state held in a comfortable posture. Physiologically, yoga activities respect the stretch reflex phenomenon called the *myotatic reflex* that allows a muscle to relax without triggering an involuntary reverse nervous system response of muscle contraction. Quick, jerky types of bouncing exercises may involve undue contractions that interfere with the enhancement of stretching and relaxation. A firm steady static stretch similar to yoga exercises calls forth an inverse neural reflex that prevents muscle shortening.

The practice of yoga also may reduce involuntary muscle tension by altering other bodily systems. The expert practitioner of shavasana (yoga relaxation) is said to be able to reduce his or her oxygen consumption by as much as 50 percent with parallel reductions in heart rate, respiratory rate, blood cholesterol, and blood sugar.[46]

Other types of exercises and sport activities also contribute to relaxation. Clues to relaxation activities are provided by Byrd, who conducted a survey of psychiatrists on the relief of tension by exercise.[47] Polling 54 psychiatrists, he found that 90 percent of these medical experts believed that

moderate exercise helps to give relief from tension, and 81 percent prescribed walking, swimming, bowling, or golf (in that order) for the reduction
of stress. In a follow-up study, using questionnaires involving 263 bowlers,
he found that the most frequent reasons cited for the easement of tension by
participants were: (1) physical activity, (2) companionship of friends, and (3)
distraction from thinking about problems.

Some recent evidence provides an objective rationale on the value of
moderate exercise in producing a tranquilizing effect among older persons.
DeVries tested a group of elderly persons using an electromyographic technique (recording electrical properties of muscle), and found that rhythmic
exercise such as walking, jogging, cycling, and bench stepping for periods
from 5 to 30 minutes at 30 to 60 percent of maximum intensities effectively
reduced neuromuscular tension.[48]

An interesting study by Bennett et al. offers further evidence of the
value of an exercise program as a treatment modality for reducing depression among the elderly.[49] These investigators studied 35 females and 3 males
ranging from 50 to 98, with a mean age of 75.7 years. Half the subjects were
residents of a nursing home and half were participants in a community
center. Subjects at each site were assigned to one of two groups, either an
exercise or control group.

The exercise program consisted of two 45-minute sessions per week for
eight weeks, during which subjects in the exercise group participated in
exercises designed to maintain or restore muscle tone, flexibility, and balance. Subjects in the control group were afforded similar social opportunities for the same period but did not participate in the exercises.

A Zung Self-Rating Depression Scale (Zung SDS) was administered to
each person at the beginning of the program, and a posttest was given on the
last day of the eight-week period. The results indicated that among the
elderly who exhibited symptoms of depression, there was a significant improvement in depression level following participation in the organized physical exercise program. In contrast, no significant improvement was found
among the depressed nonexercise control group.

Such findings certainly lend credence to the probable positive role that
exercise can play in the relief of depression among senior adults. More
research with respect to low-level exercise programs and their impact on
depression is needed.

Endorphins and Exercise

Recent findings have shown that a morphine-like substance called *endorphin* is found in the blood after various episodes of running exercises.[50]
Specifically, these substances are known as *beta-endorphins,* which are re-

leased by the pituitary gland in response to exercise and appear to invoke the "runner's high," or a feeling of euphoria. While at the present time, research studies have discovered relationships between endorphins and increased exercise, the exact function of these substances is unknown. Whether this hormone acts independently or in concert with other endocrine secretions has yet to be determined.

INDICATIONS AND CONTRAINDICATIONS OF ACTIVITIES FOR THE AGING

Throughout our discussion, we have advanced the concept that physical activity is essential for enhancing human efficiency. As research evidence mounts in support of exercise and sports for healthy bodies in the mature years, well-meaning professionals who are working with senior citizens, and who are knowledgeable about social and psychological aspects of gerontology, often embark on activity and exercise programs without understanding the anatomical, physiological, and kinesiological benefits or limitations.

Certain types of activities are indicated for some individuals but contraindicated for others. The principle of specificity of conditioning and law of individual differences must be respected. For example, jogging does very little to develop the muscle strength of the shoulder girdle and pectoral muscles.

Is jogging a suitable exercise modality for everyone? A person who is in the 250 to 300-pound weight range and/or afflicted with inflammatory arthritis of the knees should not engage in such an activity because insult and further aggravation to body joints may result.

Any conditioning program for older persons should begin with an assessment of their medical status. Prescribed activities, based upon scientific evidence, relative to type, frequency, and dosage, should be selected according to individual needs and capabilities. Piscopo and Baley have selected 26 contraindications and indications with a rationale drawn from kinesiological and physiological foundations. Although research is continually advancing knowledge about the effects of physical activity upon the human organism, the contraindications and indications given in Tables 4.3 and 4.4 should be taken into account.

Summary

Fitness is a dynamic quality with different meanings to different individuals embracing various aspects of physical, mental, emotional, social, and spiritual well-being. Physical fitness is affected by irreversible factors of genetics

Table 4.3 Contraindications and Indications for Various Exercises, with Kinesiological Rationale

Contraindication	Indication	Rationale
1. Fix or stiffen joints such as trying to touch toes with knees locked.	1. Swing free; bend knees, and move in a comfortable manner.	1. Respects bone, joint, and muscle changes; less danger of joint sprains and muscle strain.
2. Perform trunk twisting in standing position.	2. Perform trunk twister in sitting position on bench or chair.	2. Respects the basic structure and function of the joint, which is essentially a ginglymus or hinge joint. Torque generated by the twisting action of the trunk can be absorbed by the knee when flexed because of its greater capacity for rotation in sitting position.
3. Circumduction of head or head-rolling exercises.	3. Slowly rotate or turn head to left and right; flex and extend head up and down, without jerky movements.	3. Lessen the danger of "grinding" the first two cervical vertebrae (atlas and axis), which may be damaged because of the natural "thinning out" of the intervertebral disks.
4. Jog or run when such conditions as arthritis are present.	4. Utilize bicycle ergometer or pool for swimming activities.	4. Weight which creates pressure upon knee and ankle joints is removed; buoyancy of water has hydrotherapeutic effect on muscles and joints.

Table 4.3 *Continued*

Contraindication	Indication	Rationale
5. Quick flexion of trunk on thigh in supine position (sit-up) with legs straight.	5. Perform sit-up with legs bent at least 60 degrees.	5. Lessens probability of increasing lordosis angle of spine and allows greater intensity of contraction upon the abdominal muscles, and less on iliopsoas (hip flexors).
6. Double leg raising exercise to angular hold position off the floor.	6. Raise legs to 45 degree angle without hold position, with back flat on floor.	6. Lessens the risk of spinal hyperextension and resultant low back strain.
7. Continuous fast "swirling" and "whirling" movements of the body.	7. Slow rotary and/or circumducting limb movements.	7. Postural changes may induce vertigo or dizziness and loss of balance.
8. Activities that require fast reaction time and explosive power movements, such as trampoline bouncing and vaulting events with springboard.	8. Modify and adapt activities so that success in performance does not require quick or extreme bursts of power, e.g., playing doubles badminton, dancing.	8. Reaction time, perception, and neuromuscular response generally decline; activities that demand high levels of neural acuteness are threats to the mature person's safety.
9. Full flexion of the knee joint from standing position (deep-knee bends).	9. Half-knee bends from stand position.	9. May overstretch and injure supporting structure of knee, including ligaments, cartilages.
10. Stressing static balance hold positions without use of arms or visual clues, such as, standing on one leg with arms along thighs, with eyes closed.	10. Walking wide balance beam (12- to 15-inch width) with arms abducted in frontal plane and eyes focused at end of beam.	10. Improves functional balance in upright position, uses mechanical principle of extending the horizontal distance from the center of gravity with arms, and utilizes vision to establish point of reference in maintaining dynamic balance skills.

144

11. Flexing elbow exercises with hands in pronated position (palms down).	11. Flexing elbow with hands in supinated position (palms up).	11. More strength can be applied in elbow flexion with hand in supination because of favorable mechanical advantage.
12. Present exercises and game instructions quickly without loss of time.	12. Present instruction with slow pace and concrete demonstration: allow for self-pacing of motor skills.	12. Neural information, reception, and capacity for processing decreased; instructional material presented must be reduced accordingly.
13. Execute exercises in a "slump posture" stance.	13. Perform exercises in erect posture (not stiff) with attention to activation of antigravity postural muscles.	13. Lessens tendency toward kyphotic (hump-back) and postural fatigue in body alignment.

Source: Piscopo and Baley, *Kinesiology*, pp. 528–529. Used with permission.

Table 4.4 Contraindications and Indications for Various Exercises, with Physiological Rationale

Contraindication	Indication	Rationale
1. Holding breath during exercise.	1. Breathing rhythmically; with expiration at the end of the effort.	1. Holding breath decreases venous return of blood to the heart; may cause dizziness or fainting.
2. Using heavy weights with fast repetitive movements.	2. Use light weights with slow repetitive movements.	2. Heavy weights impede blood circulation to the extremities. [Small size soup cans (8 oz.) excellent for hand weight in shoulder girdle exercises.]
3. Accent overwork and stressful movements of arms in calisthenics.	3. Stress activity of big muscles of trunk and legs.	3. Arm exercises increase blood pressure at higher levels than trunk and leg workouts.
4. Take hot shower after exercise.	4. Take warm shower after exercise, slowly cooling water temperature.	4. Hot shower may elevate blood pressure.
5. Start vigorous movements with-out warm-up.	5. Always warm up 5 to 7 minutes before jogging, playing sports, etc.	5. Ischemic effect (inadequate blood flow to tissues) may result without warm-up.
6. Immediate rest after exercise.	6. Walk after jogging, or loosen up with calisthenics.	6. Fosters cool-down of the body and allows a natural transition of blood pumping action from muscles to the heart without undue stress.
7. Stress resistive and anaerobic (without O_2) exercises and activities.	7. Accent isotonic and aerobic (with O_2) exercises and activities.	7. Aerobic-type exercises enhance the function of cardiovascular system, whereas resistive work is of little value for heart and lung efficiency.

8. Work out in rubberized clothing in hot weather.	8. Work out in cool perspiration-absorbing type shirt and trunks.	8. Rubberized clothing prevents normal functioning of perspiration mechanism and constricts necessary body cooling process during exercise and after workout.
9. Stretching muscle to extreme range.	9. Stretch to full range without strain or discomfort.	9. Extreme stretching may induce muscle spasm and undue soreness or strain.
10. Short "jerky" or "bouncing" stretching movements.	10. Slow nonballistic, static stretching.	10. Jerky and/or bouncing movement may invoke a myotatic reflex in the muscle spindle, which opposes the desired stretching.
11. Sit-up exercises on inclined plane or board.	11. Sit-ups parallel with floor, back firmly on the mat.	11. Places undue strain on hip flexors, primarily iliopsoas muscle and resultant soreness to low back.
12. Perform exercises that develop muscle bulk only.	12. Perform exercises that stimulate flexibility, strength, and endurance through stretching, light resistance work, and repetitive movements.	12. Exercises that are directed toward increasing muscle bulk do not contribute to cardiovascular fitness.
13. Perform daily high-intensity workouts.	13. Generally, gear exercise intensity to low and moderate levels dependent upon medical and dynamic fitness status.	13. Body needs a minimum of one day's rest for adaptive homeostasis adjustment and avoidance of activity "staleness."

Source: Piscopo and Baley, Kinesiology, pp. 530–531. Used with permission.

and inherited characteristics, and reversible elements of lifestyle and environmental circumstances. Locomotion and the ability to move safely and efficiently in work and play without undue fatigue is essential for the maintenance of independence in older persons.

Four important biological fitness goals affecting locomotion are: (1) muscular strength and endurance, (2) flexibility, (3) cardiovascular-respiratory efficiency, and (4) balance and equilibrium. The discussion of available exercise types and systems to improve the muscular component of fitness described the advantages and disadvantages of isotonics, isometrics, free weights, the Universal Gym, the Nautilus system, and isokinetics.

The nature and functional characteristics of both passive and active flexibility were then presented. Changes in structure and function of joints, ligaments, cartilage, fascia, and tendons all affect flexibility in older persons.

The cardiovascular-respiratory systems combine to transport vital oxygen and nourishment to all body cells. The relationships between heart, lungs, and blood circulation and the limitations affecting aging were described and the effects of exercise on the heart, blood pressure, and peripheral vascular circulation explained, with recommended guidelines for exercise. Aerobic and anaerobic exercises were discussed with implications for older persons. Changes in typical heart rate and cardiac output that occur with age then were explained with suggestions for exercise and activity prescription.

Stationary and dynamic balance skills entail internal and external mechanisms. Although gradual changes in the acuteness of internal mechanisms controlling balance normally occur, practicing appropriate skills helps to sharpen the kinesthetic sense necessary to maintain balance. Maintaining balance and equilibrium follows the basic laws of motion. Seven principles of balance control were listed with specific activity examples for older adults.

A new class of senior adults—the super old—has emerged demonstrating high-level athletic skills in tennis, swimming, marathon running, golf, track, and field. It is not unusual to find 60- to 80-year-old individuals participating in competitive events that require vigorous training. Senior athletes exhibit physical characteristics similar to those of youth, and biological decrements of the aging process are slowed by continued sport participation.

Exercise has undeniable value in lessening tension, stress and depression. Recent findings about the chemical endorphins indicate their probable relaxing effect, especially in individuals who experience a "runner's high."

The chapter concluded with specific indications and contraindications of exercises for the aging delineating a rationale based on kinesiological and physiological foundations.

REFERENCES

1. Howard S. Hoyman, "Rethinking an Ecologic-System Model of Man's Health, Disease, Aging, and Death," *Journal of School Health* 45 (1975): 509–518.
2. Ibid., p. 513.
3. U.S. Senate, Subcommittee on Aging of the Committee on Labor and Public Welfare, Testimony on Physical Fitness for Older Persons, from Selected Hearings, 23 April 1978, Washington, D.C., pp. 713–899.
4. John Piscopo, "Selected Research on Various Programs to Develop Strength" (Paper presented at the Research Section of the New York State Convention for Health, Physical Education and Recreation, Syracuse, New York, January 1975).
5. John Piscopo and James A. Baley, *Kinesiology: The Science of Movement* (New York: John Wiley & Sons, 1981), p. 26.
6. Per-Olof Astrand et al., "Intra-arterial Blood Pressure during Exercise with Different Muscle Groups," *Journal of Applied Physiology* 20 (1965): 253–256; Sture Bevegard, Ulla Freyschuss, and Tore Strandell, "Circulatory Adaptation to Arm and Leg Exercise in Supine and Sitting Position," *Journal of Applied Physiology* 21 (1966): 37–46; Paul S. Fardy, "Isometric Exercise and the Cardiovascular System," *The Physician and Sportsmedicine* 9, no. 9 (1981): 43–56; and American College of Sports Medicine, *Guidelines for Graded Exercise Testing and Exercise Prescription*, 2d ed. (Philadelphia: Lea & Febiger, 1980), p. 39.
7. Robert R. Spackman, *Conditioning for Senior Citizens* (Carbondale, Ill.: Hillcrest House, 1981), pp. 12–14.
8. Ibid.
9. For further information about the system, see James A. Peterson, *Total Fitness: The Nautilus Way* (West Point, N.Y.: Leisure Press, 1978).
10. Thomas V. Pipes and Jack H. Wilmore, "Isokinetic vs. Isotonic Strength Training," *Medicine and Science in Sports* 7, no. 4 (1975): 262–274; David H. Clarke, "Adaptations in Strength and Muscular Endurance Resulting from Exercise," in J. H. Wilmore, ed., *Exercise and Sport Sciences Reviews* I (1978): 73–102; and Thomas V. Pipes, "Strength-Training Modes: What's the Difference?" in E. J. Burke, ed., *Toward an Understanding of Human Performance* (Ithaca, N.Y.: Movement Publications, 1977), pp. 17–24.
11. David H. Clarke, *Exercise Physiology* (Englewood Cliffs, N.J.: Prentice-Hall, 1975), p. 49.
12. Lois C. Perkins and Helen L. Kaiser, "Results of Short Term Isotonic and Isometric Exercise Programs in Persons over Sixty," *The Physical Therapy Review* 41, no. 9 (1976): 633–635; H. Suominen, E. Heikkinen, and T. Parkatti, "Effect of Eight Weeks' Physical Training on Muscle and Connective Tissue of the M. Vastus Lateralis in 69-Year Old Men and Women," *Journal of Gerontology* 32, no. 1 (1977): 33–37; and Toshio Moritani and Herbert A. deVries, "Potential for Gross Muscle Hypertrophy in Old Men," *Journal of Gerontology* 35, no. 5 (1980): 672–682.
13. Roy J. Shephard, *Physiology and Biochemistry of Exercise* (New York: Praeger Publishers, 1982), p. 389.

14. H. Harrison Clarke, *Muscular Strength and Endurance in Man* (Englewood Cliffs, N.J.: Prentice-Hall, 1966), p. 1.

15. David Hall, *The Ageing of Connective Tissue* (London: Academic Press, 1976), p. 62.

16. E. Gutman, "Muscle," in C. E. Finch and L. Hayflick, eds., *The Biology of Aging* (New York: Van Nostrand Reinhold, 1977), pp. 445–469.

17. R. V. Dickinson, "The Specificity of Flexibility," *Research Quarterly* 39 (1968) 792–794; Charles B. Corbin and Larry Noble, "Flexibility," *Journal of Physical Education and Recreation* 51, no. 6 (1980): 23–60; and Marlene J. Adrian, "Flexibility in the Aging," in E. L. Smith and R.C. Serfass, eds., *Exercise and Aging* (Hillside, N.J.: Enslow Publishers, 1981), p. 53.

18. Edward B. Elkowitz, *Geriatric Medicine for the Primary Care Practitioner* (New York: Springer Publishing, 1981), p. 5.

19. Harrison H. Clarke, "Exercise and Aging," *Physical Fitness Research Digest*, President's Council on Physical Fitness and Sports, Series 7, no. 2 (Washington, D.C.: April 1977).

20. Rudolph H. Dressendorfer, "Physiological Profile of a Runner," *The Physician and Sports Medicine* 8, no. 8 (1980): 49–52.

21. Howard G. Knuttgen, "Development of Muscular Strength and Endurance," in H. G. Knuttgen, ed., *Neuromuscular Mechanisms for Therapeutic and Conditioning Exercise* (Baltimore: University Park Press, 1976), p. 108.

22. Shephard, *Physiology and Biochemistry,* p. 343, and Clarke, *Muscular Strength and Endurance,* p. 9.

23. Herbert deVries, *Physiology of Exercise* (Dubuque, Ia.: Wm. C. Brown, 1981), p. 121.

24. Bud Getchell, *Physical Fitness: A Way of Life,* 2d ed. (New York: John Wiley & Sons, 1979), p. 27.

25. M. Brandfonbrener, M. Landowne, and N. W. Shock, "Changes in Cardiac Output with Age," *Circulation* 12 (1955): 567–576.

26. Raymond Harris, "Cardiac Changes with Age," in R. Goldman and M. Rockstein, eds., *The Physiology and Pathology of Human Aging* (New York: Academic Press, 1975), p. 118.

27. Andrew A. Fischer, "The Effect of Aging and Physical Activity on the Stabile Component of Arterial Distensibility," in R. Harris and L. J. Frankel, eds., *Guide to Fitness after Fifty* (New York: Plenum Press, 1977) pp. 81–94.

28. Roy J. Shephard, *Physical Activity and Aging* (Chicago: Year Book Medical Publishers, 1978), pp. 245–247; and G. S. Thomas et al., *Exercise and Health* (Cambridge, Mass.: Oelgeschlager, Gunn & Hain Publishers, 1981), pp. 55–74.

29. Clarke, "Adaptations," p. 215.

30. John Wahren and Stellan Bygdeman, "Onset of Angina Pectoris in Relation to Circulatory Adaptation during Arm and Leg Exercise," *Circulation* 44 (1971): 432–441.

31. Marjorie W. Allshouse, "The Rate of Adjustment of Oxygen Transport at the Onset of Submaximal Leg and Arm Exercise in Older Adults" (Master's thesis, State University of New York at Buffalo, 1982).

32. Piscopo and Baley, *Kinesiology,* p. 289.

33. Alfred Kamm, "Senior Olympics," *Journal of Physical Education and Recreation* 50, no. 7 (1979): 32–33; and Steven L. Yasgur, "The Senior Olympics: Games for Adults Who Won't Quit," *Geriatrics* 30 (January 1975): 120–125.
34. Roy J. Shephard and Terence Kavanagh, "The Effects of Training on the Aging Process," *The Physician and Sportsmedicine* 6, no. 1 (1978): 33–40; and John Piscopo, "Fitness and Aging," *The Easterner* 7, no. 1 (1982): 2–6.
35. R. James Barnard, Glen K. Grimditch, and Jack A. Wilmore, "Physiological Characteristics of Spring and Endurance Masters Runners," *Medicine and Science in Sports* 11, no. 2 (1979): 167–171.
36. Michael Pollock, "Physiological Characteristics of Older Champion Track Athletes," *Research Quarterly* 45, no. 4 (1974): 363–373; and Shephard and Kavanagh, "Effects of Training on Aging."
37. E. Asmussen, K. Fruensgaard, and S. Norgaard, "A Follow-Up Longitudinal Study of Selected Physiologic Functions in Former Physical Education Students—After Forty Years," *Journal of the American Geriatrics Society* 23, no. 10 (1975): 442–450.
38. M. Hebbelinck, "Kinanthropometry and Aging: Morphological Structural Body Mechanics and Motor Fitness Aspects of Aging," in F. Landry and W. Orban, eds., *Physical Activity and Human Well-being* (Miami: Symposia Specialists, 1978), p. 106.
39. deVries, *Physiology of Exercise,* p. 362.
40. Henry J. Montoye, Wayne Van Huss, and Marvin Zuidema, "Sports Activity of Athletes and Non-Athletes in Later Life," *The Physical Educator* 16, no. 2 (1959): 48–51.
41. "America Shapes Up," *Time* 1981 November 2, pp. 94–106.
42. Personal interview with director of American Fitness Center, Buffalo, New York, April 1982.
43. Josephine Rathbone, *Relaxation* (New York: Bureau of Publications, 1943), p. 19.
44. Kurt Bowman, "Effect of Emotional Stress on Spasticity and Rigidity," *Journal of Psychosomatic Research* 15 (1971): 107–112.
45. Roland H. Vines, "The Influences of Race and Anxiety Level upon Performance of Novel Motor Tasks under Varying Stressful Conditions," *Dissertation Abstracts International* 32, no. 7-A (January 1972): 3770.
46. Shephard, *Physiology and Biochemistry,* p. 278.
47. Oliver E. Byrd, "A Survey of Beliefs and Practices of Psychiatrists on the Relief of Tension by Moderate Exercise," *Journal of School Health* 33, no. 9 (1963): 426–427.
48. Herbert A. deVries, "Tranquilizer Effect of Exercise: A Critical Review," *The Physician and Sportsmedicine* 9, no. 11 (1981): 47–53.
49. Jeanine Bennett, Mary Ann Carmack, and Valerie Gardner, "The Effect of a Program of Physical Exercise on Depression in Older Adults," *The Physical Educator* 1, no. 39 (1982): 21–24.
50. Mike Moore, "Endorphins and Exercise: A Puzzling Relationship," *The Physician and Sportsmedicine* 10, no. 2 (1982): 111–114.

5

Design and Conduct
of Fitness Programs
for the Aging

IDENTIFYING TARGET POPULATIONS

The design and conduct of any fitness program for older adults must consider the nature and characteristics of the specific group within the diverse populace of the over-60 category. Dissimilarity, rather than uniformity of needs, interests, and capabilities is the rule, not the exception, when planning and implementing a program. Four general groups can be identified: (1) well-aging, (2) ambulatory and wheelchair elderly, (3) frail elderly, and (4) bed patients. Each of these groups has fitness commonalities and differences, which can provide principles and guidelines when selecting and conducting activities for the improvement and maintenance of senior adult fitness levels. These categories are composed of individuals with a variety of health problems, such as sensory deficits in hearing and vision, cardiac and stroke conditions, arthritis, and mental or emotional conditions.

It is important to determine the health status of the individual prior to the start of a fitness program. The program goal should emphasize self-improvement within the medical status of the participant, rather than the attainment of fitness levels based upon norms or the achievements of population samples. Personalization of goals and the provision of fitness activities to meet the specific needs of the older adult is the sine qua non of a successful program.

Table 5.1 indicates a general description of each group from a mobility and locomotion perspective.

Table 5.1 Target Population Descriptions

Group	General Characteristics	Mobility/Locomotion Capacity
Well-Aging	General good health, free of major disabling conditions, usually independent and self-sufficient in carrying on everyday tasks	Mobility and locomotion patterns restricted only to normal biological changes that occur in cardiovascular, musculoskeletal, respiratory, and nervous systems
Limited Ambulatory and Wheelchair Elderly	Conditions that restrict movement for normal walking or jogging, bending, turning, or twisting due to disabilities that may be caused by cardiac constrictions, orthopedic deviations, respiratory or musculoskeletal problems	Mobility goals accent flexibility, maintenance of muscular and postural tone, toward the specific objective of moving the participant from the wheelchair to the freedom of independent walking, unless medical conditions such as, stroke, amputations, etc., preclude the attainment of this goal
Frail Elderly	Conditions that result in major deficiency in muscular strength and cardiovascular performance; individual cannot bear any strain, stress, or pressure on any of the biological systems; usually weak and may or may not be institutionalized depending upon the degree of frailty	Activities geared to increasing joint ranges of motion (flexibility); relaxation; posture; reinforcing walking skills; assistive type fitness activities whereby instructor aids the individual in performing an exercise
Bed Patients	Conditions that confine the individual to bed because of inability to walk; patient can usually sit up, may be alert and well oriented to his or her surroundings, is not incontinent and does not manifest serious mental or emotional problems	Activities that maintain integrity of muscle mass through controlled dynamic and isometric exercises; prevention of muscular atrophy, and joint contraction; minimizing development of pressure sores

153

PROGRAMS FOR THE WELL-AGING

This particular segment of older adults contains by far the greatest number of persons within the over-60 population. A persistent myth exists about infirmity and older people. Many have the notion that most of our elderly are ill and reside in institutions such as nursing homes and segregated geriatric facilities. This is not the case—95 percent of the elderly, old, and very old live in the community, either independently or with their families. Therefore, we are referring to over 30 million independent people past 60, free of serious disabling disease, and able to function without assistance.[1] In other words, these individuals are noninstitutionalized and reflect similar patterns of fitness levels as found among other age groups, with the exception of greater frequency in heart conditions, arthritis, and rheumatism, accompanied by some decline in visual or hearing acuity.

Fitness programs for the well-aging adult exist in a variety of settings: multipurpose senior centers; YMCAs and YWCAs; Golden Ager–type organizations; private organizations affiliated with churches; community-related college and university programs; and commercially operated health spas and fitness centers. Program offerings range from low-stress-level types to sports for the elite "young-old" participating in senior amateur athletic organizations. The content and method of a specific program depend upon caliber of professional leadership, budgetary allowances, and availability of facilities and equipment.

PRINCIPLES AND GUIDELINES: ORGANIZATION AND ADMINISTRATION

Although programs for the well-aging are found in various organizational environments, five important principle and guideline components apply to all groups seriously interested in pursuing excellence in program operation: (1) program philosophy and goals, (2) personnel and management, (3) budget and finance, (4) facilities and equipment, and (5) program evaluation and assessment.

Philosophy, Goals, and Objectives

A point of view, an attitude about an endeavor or undertaking, a belief in worth—each relates to a philosophy that subsequently gives direction to program design and conduct. For example, adopting the concept of health and fitness of the World Health Organization, which interprets health as a state of complete physical, mental and social well-being, and not merely the absence of disease or infirmity, accepts the idea of organismic unity and the totality of man, and the belief that the individual should be considered as an indivisible unit, the parts acting as an integrated whole. This basic premise relies on the philosophy that any approach to the conduct of program activities must involve the mental, emotional, social, and physical components, all interacting and simultaneously affecting the physical performance and behavior of the senior adult.

Another basic philosophic premise deals with the phenomenon of aging itself. For example: "Aging is a normal process of maturational changes, and not a disease or pathology." This assumption implies that long-living adults are a normal, vital, and integral part of society and have the right of maintaining their dignity, self-worth, and participation in decisions that affect their interests and destiny.

Following the establishment of philosophy and a viewpoint about aging and the older adult, general goals and objectives must be formulated for the attainment of a stated philosophic stance. Goals are long-term intentions expressed in general and broad terms. Objectives may be long- or short-term, but differ from goals in their greater degree of specificity. For example, a goal of a multipurpose senior center may be that "the senior adult will be provided with experiences and activities that will improve his or her quality of life." Such a statement is long-range and represents a continuum of effort that in a sense is timeless but nevertheless provides a perception of direction for program directors and planners.

Objectives reflect greater precision, and concepts that can be accomplished over a long period of time (several years) or within a short time frame (one month). For example, a general fitness objective may be "to enhance the mobility and locomotion of participants by providing physical activities and experiences that increase flexibility." A statement that gives further specificity to this objective might be: "to increase the range of motion of the back, arms, and legs by 10 percent at the conclusion of the fall exercise session." Thus, it can be seen that philosophy, goals, and objectives follow a sequential plan in setting the direction and design of a program. The following statement reflects the philosophy and goals of the Town of Amherst Senior Center, New York:

The purpose of the Town of Amherst Senior Center is based on the premise that aging is normal; that human beings need peers with whom to interact, and who are available as a source of encouragement and support; and that older adults have a right to determine matters in which they have a vital interest. In accordance with this philosophy, the Town of Amherst Senior Center is a multipurpose facility committed to:

PROVIDE an atmosphere that recognizes the value of human life, and where adults can maintain their dignity, self-worth, and well-being,

PROVIDE a program of meaningful educational, cultural, social, recreational, and volunteer activities which will foster continued personal and group development,

PROVIDE opportunities for personal choices and decision making, for demonstrating individual capacities, creative potential, and uniqueness for developing attitudes of caring, sharing, supporting, and rendering service to others,

ACT as a provider of information, referral, counseling, and nutritional needs that will encourage independence and community involvement, and

TO BE RESPONSIVE AND ACCESSIBLE to the changing needs of the elderly in the community regardless of color, national origin, race, religion, sex, or physical handicap.[2]

This statement is broad in context, aimed at improving the quality of life of participants, and allows for considerable flexibility in the design, content, and conduct of program activities.

Personnel and Management

The key to a successful activity program in a governmental or private setting is personnel. The program director or coordinator establishes the tone and ambience of the environment. The director is viewed as a supervisor and resource consultant, serving as a facilitator of physical, social, and intellectual recreational experiences for program participants.

Professional Preparation of Staff. Many activities in organizational settings are conducted by volunteers (often, senior adults within the organization); however, even though these individuals perform admirably in terms of the technical skills required in the conduct of activities, congnitive information about the activity is usually deficient. For example, volunteer leaders can conduct calisthenics with enthusiasm and vigor without necessary information about the anatomy and physiology of the body or its exercise effects. This is acceptable provided the program of exercise prescription testing, assessment, and overall supervision is under the leadership of a professional staff member with a background in health, physical education, recreation, or one of the allied health fields that includes a solid grounding in biological, sociological, and psychological functioning of the human body.

The ideal professional staff member should hold an undergraduate degree in a health-related area with an emphasis in gerontology. Figure 5.1 illustrates a recommended four-year geriatric fitness and recreation curriculum that blends a general and liberal education with core and specialized courses.

The professional core is viewed as central for students concentrating on fitness and recreation programs for special populations. Core courses are included to allow beginning specialization in areas where particular and unique groups, including the aged, are served. The specialized professional education component shown in Figure 5.1 exhibits specific courses and experiences germane to gerontological fitness and recreation. The specialized Tier III allows the student to further study his or her subdivision of interest after completing required courses appropriate for special populations. Community field exposure is initiated at the sophomore or junior level. This early community "on-the-job" opportunity nurtures a natural transition to full-time clinical internship experiences usually scheduled during the senior year.

The entire curriculum emphasizes an interdisciplinary approach which focuses upon individuals as total entities, rather than being compartmentalized into health, physical education, and recreation characteristics. Commonalities of each discipline, instead of differences, are advanced.

Basic qualifications for successful leadership in working with older adults also include desirable personality and temperament characteristics. The staff member (professional and volunteer) should possess a strong desire to work with, and an appreciation of, older adults. Such characteristics as friendliness, conscientiousness, and warmth, combined with appropriate professional preparation foster enthusiasm and sincerity on the job and translate into motivating seniors toward greater participation in program activities.

Program Personnel. In addition to the general professional preparation discussed earlier in this chapter, a fitness program that includes circulorespiratory maintenance and improvement should have two key professionals on staff: a medical director or consultant and a health and physical director. These professionals provide the necessary leadership expertise in the design and conduct of all activities within the program. The medical director should be a licensed physician, preferably a cardiologist. The health and physical director should be a graduate of a four-year accredited college or university with a major in physical education or allied health-related area. Such an individual is considered a fitness specialist, with special training in anatomy, physiology, of exercise, kinesiology, and gerontology. The roles of each specialist include the following:

MEDICAL DIRECTOR

1. Interpret medical information.
2. Supervise stress testing evaluations.

I. GENERAL AND LIBERAL EDUCATION[a]

Mathematics		Sciences		Humanities		Social Sciences		English		Electives	
Electives	(3)	Biology, Physics or Chemistry	(8)	Literature, Philosophy or the Arts	(3)	General Psychology	(6)	English Composition	(6)	Liberal Studies Electives	(12)
			(4)			Sociology	(6)	Speech Communication	(6)		
		Physiology	(4)			Psychology Electives					
	3		16		6		18		6		12

Total = 61 hours

II. PROFESSIONAL EDUCATION CORE[b]

Foundations of Physical Education	(3)	Kinesiology	(4)
Foundations of Recreation	(3)	Measurement and Evaluation in Physical Education	(3)
Introduction to Health Education	(3)	Sociology of Leisure	(3)
Community Field Experience[c]	(2)	Recreation for Special Populations	(3)
	11		13

Total = 24 hours

III. SPECIALIZED PROFESSIONAL EDUCATION[b]

Applied Sciences		Technical Specialists		Curriculum and Instruction		Internship		Activity Leadership	
Gross Anatomy	(4)	Motor Learning	(2)	Adaptive Physical Education	(3)	Clinical Internship (consortia of community agencies and college/university)	(6)	Low and Moderate Stress Activities for the Aging	(1)
Physiology of Exercise	(4)	Biological Aspects of Aging	(2)	Recreational Leadership	(3)			Bowling	(1)
Neurophysiology	(3)	Psycho/social Aspects of Aging	(2)	Organization, Administration, and Supervision of Geriatric Fitness Programs	(3)			Folk/Square Dancing	(1)
Nutrition	(2)	Principles of Therapeutic Exercise	(2)					Aquatics	(1)
		Introduction to Rehabilitation and Counseling	(3)					Yoga	(1)
								Quiet Games	(1)
								Electives	(2)
	13		11		9		6		8

Total = 47 hours

Grand Total = 132 hours

[a] Includes Life Support Services Certification as prescribed by the American Heart Association.

[b] Credit hours for specific courses may be adjusted to individual college/university credit hour allocation designs.

[c] Sophomore or junior level supervised observation experience in: retirement center, YM/WCA, Golden Ager organizations, Veteran's Administration Hospital, and such other community organizations offering programs for the elderly.

Source: J. Piscopo and C. Lewis, "Preparing Geriatric Fitness and Recreation Specialists," Journal of Physical Education and Recreation 48 (1977): 51. Used with permission.

Figure 5.1 Geriatric fitness and recreation concentration (from J. Piscopo and C. Lewis, "Preparing Geriatric Fitness and Recreation Specialists," Journal of Physical Education and Recreation, 48:51, 1977.

3. Assume responsibility in establishing policies for safety and well-being of participants.
4. Establish policy for emergency management and procedures.
5. Determine medical status and clearance for exercise participants.
6. Serve as medical counselor to other program personnel.

HEALTH AND PHYSICAL DIRECTOR

1. Devise program development and implementation.
2. Set up exercise prescriptions with the program medical director.
3. Supervise exercise leaders conducting activities in the program.
4. Coordinate the program with physician and organization director or manager.
5. Serve as a chief public relations officer for the program.
6. Possess competencies in following areas: stress testing, electrocardiography, exercise prescription, exercise leadership, gerontological fitness, program administration, emergency procedures (CPR certification), and psychological and human factors of exercise and related activities affecting the senior adult.

The above responsibilities require a positive, close relation between the physician and health-fitness education director. Their roles should be ones of mutual respect for one another with the central focus of attention on the health and well-being of the senior adult.

Another important individual in the prgram is the exercise leader—the person who actually leads the physical activity or calisthenics for the group. Such qualities as a caring temperament, understanding of exercise progressions, leadership ability, and understanding of emergency procedures are essential leader competencies. Leaders may be full-time or part-time staff members or volunteers who serve directly under the health and physical director. The Guidelines for Graded Exercise Testing and Exercise Prescription of the American College of Sports Medicine contain further details and specific information about desired competencies of various personnel involved in organized adult fitness programs.[3]

Administrative Structures. A wide variety of administrative structures exist which provide for fitness and recreational programs for the senior adult. As noted earlier, programs are found in voluntary organizations, commercial operations, community organizations, and public agencies. Each group operates according to its overall purpose, available funds, and facilities.

Perhaps the fastest growing type of organization in the United States is the multipurpose senior center–type structure. These centers are springing up in most major cities and metropolitan suburban areas in response to the increasing number of individuals 60 and over seeking social and recreational outlets. Usually this type of organization is sponsored by the local community with funding from a number of sources. For example, it is not uncommon to find a local multipurpose center receiving monies for its operation from the city or town, county office of the aging, United Way, state and federal agencies, and private foundations. Centers may be programmed under the aegis of the city recreation department or exist as autonomous units within the administrative structure of the municipality, funded by separate budget.

An organizational structure whereby a duly designated department of senior services, under the sponsorship of a town or municipality, is directed by a professional gerontologist would be an ideal administrative plan for maximizing the delivery of services to older adults. Funding and budgeting for the department should be derived from the local community with ancillary support from state and federal agencies. Given this kind of an administrative and funding resource, community centers can plan and conduct their activities with stability and in a professional manner without the threat of losing monies that depend on sporadic state and federal grants. Figure 5.2 illustrates a model organizational plan for a multipurpose senior center which allows a full range of activities with a professional staff. From an ideal viewpoint, the center should serve as a focal point where older adults can secure the counseling and other services they need, as well as providing environmental contact opportunities with people of all ages.

Every administrative unit that includes an older adult fitness program should have a medical advisory board. The board should consist of four to five members and include at least two physicians, preferably a cardiologist and orthopedist. Other members of the board should be a program director and one or two adult program participants. The principal purpose of the board is to establish medical guidelines for the fitness programs. Such matters as medical prerequisites for fitness program entrance, contraindications of certain fitness activities, stress testing advisability, and general overall health effects of program activities fall within the purview of the board's concerns. It is essential that an amiable and cooperative relationship be established between the board and program director in order to maximize the effectiveness of the program and safety of its participants.

Budget and Finance. The type of program, services, and support costs of building maintenance and equipment will determine the amount of funds needed to operate a multipurpose senior center. The largest single factor in an operating budget is usually the salaries of personnel. This supports the philosophy that "people make programs" and the belief that professional, and dedicated workers can produce creative and imaginative programs. In

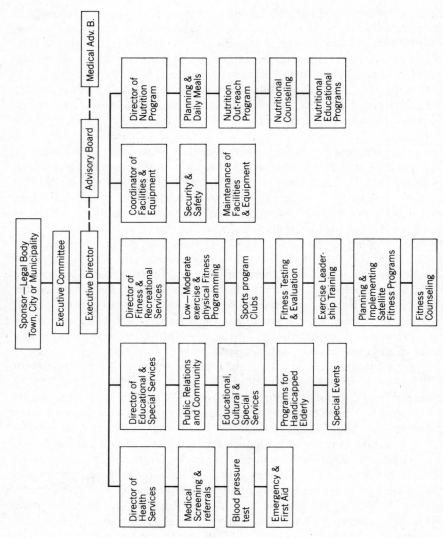

Figure 5.2 Suggested model for a multipurpose senior center.

addition to basic funding from the legal sponsoring body, program activities can be enriched by income raised through special events and by donations of civic organizations and voluntary groups. Such supplemental income should complement the program of activities, not serve as a substitute for budget requirements.

The cost of operating a senior center reflects the scope of the program. Fitness related equipment ranges from sticks used as wands in exercises to sophisticated electronic cardiac monitoring instruments. Complex medical equipment such as stress testing equipment requires qualified fitness specialists working in concert with a physician—and obviously entails greater costs. In certain cases where the senior center has an arrangement with a local hospital and its medical staff, such evaluative procedures can be secured at a reasonable charge. For example, in a community-university program at the University of Southern Maine, stress testing can be offered because the costs are shared by the sponsor (university facilities), Maine Medical Center (medical personnel), private insurance corporation (donated testing instruments—see Fig. 5.3), and the senior participants (modest testing fee).

Ideally, a completely equipped senior center should contain a gymnasium, areas for walk-jog activities, several activity rooms for assorted leisure and crafts, comfortable sitting rooms for reading and intellectual activities, complete kitchen for implementation of a nutrition program, and a swimming pool. The last item is the most costly; however, provision for swimming is very important since many older persons develop arthritis and limiting orthopedic conditions. Most senior centers interrelate swimming programs with local schools or Ys. Such arrangements can be set up with some of the cost shared by the membership. However, even though this system is common, the inclusion of a pool on the premises is more desirable because of its great value as a fitness activity for older adults.

The director or administrator of a senior center is usually responsible for preparing a budget. There is nothing mysterious about constructing a budget provided three basic principles are followed: (1) collect the necessary information about the center's operation; (2) classify the information; and (3) present the adopted budget to the appropriate sponsoring body of the organization.

Collecting information entails an estimate of income and expenditures including membership fees and other sources of income from special events and private donations. Expenditures involve a tabulation of all costs of operating and maintaining the organization. This includes salaries, building operations, and maintenance.

After the information has been gathered, classification follows. This process assures uniformity of presentation and fosters accuracy in planning.

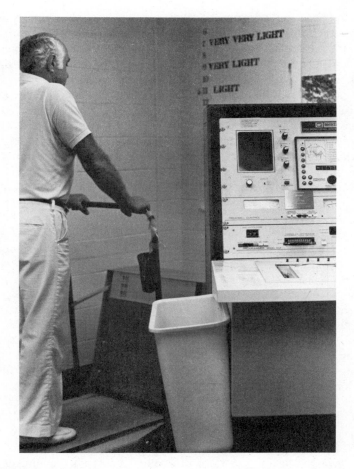

Figure 5.3 Stress testing equipment: a viable program component. (Courtesy of Lifeline Program, University of Southern Maine.)

Such items as personnel salaries, travel, equipment, office supplies, and repairs are typical categories.

The presentation of the budget is usually done once each year, and it follows a hierarchical sequence from the executive committee of the organization to the final legislative approval body of the city or municipality. For sound fiscal practice, it is important to remember that purchases or expenditures should not be made until the budget is approved and adopted.

Facilities and Equipment. Several principles and guidelines relevant to organization and administration are listed in this section. Chapter 8 contains a detailed presentation on types, use, and appropriateness of facilities and equipment designed to maximize the benefits of fitness programs. The following principles are suggested when planning and implementing the administrative elements of facilities and equipment:

1. Areas and facilities should be planned with concern of *full use* of physical resources.
2. Facilities should provide for program activities that serve the *needs* and *interests* of older persons.
3. Facilities and space areas should conform to *standards* established for the sport or activity, as well as to local or state *building regulations* where applicable.
4. All interested *organizations, individuals,* and *groups* who intend to use the facilities should be included in planning aspects.
5. Experience and expertise of *qualified persons* should be utilized in planning activity areas and facilities.
6. *Safety* and *welfare* of the person must be foremost in the selection and care of equipment.
7. A complete and accurate *inventory* of all equipment should be maintained in order to preserve fiscal integrity of acquisition and maintenance costs.
8. *Quality equipment* should be purchased from reputable firms.
9. Equipment should be *inspected* periodically to keep items in a safe and sanitary condition, and to expedite repairs when needed.

Administrators are frequently judged by the competence with which they perform their fiscal duties. Successful programs cost money to operate. Therefore, careful attention to the management of expenditures, with complete and accurate records, is essential. Directors of senior centers should strive to end each year with a balance rather than a deficit in operating funds.

Program Evaluation and Assessment. A fundamental purpose of evaluation and assessment is to determine the effectiveness of the program of experiences and activity. Program evaluation leads to assessment, which provides the director of the program with clues to strengths and weaknesses of program content and environment. Evaluation may be both subjective and objective. Such testing procedures as checklists, observations, and interviews are generally classified as subjective techniques because responses are based upon opinions. This approach to evaluation is important when seeking feedback about attitudes and practices. Objective evaluation procedures involve the documentation of discrete facts and data such as attendance, frequency of participation in various activities, expenditures, and measurements of participant physical fitness variables (strength, flexibility, balance, etc.).

Evaluation also may be informal or formal. For example, casual observation and discussion of an activity with an involved senior adult is really an informal evaluation technique. On the other hand, asking a class of exercise participants to complete a written questionnaire about the activity is considered a formal measurement procedure. Informal evaluations should be a continuous and ongoing process, while formal techniques may be applied at specific intervals, usually after an activity unit is completed. Effective evaluation entails the use of both modes.

Actually, informal program evaluations should be an everyday affair. The program director should subjectively evaluate the behavioral responses frequently through observations, individual discussions, anecdotal records, and small group discussions. The following items may be incorporated into informal or formal evaluation procedures:

A. Individual Senior Adult
   1. Attendance record
   2. Types of activities involved
   3. Behavior responses such as friendliness, cooperation, general attitude
   4. Development of new skills or interests

B. Program Content
   1. Wide scope of activities
   2. Activities that meet the needs, interests, and capabilities of participants
   3. Effectiveness of program leaders—personality, knowledge of subject, and presentation ability
   4. Relevance and meaningfulness of activities
   5. Degree of potential satisfaction and pleasure from the program

C. Relations with Agencies outside the Organization
   1. Degree of support from legislative bodies (city, town, or municipality)
   2. Public relations with local media, e.g., newspaper, radio, and television
   3. Interest of other civic groups in the community, e.g., Rotary, Kiwanis Club, etc.

Physical fitness and motor skills such as muscular strength, flexibility, endurance, balance, and equilibrium are best evaluated using discrete objective tests. Chapter 9 contains specific examples of fitness and program tests.

MULTIPURPOSE SENIOR CENTER AND OTHER NONINSTUTIONALIZED SETTINGS

As the name implies, "multipurpose senior center" signifies a place where persons (usually 60 and over) participate in a variety of social, physical, and cultural activities and programs. Thousands of senior centers are found throughout the nation, usually in urban areas. A report from a national survey of 472 senior centers provides insight to the nature and characteristics of senior center participants.[4] Several highlights of the report were the following findings:

1. About half of center participants were 65–74 age bracket; nearly one quarter were between 75 and 84 years of age.
2. Three of every center participants were women; relatively few center users came from professional and managerial work backgrounds.
3. Almost 60 percent of those who came to the center lived alone.
4. Tours and trips were among the most popular reasons for coming to the center. Table games were highly popular. Sedentary recreation activities contained more participants than active recreation activities.
5. Loneliness and desire to meet others were a prominent reason given for attendance; others came because of services and meals.

That report provides some clues for the design and conduct of activity programs. Essentially, we are dealing with a well-aging population consisting primarily of women between the ages of 65 and 74 from a middle-class background participating mainly in myriad sedentary recreational activities. Nevertheless, the mix of people warrants a great and diverse number of different activities to satisfy the needs of all participants. Figure 5.4 illustrates a sample monthly program of activities.

This program serves approximately 8000 members and has expanded its operation to include satellite centers to accommodate the growing number of eligible persons 60 and over. Figure 5.4 reveals that senior centers provide meaningful services that offer satisfying individual and group experiences through arts, music, drama, dance, exercise, sports, travel, lectures, special classes, games, special events, counseling, nutrition, hobbies, special clubs, crafts, and current events. The list can be endless, depending upon the interests and needs of the particular neighborhood the center serves.

Although senior centers have contributed immeasurably to the enrichment of life experiences in the mature years of participating older adults, considerable improvement is needed in the area of fitness programming.

March

Monday	Tuesday	Wednesday	Thursday	Friday
ROOM CODES CL - Classroom CR - Craftroom DA - Dining Room A - Auditorium L - Lounge NC - Nurses Clinic IR - Into & Referral ACC - Amherst Community Church, 77 Washington Hwy.	**SPECIAL T.V. PROGRAMS** A program entitled "Aging is for Everyone" is broadcast on Channel 7 at 1 p.m. the 4th Saturday of each month. "Over 50" is a new program on Channel 17. Sundays at 1 p.m. Chuck Healy is the host of this show aimed at Senior Citizens. You may recognize people you know on various programs.	**FOSTER GRANDPARENT PROGRAM** Catholic Charities of Buffalo is recruiting persons over age 60, with low income. This program provides an opportunity to establish an ongoing, one-to-one relationship with two children with special or exceptional needs. Foster Grandparents receive a stipend plus other benefits. Eligible persons should contact: Mimi Ferraro Smith, Project Director at Catholic Charities at 856-4494 for more information.	**1** 9:00 M.O.W. Bookkeepers - CL 9:15 "Swingers' Sq. Dance Class - A 9:30 Beg. Ceramics - CR 11:00 Weekly Walk 12:30 Adv. Ceramics - CR 1:00 Yoga - A 1:30 Calligraphy I - DA 1:30 Square Dance Club - A	**2** Exercise at ACC Cancelled 9:30 Recorder Group - CL 10:00 Am-Center Seminar - A 1:30 Bridge Club - A 1:30 Calligraphy II - CR 2:00 Bridge Class - DA
5 9:30 Exercise Class - A 9:30 Stamp Club - DA 9:30 Organ - L 9:30 Community Service - DA 9:30 Quilting - CR 10:00 Beg. Cross Stitch 1:00 Cross Stitch (adv.) 1:00 Painting - CR 1:30 Am-Tones - A 1:30 Community Service - A 1:30 Ballroom Dancing - DA 1:30 Garden Club - CL	**6** 9:00 Tap Dancing - A 9:00 Woodcarving - CL 9:30 Knitting Club - L 9:30 Looking Thru the Papers - CR 12:00 Beg. China Painting - CR 1:00 Alumni Club - A 1:30 Slim Down - DA 2:30 Adv. China Painting - CR	**7** 9:00 Knitting Class - CR 9:30 Pinochle Class - CL 9:30 Exercise Class - A 1:00 Community Service - CR 1:15 French Class - CL 1:30 Men's Club - A 1:30 Pinochle Club - A	**8** 9:00 M.O.W. Bookkeepers - CL 9:15 "Swingers' Sq. Dance Class - A 9:30 Beg. Ceramics - CR 11:00 Weekly Walk 12:30 Adv. Ceramics - CR 1:30 Book Review - L 1:30 Calligraphy I - DA 1:30 Square Dance Club - A Yoga Cancelled Today	**9** 9:30 News That Was - CR 9:30 Recorder Group - CL 9:30 Exercise Class - ACC 1:30 Bridge Club - A 1:30 Calligraphy II - CR 1:30-4:30 Income Tax Assistance - CL 2:00 Bridge Class - DA
12 9:30 Exercise Class - A 9:30 Organ - L 9:30 Community Service - DA 9:30 Quilting - CR 10:00 Beg. Cross Stitch 1:00 Cross Stitch (adv.) 1:00 Painting - CR 1:30 Am-Tones - A 1:30 Community Service - A 1:30 Ballroom Dancing - DA	**13** 9:00 Tap Dancing - A 9:00 Woodcarving - CL 9:30 Vision/Glaucoma Screening - CL 9:30 Knitting Club - L 9:30 Looking Thru the Papers - CR 12:00 Beg. China Painting - CR 1:30 Camera Club - A 2:30 Adv. China Painting - CR 6:00 Couples Club	**14** 8:00 Advisory Board - DA 9:00 Knitting Class - CR 9:30 Pinochle Class - CL 9:30 Exercise Class - A 12:30 What is Cardio-Pulmonary Resuscitation? - A 1:00 Community Service - CR 1:15 French Class - CL 1:15 Nutrition/Hospitality Mtg. - L 1:30 Pinochle Club - A	**15** 9:00 M.O.W. Bookkeepers - CL 9:15 "Swingers' Sq. Dance Class - A 9:30 Beg. Ceramics - CR 11:00 Weekly Walk 12:30 Adv. Ceramics - CR 1:00 Yoga - L 1:30 Calligraphy I - DA 1:30 Square Dance Club - A	**16** 9:00-11:00 Groove Your Swing - A 9:30 News That Was - CR 9:30 Recorder Group - CL 9:30 Exercise Class - ACC 12:00 St. Patrick's Nutrition Luncheon Wearing of the Green Contest 1:30-4:30 Income Tax Assistance - CL 1:30 Senior Jobs - IR 1:30 Bridge Club - A 1:30 Calligraphy II - CR 2:00 Bridge Class - DA
19 9:30 Exercise Class - CL 9:30 Stamp Club - DA 9:30 Organ Club - L 9:30 Community Service - DA 9:30 Woodcarving - CL 10:00 Beg. Cross Stitch 1:00 Cross Stitch (adv.) 1:00 Painting - CR 1:30 Am-Tones - A 1:30 Community Service - A 1:30 Ballroom Dancing - DA	**20** 9:00 Tap Dancing - A 9:00 Woodcarving - CL 9:30 Knitting Club - L 9:30 Looking Thru the Papers - CR 12:00 Beg. China Painting - CR 1:30 Camera Club - A 1:30 Travel Club - A 1:30 Sewing - CL 2:30 Adv. China Painting - CR	**21** 9:00 Knitting Class - CR 9:30 Pinochle Class - CL 9:30 Exercise Class - A 1:00 Community Service - CR 1:15 French Class - CL 1:30 Men's Club Business Mtg. - DA 1:30 Pinochle Club - A 7:30 Senior Nightclub	**22** 9:00 M.O.W. Bookkeepers - CL 9:15 "Swingers' Sq. Dance Class - A 9:30 Beg. Ceramics - CR 11:00 Weekly Walk 12:30 Adv. Ceramics - CR 1:00 Yoga - L 1:30 Calligraphy I - DA 1:30 Square Dance Club - A	**23** 8:00 Community Relations Special Committee Mtg. 9:30 News That Was - CR 9:30 Recorder Group - CL 9:30 Exercise Class - ACC 1:00 Humanities "Heritage of the Future" - CR 1:30 Senior Jobs - IR 1:30 Bridge Club - A 1:30 Calligraphy II - DA
26 9:30 Exercise Class - A 9:30 Organ - L 9:30 Community Service - DA 9:30 Quilting - CR 10:00 Beg. Cross Stitch 1:00 Cross Stitch (adv.) 1:00 Painting - CR 1:30 Am-Tones - A 1:30 Community Service - A 1:30 Ballroom Dancing - DA	**27** 9:00 Tap Dancing - A 9:00 Woodcarving - CL 9:30 Knitting Club 9:30 Looking Thru the Papers - CR 12:00 Beg. China Painting - CR 1:30 Birthday Party, free for those born in Feb. or Mar. - A Reserve at the switchboard 1:30 National Council of Senior Citizens - L 2:30 Adv. China Painting - CR	**28** 9:00 Knitting Class - CR 9:30 Pinochle Class - CL 9:30 Exercise Class - A 1:00 Community Service - CR 1:15 French Class - CL 1:30 Men's Club - A 1:30 Pinochle Club - A 7:30 Camera Club	**29** 9:00 M.O.W. Bookkeepers - CL 9:15 "Swingers' Sq. Dance Class - A 9:30 Beg. Ceramics - CR 11:00 Weekly Walk 12:30 Adv. Ceramics - CR 1:00 Yoga - L 1:30 Calligraphy I - DA 1:30 Square Dance Club - A	**30** 9:00-11:30 Groove Your Swing - A 9:30 News That Was - CR 9:30 Recorder Group - CL 9:30 Exercise Class - ACC 1:00 Humanities "Heritage of the Future" - CR 1:30 Senior Jobs - IR 1:30 Bridge Club - A 1:30 Calligraphy II - DA

Figure 5.4 Monthly activity program. (Courtesy of Town of Amherst Senior Center, Williamsville, N.Y.)

Most centers conduct a variety of low-level exercise classes and offer some activity in bowling, swimming, and table tennis. However, few provide professional leadership in this vital health area. Programs of exercise and sport activities should be based upon a sound framework of anatomical, physiological, psychological, and kinesiological principles and approved by a medical advisory board of the program administrative unit. The following section deals with the health-fitness program components of multipurpose centers and similar organizations.

Exercise and Fitness Program

Exercise-activity experiences can provide assorted benefits and serve different purposes, depending upon type or mode, frequency, duration, and intensity. The overload principle and specificity of exercise principle discussed in Chapter 4 should be applied with disciplinary rigor if improvement of health-fitness and the prevention of immobility is expected. As with other age groups, exercise programs can be conducted at low, moderate, or high stress levels depending upon the general organic (medical) and dynamic (performance) condition of the participants.

In most cases, fitness programs for older persons are geared to low and moderate levels. Therefore, our discussion deals primarily with the deconditioned individual seeking fitness and greater mobility in his or her living environment as well as reinforcing the probability of slowing the overall aging process itself.

Before a specific program or curriculum of activities is presented, the physical director should select target fitness goals. Although many factors of fitness can be identified, the components of muscular strength and endurance, flexibility, cardiovascular-respiratory efficiency, balance and equilibrium, and body composition are most relevant for persons past 60. Such factors as power, speed, and high-level athletic skills are also part of fitness, but these parameters are secondary in importance to the above five components for the older adult.

Safety Considerations. Safety of the participant is a prime qualification in the conduct of fitness activities. Therefore, each senior should have medical clearance before beginning a conditioning regimen. Figure 5.5. illustrates a sample format that can be used. Completing a clearance form serves as a safeguard for participant and helps the program director to establish guidelines concerning modification or adaptation of specific sports and exercises for individuals who may have limiting health conditions.

The question of whether the participant should be required to have a medical examination before participation in a low stress level exercise pro-

Figure 5.5 Physical and laboratory examination form.

Name _____ Tel. _____ Date _____

Street _____ City _____ Zip _____ Age _____

Physical Examination

Thyroid abnormal?	Yes	No		
Chest auscultation abnormal?	Yes	No		
Heart size abnormal?	Yes	No		
Peripheral pulses absent?	Yes	No		
Gallops, abnormal heart sounds?			Yes	No
Any joints abnormal?			Yes	No
Abnormal masses?			Yes	No

Resting Blood Pressure _____

Present medication _____

Limitations _____

Laboratory Examination (within 1 year of present date)

Resting ECG rate _____ Rhythm _____

axis _____ interpretation _____

S.M.A.–12 Profile

cholesterol _____ blood sugar _____

Summary Impression of Physician

1. Comments of any history or physical finding (especially "YES" answers)

_____

Diagnoses: _____

2. Recommendations: (check one)

☐ there is *no contraindication* to participation in moderate exercise program.

☐ because of the above diagnosis, participation in a moderate exercise program *may be advisable* but further examination or consultation is necessary—namely: STRESS EKG, OTHER.

☐ because of the above diagnosis, my patient *may participate only under direct supervision of a physician* (Lifeline Cardiac Rehabilitation Program).

☐ because of the above diagnosis, participation in a moderate exercise program is *inadvisable*.

3. This patient has my permission to receive nutrition counseling under the supervision of a registered dietitian in conjunction with the Lifeline program. ☐ YES ☐ NO

Physician _____ Signed _____
                (please print)   (physician)

Physician's Address _____

Release: I hereby release the above information to the Exercise Program Director.

Consent: I agree to see my private physician for medical care and agree to have an evaluation by him once a year.

Signed _____
                              (patient)

Source: Courtesy of Senior Lifeline Program, University of Southern Maine.

gram is frequently asked. Minimizing the risks through proper screening and individualized exercise prescription can decrease the probability of cardiorespiratory or orthopedic accidents.

The committee on aging of the American Alliance of Health, Physical Education, Recreation, and Dance recently adopted the following guidelines for exercise programs for older persons (50 and older), which can be valuable in conduct of exercise activities:

> For programs involving vigorous exercises (i.e., exercises that exceed the level of intensity encountered in normal daily activities such as walking and climbing stairs), the medical evaluation should insure that the individual can participate in vigorous exercise without any undue risk to the cardiovascular and other bodily systems. Normally, a test that ascertains an individual's cardiorespiratory adjustment to the stress of exercise is an advisable part of the examination. Minimally it should ascertain if the cardiovascular system, by such appropriate indicators as heart rate and blood pressure, can adequately adjust to vigorous exercise.
>
> For exercise programs involving low intensity exercises (i.e., exercises that do not exceed the level of intensity encountered in normal daily activities), participants should have their personal physician's approval.
>
> Regardless of whether or not a program of exercises is vigorous or of low intensity, the following guidelines to insure the safety of the participants are offered:
>
> 1. In that each person's response to the stress of exercise is specific to that individual, it is important that each person's response to exercise be monitored periodically for signs of undue stress (unduly high heart rate, nausea, dyspnea, pallor, pain). Participants should be taught to monitor their own heart rate and to recognize these indicators of stress. Unusual responses should be reported to the exercise leader immediately. Exercise leaders also should be vigilant of these warning signs.
>
> 2. Every exercise program must have a well-defined emergency plan for exercise leaders to follow in the event of cardiac arrest or other accidents.
>
> 3. Exercise programs must have adequate supervision. Exercise leaders should be trained in cardio-pulmonary-resuscitation (CPR) techniques. At the very minimum, CPR trained personnel should be present during every exercise session or in close proximity to the exercise program.[5]

These guidelines imply active involvement of the participant's personal physician or a medical specialist connected in the fitness program. Guidelines for programs that involve specific conditions such as cardiac rehabilitation or with obese individuals, orthopedic aberrations, or atypical states should be drawn up under the advice of a physician with regard to contraindications.

The concept that "the higher the risk—the greater the supervision and control of the activity'' is sound and should be applied when working with a diversity of individuals in a senior population. Dr. Betty Van der Smissen, an expert on legal liability in Health, Physical Education and Recreation points out that it is not only vital to have professional and competent personnel leading adult fitness programs, it is also essential that the exercise specialist keep abreast of the latest developments in the field of fitness and emergency care and make use of them in programming.[6]

APPLYING FITNESS PRINCIPLES AND GUIDELINES

We have discussed the anatomical and physiological changes that occur with the aging process, pointing out that such structural and functional alterations directly affect human performance and effectiveness. This section examines the specific application of fitness principles. Program content and modes are described with emphasis upon usability and practice for program directors and exercise specialists in a noninstitutional setting such as a multipurpose senior center or similar organization where structural programs are offered.

Developing Muscular Strength and Endurance

The need for maintaining muscular strength and endurance is important at all age levels; however, this fitness component has special meaning for older persons because it is the source of energy and force necessary for the maintenance of good posture and proficient movement skills, as well as a protective buffer for bones and soft tissues. Decline in strength occurs steadily with age, but muscle hypertrophy can be maintained longer and fulfill the strength needs of older adults quite adequately provided a progressive and systematic exercise plan is followed at least three times per week for a minimum of 30 to 40 minutes each session.

Specific Muscle Strengthening Plan. Exercise patterns and descriptions are abundant in the literature, ranging from sophisticated textbooks for research scientists to popular magazines for laypersons. Many primers present activities for various regions of the body, from shoulder girdle exercises of push-ups to full body movements of jumping jacks. It is important that exercises be carefully prescribed with the following considerations: (1) age and medical/dynamic fitness condition, and (2) prescribed kinesiological movements. The ensuing exercises and activities are recommended specifically for the purpose of strengthening areas of the body that are generally weak among persons over 50.

Pectoral Muscles (Anterior Chest Region). Arm throwing movements—for example, overhead throwing of a ball or other object, or a calisthenic exercise of thrusting arms across the chest (adduction in horizontal plane)—will activate the pectoral muscles. These muscles are important for maintaining strength of the upper body and are particularly vulnerable to flaccidity and sagging from the constant downward pull of gravity. Disuse further hastens the "posture fatigue" appearance of forward body flexion in advanced age. Crawl stroke swimming, racquet sports utilizing a variety of overhead arm movements, and specific calisthenic exercises—moving arms across the chest toward the body midline—are excellent activities for maintaining sufficient muscle tone and hypertrophy.

Abdominal Muscles (Rectus Abdominus, Transversalis, External and Internal Oblique Group). Ptosis (sagging abdominal wall) is a common condition among adults of all ages, whereby the waistline is larger than chest girth. The ptosis effect is usually due to an accumulation of subcutaneous tissue (predominantly fat) ranging from two to six inches or more in extreme cases of obesity. The need for maintaining tone and functional strength of the abdominal group probably has as much basis in aesthetics as in movement efficiency. A protruding waistline affects the anterior-posterior lumbar spinal curvature and presents a striking postural image. Excessive protuberance can cause a forward shift of the body weight, forcing the head and upper trunk backward to maintain standing equilibrium. This compensating backward movement often results in *lordosis,* or swayback.

Improved strength of the abdominals can be developed by assorted types of sit-ups. In addition to the individual's adipose status, force requirements for this exercise also depend upon weight and length of the trunk (distance from the hip joint to the head). Individuals with heavy and long trunks must exert a greater force than persons with lighter and shorter upper bodies because of the mechanical disadvantage of longer resistance arms inherent in their internal lever structure. Twenty-five sit-ups may be a reasonable sum for a person of short stature, but the same count will require more force and work for an individual over 6 feet in height. This kinesiological fact should be considered before establishing a target number of sit-ups as a goal for all participants. Certain men and women are unable to perform even one sit-up. These individuals should be taught how to execute this movement by using the arms and legs as auxiliary aids. A downward thrust of the legs with a push from the palm of the hands facing the floor will allow most persons to lift the trunk to an upright sitting position.

Number of repetitions and types of sit-up styles should be prescribed according to the individual's somatotype and conditioning objectives. Participants should be encouraged to perform trunk-twisting movements in order to activate the external and internal oblique muscles to supplement the regular sit-up. Exaggerated breath expiration (without strain) is beneficial for toning the transversalis muscle of the abdominal group.

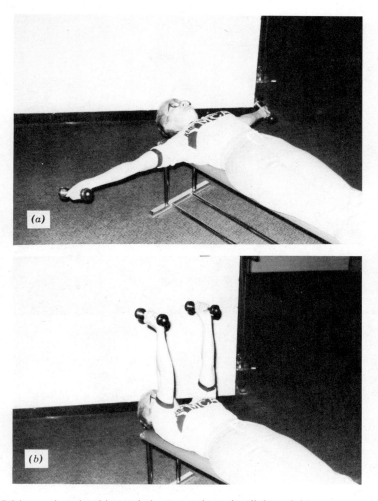

Figure 5.6 Improving shoulder and chest muscles using light weights.

Pelvic and Hip Extensor Muscles (Gluteus Maximus, Medius and Minimus).
These extensor muscles tend to decrease in resiliency and increase in flaccidity with the aging process. Hip girth is usually greater due to excessive
adipose tissue and more time spent sitting. This condition, characterized by
loss of spring and strength, often results in the body literally sinking within
the pelvic basin.[7] This sinking effect, coupled with weakness, impedes the
extensor mobility movements of the hips and contributes to the gradual loss
of standing height as age advances. Firm gluteal muscles play an important

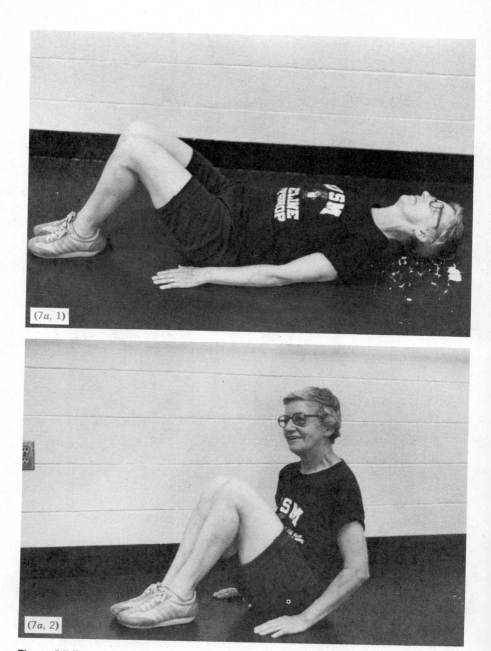

(7a, 1)

(7a, 2)

Figure 5.7 Four methods of performing a sit-up, in progressive order of difficulty.

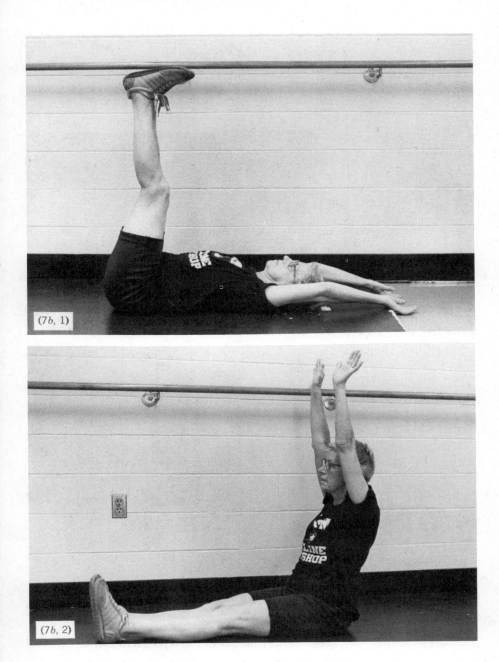

(7b, 1)

(7b, 2)

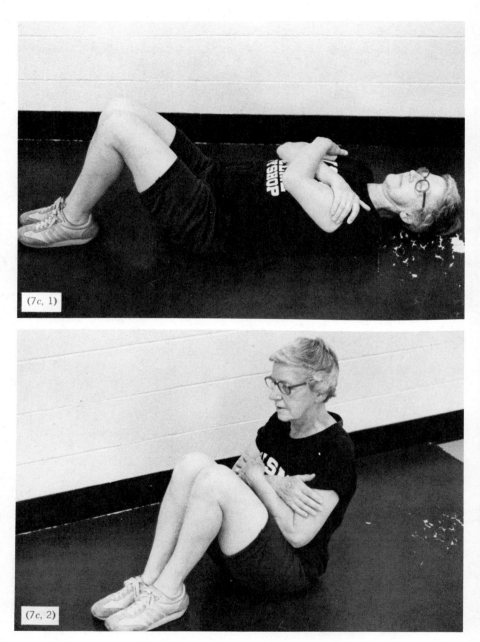

Figure 5.7 (Continued)

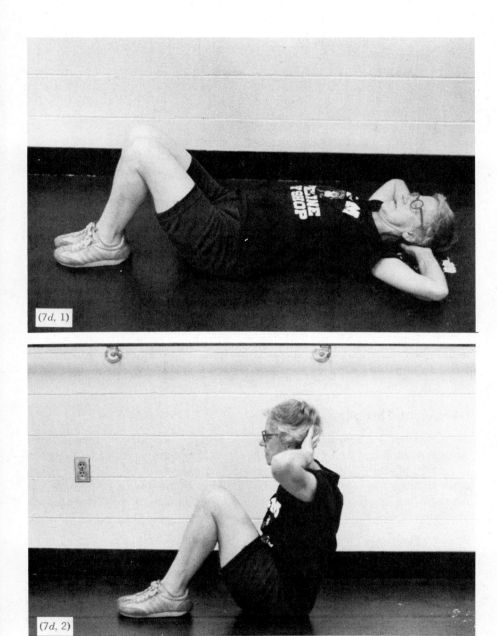

Figure 5.7 (Continued)

role in preventing sagging of the pelvis in the propulsive phase of walking and running, and these muscles can be strengthened by brisk walking, hopping, and jogging. When certain arthritic and lower joint anomalies are present, however, these exercises may be contraindicated. Hip extensor actions, with the individual either standing or lying prone, also are excellent for the gluteal muscles. Figure 5.8 illustrates specific movements designed to strengthen the extensors of the hip.

Shoulder Blades and Extensor Muscles of Upper Back (Rhomboids and Erector Spinae). The constant pull of gravity tends to create an overstretching of the rhomboid muscles (muscles that contract the shoulder blades). This overstretching, coupled with weaknesses of age changes in the posterior lumbarthoracic spine muscles (erector spinae), hastens the kyphotic or excessive round upper back commonly called the "dowager's hump" in older women. Exercises that contract the rhomboids and erector spinae, similar to the back arch shown in Figure 5.9, are beneficial in preserving upright posture.

Although exercises and physical activities that activate other body muscles are desirable, pectoral, abdominal, gluteal, and upper back muscles are notably weakened with age past maturity. These muscles significantly affect posture and appearance, as well as the mobility of older persons. Adequate levels of muscular strength of these particular muscle groups should be maintained throughout life. Appendix B provides a sample program of strength-building exercises appropriate for older persons.

Developing Flexibility

As mentioned earlier, flexibility is quite different among youths and older adults. Anatomical and physiological changes generally decrease the range of motion of all body joints; however, the decline is slowed when the senior adult practices prescribed stretching activities regularly. Everyone can improve his or her flexibility provided he or she is free of serious pathology involving bones or joints.

Specific Flexibility Plan. How can flexibility be improved? Do we need more flexibility of certain joints over other joints? What is the best method of developing flexibility? Is slow-hold stretching more effective than fast-bouncing-type stretching exercises? Before discussing various techniques used to improve flexibility, a brief neurophysiologic review of stretching is necessary, because what happens to an elongated muscle and joint depends upon the natural interplay of the body's nervous and muscular systems.

Myotatic Reflex. The muscle fibers contain sensitive nerve ending receptors called the *Golgi tendons* at the connection of the tendon with the muscle.

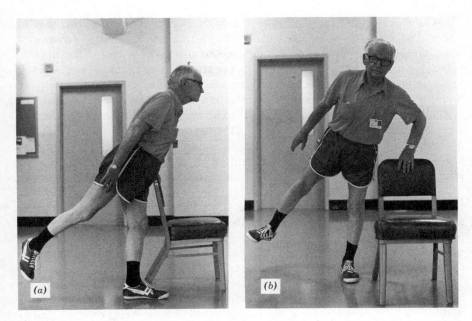

Figure 5.8 Strengthening pelvic and hip extensors: (a) hip extensors; (b) hip abductors.

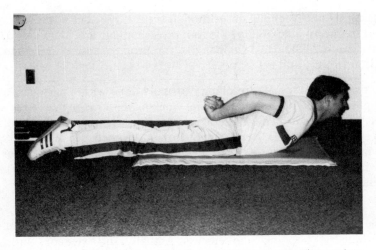

Figure 5.9 Improving posture by strengthening posterior upper trunk muscles.

The Golgi organs are responsive to the degree of tension within the muscle fibers. The *myotatic reflex,* also called the stretch reflex, occurs whenever a muscle is lengthened; that is, a reflex mechanism is fired within the muscle spindle which excites the muscle to contract automatically. The stretch reflex is sensitive to fast-bouncing-type and slow-hold stretching; however, if a muscle is extended quickly, the resulting amount and rate of contraction elicited from the stretch reflex is likely to be more forceful than if the muscle were lengthened gently and slowly.[8] DeVries' research points out that the quick jerky type of stretching exercises called ballistic stretching may invoke undue contractions that interfere with the development of flexible joints and muscles and is more likely to induce muscle soreness.[9]

Both methods of stretching can improve joint flexibility, but most authorities agree that it is prudent to use static-type exercises. Bouncing-type stretching, if used, should be done with control—that is, the speed of return to the starting position after a stretching movement should be regulated by the exerciser. This procedure can minimize the myotatic reflex effect and foster greater flexibility of the exercised joint.

A slow-static stretch is generally held between 10 to 30 seconds or more before release. Beginners and those individuals not training for athletic competition can receive effective stretching benefits from everyday functional tasks, with shorter hold periods, whereas elite older athletes will require longer static hold postures for maximum advantages.

Specific Stretching Techniques. Although several types of stretching modes are used to improve flexibility, the four most popular are: (1) passive (slow-stretch), (2) ballistic (fast-bouncing), (3) proprioceptive neuromuscular facilitation (PNF), and (4) static.

Passive Type. This type of stretching is usually done with a partner. Another person exerts force beyond the normal working joint range in a slow, steady manner without pain. This method is effective when the individual needs help to stretch a joint. Extreme care must be taken because of the possibility of moving a joint beyond its limit. Nevertheless, the procedure does have value when done properly, and when the older individual is unable to move a particular limb or joint under his or her own power.

Ballistic (Fast-bouncing). This type of stretching entails bouncing or jerky movements, such as standing with feet apart, legs straight, and attempting toe touching by "bobbing" movements. Actually, the extensor (hamstrings) muscles are stretched as the flexor (quadriceps) group contract. Quick uncontrolled movements, forcing muscles to stretch, trigger the stretch reflex, and result in shortening rather than stretching the muscle under exercise.

Research has shown that the amount of tension developed for a stretch

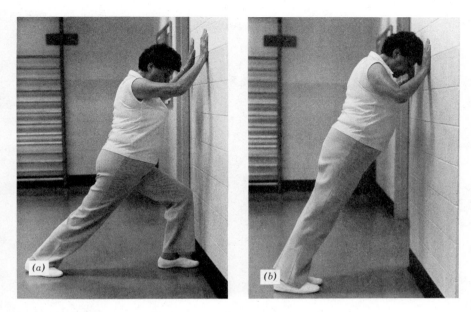

Figure 5.10 Slow-hold stretching technique applied to calf and Achilles tendon.

created is more than doubled by a fast stretch as compared to a slow, gentle stretch through the same range of motion.[10] Therefore, deconditioned persons should avoid this type of flexibility exercise procedure. Dynamic or active techniques, if used, should be done *slowly* and carefully with controlled bobbing motions, after the older adult has practiced static forms of flexibility exercises. For example, rhythmic exercises accompanied with slow music in which the participant does not move to extreme joint ranges and exercises in a gentle manner are recommended. Many people find this kind of stretching less boring than the static-hold type. Such a program was analyzed in a study by Lesser involving 60 volunteer subjects from 61 to 89 years of age, using rhythmic exercises performed with music for a period of ten weeks, twice a week for half an hour.[11] Her findings showed that significant gains in flexibility of shoulder, elbow, wrist, hip, knee, and ankle joints occurred relevant to performing everyday self-care activities.

Proprioceptive Neuromuscular Facilitation (PNF). A well-known technique commonly used by physical therapists with paralytic patients to improve flexibility is *proprioceptive neuromuscular facilitation (PNF)*. PNF uses the neurophysiological principle of reciprocal innervation and inhibition, which indicates that when agonist muscles are stimulated, inhibited action of the opposing or antagonist muscles occurs. In other words, muscles work in

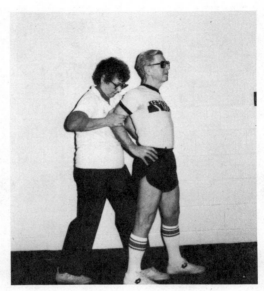

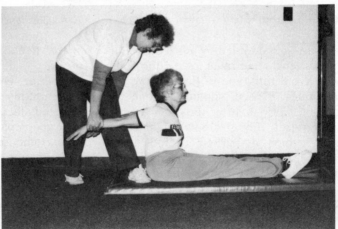

Figure 5.11 Passive stretching of the pectoral muscles.

pairs—when one group is contracting, the opposing set is relaxing. For example, when one flexes the elbow joint, biceps are flexing while triceps are relaxing.

This procedure, described by Kabat in a study of paralyzed patients, combines reciprocal innervation with voluntary relaxation of spastic antagonists.[12] The spastic muscle is placed in a lengthened range and is contracted voluntarily against manual resistance great enough to prevent motion. The patient is then requested to relax and follows this with voluntary contractions of the agonist against resistance. This procedure has also been used with individuals without neuromuscular dysfunctions. Those who endorse the procedure suggest that PNF, because of the myotatic reflex, the reciprocal innervation-inhibitory impulses from the Golgi tendon organ, and the resultant muscle relaxation, enhances the benefits of static muscle lengthening exercises.[13] Actually, PNF is a form of static stretching, and is effective in increasing flexibility.

Static Type. Static styles of stretching are a slow-hold form of movement, as shown in Figure 5.13. Static stretching differs from passive stretching because the movement is performed by the exerciser without the aid of a partner. This type of stretching is more desirable for older persons who can move under their own volition, since it resembles the active motions required in natural living patterns. Passive stretching has greater therapeutic value when the person is unable to exercise singly. The specific procedure for active static stretching is as follows:

1. Move to a position of stretch gradually and slowly.
2. Hold a comfortable stretch (not to extreme range) without pain or discomfort for a period of 10 to 12 seconds. This time interval can be increased as the joint becomes more flexible.
3. Relax the extensor muscle to allow the inverse stretch reflex to become operative.
4. Repeat the procedure six to eight times. Best results are achieved when stretching of the exercised joint is done daily.

Figure 5.13 illustrates a static stretching exercise designed to increase the range of motion of the back hips and knees. The exerciser should reach forward and drape fingers close to the toes without pain or discomfort. A slow pull of low back, hamstrings, and calf muscles results as the movement is completed and held for a period of 10 to 12 seconds.

Planning a Stretching Program. How stretching exercises are incorporated into an exercise regimen depends upon the purposes of the participant. For example, if the senior adult is seeking better athletic performance in a selected sport such as jogging, swimming, track and field, bowling or some

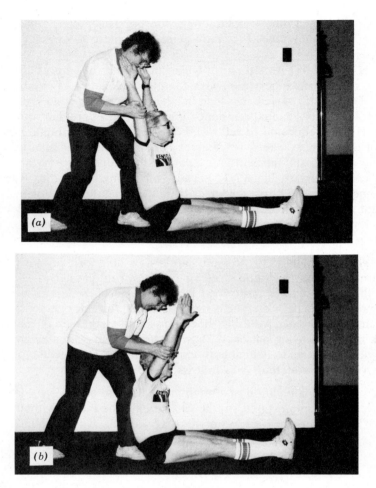

Figure 5.12 Improving shoulder flexibility using PNF technique.

other specialized motor skill, a specific set of flexibility exercises to parallel the movements of the required sport should be practiced, because flexibility is a specific factor, and not a general trait. When greater proficiency in swimming the crawl stroke is desired, then special static exercises that increase ankle flexibility and shoulder range of motions are appropriate, because high flexibility levels of these joints are related to superior performance in crawl stroke swimming. A sample regimen sequence for an elite senior swimmer follows:

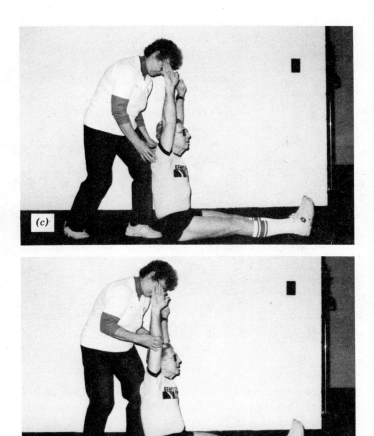

1. *Warm up*—with mild static flexibility exercises focused upon ankle, shoulders, hips, and knees. Alternate body positions, moving slowly and progressively from moderate stretching to maximum stretching hold positions.

2. *Work-out core*—according to the exercise prescription of the sport. For example, a swimming workout may include swimming 20 lengths, kicking 10 lengths with kickboard, and pulling 20 lengths using arms alone, followed by 10 lengths of swimming using combined leg kick and arm stroke.

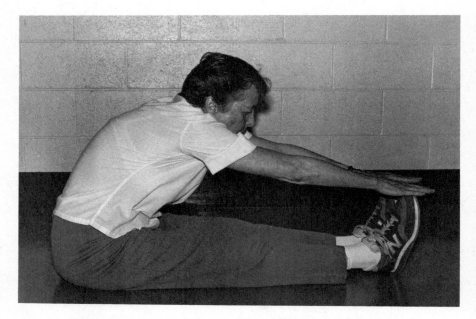

Figure 5.13 Static stretching of the back, hips, hamstrings, and calf muscles.

3. *Cool-down*—perform similar flexibility exercises done before work-out core. This procedure allows the muscles to relax while they are warm and extensible.

This sequence focuses upon crawl stroke swimming. Each sport contains its own movement pattern that demands certain flexibility requirements of certain joints, and each motion configuration should be analyzed and incorporated into a specific stretching workout plan.

Maintaining good health and dynamic fitness, including adequate flexibility, are common goals sought by most people, particularly after 50. Such concerns as avoiding low back pain, sustaining good posture, and escaping muscle spasms and injury, require the maintenance of adequate flexibility. The rule of joint specificity is operative for health-fitness purposes as well as for the improvement of athletic skills. For example, if the individual is seeking relief from low back pain, flexibility exercises directed to stretching the low back, hip muscle illiopsoas, and posterior thigh muscles (hamstrings) are important in addition to strengthening the muscles surrounding the spine (see chapter 3).

When applying flexibility requirements to standing posture, stretching the pectoral muscles (chest) in conjunction with strengthening the rhomboids (muscles between shoulder blades) helps to prevent kyphosis (round-upper back) and the "postural slouch" appearance. Flexibility of the calf muscles helps to relieve muscle soreness. For example, regular static exercises such as those shown in Figure 5.14 can prevent shin splints and spasms of the gastrocnemius (calf) muscles.

When the exerciser is seeking the amelioration of a specific condition, a full work-out core of prescribed exercises for 20 to 30 minutes daily, using the specificity of joint flexibility principle, is indicated. Appendix A illustrates selected flexibility exercises designed to reach primary joints and muscles necessary to perform tasks for everyday living.

Developing Cardiorespiratory Efficiency

Central to a fitness program for senior adults are activities that will maintain and improve the participants' cardiovascular systems and ancillary mechanisms; i.e., involving heart, lungs, and circulatory functions, which interrelate to carrying out cardiorespiratory work of the body. As pointed out in Chapter 4, such factors as vascular circulation, cardiac output, lungs, metabolism, blood pressure, and the imponderables of lifestyle have a confluent and blending effect on the heart, lung, and vessel efficiency, inevitably resulting in a decline to varying degrees in older persons. The discussion here focuses primarily upon the typical senior adult who is ambulatory, is generally free of serious disease, and can function without assistance in carrying out everyday living chores.

Medical Examination and Clearance

Most authorities agree that medical clearance for senior adults by a physician is important before their participation in a cardiorespiratory exercise activity program. However, variance does exist about the type and extent of the medical examination that should be required. Should all seniors take a stress test? Is any kind of a medical examination necessary before clearance is given? The guidelines of the American Alliance for Health, Physical Education, Recreation, and Dance on page 172 offer a prudent and reasonable approach to medical clearance and exercise testing. The ideal policy would be to require the physician's approval at any entry level to an exercise fitness program. Such a policy protects the senior adult from participating in an exercise activity that may be contraindicated, as well as offering some protection to the program staff from a legal liability perspective.

Should the senior participant be required to take a medical examination? Older persons, especially those who are in a deconditioned state,

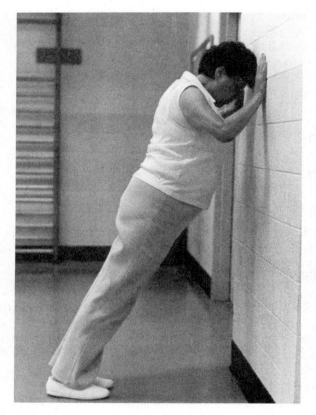

Figure 5.14 Improving flexibility of the calf muscles through static stretching.

should have a basic examination including such measurements as blood count, urinalysis, fasting blood sugar, serum cholesterol, and resting electrocardiogram.[14] The majority of adults seeking activity programs of low and moderate levels do not need extensive medical evaluations, unless some pathological condition exists or the adult is preparing for intense sport competition or seeking engagement in high-intensity-level bouts of physical exertion, such as handball or speed swimming.

In addition to the sample clearance format shown in Figure 5.5, a medical history questionnaire should be completed (see Appendix C).

Fitness Profile

In addition to receiving medical clearance from a physician, prospective participants should be evaluated to determine their state of dynamic fitness—that is, their ability to perform various everyday mobility tasks that require muscular strength, endurance, flexibility, and postural muscle tone. The results of such tests are used to prescribe type and intensity starting points. Specific body composition, strength, flexibility, cardiovascular, and balance tests are described in Chapter 9.

Activity Profile

Some form of personal contact should be made before the senior actually becomes involved in the exercise program. This program feature is usually set up as an informal interview between the program director or instructor. Necessary program forms are completed and written materials about the program are discussed to relieve any possible apprehension about the activities. This part of the program is essential to establish an initial personalized approach with the senior adult and provide the motivation impetus for new members. Such background factors as nature of employment, self-assessment of physical fitness, program expectations, and social and recreational interests are usually discussed. A sample entrance physical activity profile form with specific questions is shown in Appendix E.

Cardiovascular Workout

The core of an effective exercise class for most healthy senior adults includes a 15–20-minute aerobic-type workout that stimulates the heart, lungs, and blood vessels. When planning activities aimed at improving the cardiovascular system and cardiorespiratory efficiency, the following elements should be considered about activity quantity and quality: type of activity, intensity of exercise, duration of workout, frequency of participation, and progression rate. Each of these elements is discussed in the following section.

Type of Activity. As we have previously discussed, the specificity of training principle as applied to exercise type means that particular modes of exercises and activities contain specific purposes. In this case, exercise activity that is specifically designed to maintain and improve circulorespiratory mechanisms of the heart, lungs, and blood vessels must be used in order to receive beneficial results.

Activities that are dynamic (isotonic) in nature as contrasted with static (isometric) are necessary for the improvement of this fitness component. In general, aerobic activities that require sustained physical exertion, such as walking, jogging, bicycling, swimming, dancing, skating, and calisthenics, are preferred modes of developing a good cardiovascular system.

The American College of Sports Medicine classifies aerobic endurance activities into two groups: (1) physical activities during which the exercise intensity is easily sustained with little variability in heart rate response (e.g., walking, jogging, running, swimming, cycling, skating), and (2) physical activities in which the continuous exercise intensity is not maintained (e.g., dancing, figure skating, mountain hiking, and a variety of games and sports).[15] Both types can be used for older adults, provided the activity is adapted to the medical and physical fitness status of the individual. The college further suggests that group 1 activities be used when precise control of intensity is necessary, as in the early stages of conditioning and rehabilitation.[16] Although such activities as stationary bicycling, calisthenics, dancing, rhythmic exercises, and swimming can be conducted in group settings, participants should also be encouraged to pursue dynamic aerobic activities of their interests and enjoyment; these may include badminton, racquetball, tennis, and volleyball.

In cases of competitive games, rule modifications to keep exercise intensity within safe limits are advisable. For example, playing doubles rather than singles badminton, tennis, or racquetball automatically reduces the intensity of play, thereby decreasing the cardiovascular demand and risk of injury to the player.

Generally, deconditioned older persons should participate in exercises that are continuous and hold a steady intensity level, such as walking, jogging, cycling, or swimming. When the senior adult improves his or her cardiovascular system, then games such as tennis, racquetball, and other competitive sports that require intermittent bursts of energy and quick movements may be introduced. Such factors as medical fitness, dynamic fitness, and skill ability should be reviewed in consultation with the physical director and assessed before the senior adult engages in competitive aerobic sports.

Intensity of Activity. Sustaining energy levels to climb a flight of stairs or walk several blocks without physiological stress require threshold standards of cardiovascular fitness. In order to improve heart, lung, and circulatory (endurance) levels, the intensity of heart rate and breathing must be judiciously increased in a safe and prudent manner with minimum risk to the senior adult. Each person's response to exercise stress is *specific*; that is, one individual may engage in activities that elevate the heart rate to 125 beats per minute without stress, whereas another person may experience breathlessness, discomfort, or dizziness at the same heart rate. After the staff has reviewed the medical history and physical examination information, the participant is ready to begin a program designed to improve the cardiovascular component, provided there are no contraindications for program participation and medical clearance is given by a physician.

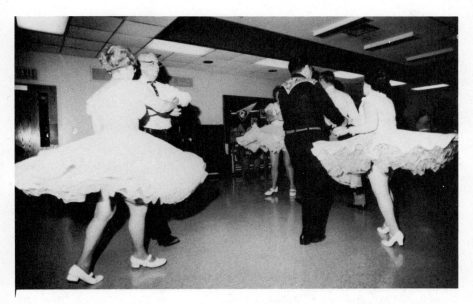

Figure 5.15 Square Dancing: an excellent aerobic activity for improvement of the circulorespiratory system.

How can the participant's exercise intensity be determined before the workout? How can it be estimated during the exercise session? For most adults, the intensity of exercise can be determined by monitoring the heart rate using the basic formula of subtracting the individual's age from 220. Complicated heart rate monitoring procedures are not essential in a field setting, but fitness and recreational specialists should be thoroughly acquainted with medical concepts and such terms as VO_2 max, aerobic capacity, oxygen intake and uptake, and MET unit, used by physiologists and cardiologists to assess cardiorespiratory performance. A system that is simple and quick should be used, whereby senior adults can learn to monitor their own heart rate.

Exercise Intensity by Heart Rate. For apparently healthy adults (free from serious disease), a linear relationship exists between heart rate (HR) and exercise intensity. When vigorous exercise is performed there is a direct rise in HR, blood flow, and metabolic chemical energizers that require more oxygen. The opposite condition prevails when the body is at rest, unless external environmental or internal pathology is present. Thus, heart rate provides a meaningful measure of exercise intensity.

When making a valid estimate of exercise training and workout load, it

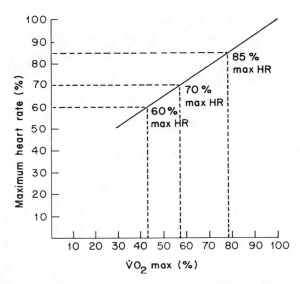

Figure 5.16 Straight line relationship between oxygen utilization and heart rate. (From M. Pollock, J. H. Wilmore, and S. M. Fox III, *Health and Fitness through Activity* [New York: John Wiley & Sons, 1978], p. 123. Used with permission.)

is important to know the individual's resting and maximum heart rates. Maximum heart rate may be estimated from results of graded stress test data or from an electrocardiogram (EKG). However, although these methods may be more accurate in quantitative terms, the 220 minus age formula offers a practical and satisfactory method of estimating workout intensity.

The following formula developed by a Finnish exercise researcher, M. K. Karvonen, illustrates the application of this basic formula using maximum and resting heart rate figures to arrive at an exercise heart rate called target heart rate:[17]

$$220 - Age = MHR$$
$$MHR - RHR = HRR$$
$$(\% \text{ of HRR}) + RHR = THR$$

MHR = Maximum heart rate (220 − age)
RHR = Resting Heart rate
HRR = Heart rate range
THR = Target heart rate (exercise heart rate)

Let us assume that Mr. Brown, a 70-year-old, with a resting heart rate of 72 and free of pathological conditions, desires a personalized exercise intensity prescription. Using the above formula, we can calculate a starting percentage exercise dosage as follows:

Mr. Brown, age 70

$$220 - \text{Age (70)} = 150 \qquad \text{(MHR)}$$
$$\text{pulse rate at rest} = 72 \qquad \text{(RHR)}$$
$$150 \text{ (MHR)} - 72 \text{ (RHR)} = 78 \qquad \text{(HRR)}$$
$$40\% \times 72 \text{ (HRR)} = 31.2 \qquad \text{(\% HRR)}$$
$$31.2 + 72 \text{ (RHR)} = 103.2$$
$$\text{THR} = 103$$

Thus, Mr. Brown is advised to begin his walk-jog or activity regimen making sure that his heart rate does not exceed 40 percent of his maximal heart rate response. This percentage can be increased gradually and progressively as he proceeds from the deconditioned to a conditioned cardiorespiratory fitness state.

DeVries investigated exercise intensity thresholds for the improvement of cardiovascular-respiratory function of men 60 to 79 years of age using the system of percentage of heart rate range in calculating exercise target points.[18] The training consisted of a run-walk program over a six-week period. He found that improvement of heart-lung-circulatory function occurred at the 40 percent level of heart rate range. On the basis of his data, men in their 60s and 70s, of average physical fitness, need only raise their heart rates above 95 and 98 respectively to provide a training stimulus to the cardiovascular system; and well-conditioned men in these age brackets need only exceed 106 and 103, respectively. Thus, for all but highly conditioned older men, vigorous walking, which raises heart rate to 100 to 120 beats per minute for 30 to 60 minutes daily, will bring about some improvement in cardiovascular-respiratory function.[19]

Adams et al. studied the trainability and effects of exercise upon women aged 52 to 79, and found that improvement in heart function among the older female is similar to that of the older male.[20] DeVries offers three reference heart rates for guiding personal progress:[21]

40% of HRR = *Minimum rate* for cardiorespiratory improvement
60% HRR = *Target heart rate* for optimal improvement
75% HRR = *Maximum* (not to be exceeded) *heart rate*

Senior Lifeline Fitness Progress Chart

Name: _____

Maximum Heart Rate = 220
                        − _____ Age

AGE	60–70%	MAX.
50	102–119 $4 \times (25-30)$	170
55	99–116 $4 \times (25-29)$	165
60	96–112 $4 \times (24-28)$	160
65	93–109 $4 \times (23-27)$	155
70	90–106 $4 \times (22-27)$	150
75	87–103 $4 \times (21-26)$	145
80	84–100 $4 \times (21-25)$	140

Date started _____
Medical form _____
Limitations _____
Training range (_____)
Fitness test _____

Figure 5.17 Senior lifeline fitness progress chart—based upon predicted maximal heart rates. (Courtesy of Senior Lifeline Program, University of Southern Maine.)

In Mr. Brown's case, an exercise heart rate of 103 beats per minute would meet a minimum threshold for improvement. Using the same formula at 60 and 75 percent levels would yield target and maximum rates of 118 and 130 respectively. A modification of the above formula, based on predicted maximum heart rates from research data, may also be used. For example, the chart and score card shown in Figure 5.17 indicates 60 to 70% maximum heart rate from age 50 to 80.

Each person should keep his or her own score card, count his or her own pulse, and exercise within the 60 to 70 percent intensity rate for a particular age range. If Mr. Brown used this chart, his maximum exercise target heart rate would be 108 beats per minute. The predicted heart sched-

	Date	Pre	Peak	Post	Distance
1.					
2.					
3.					
4.					
5.					
6.					
7.					
8.					
9.					
10.					
11.					
12.					
13.					
14.					
15.					

Figure 5.17 (Continued)

ule is designed not to exceed workout intensity of 120 beats per minute, which places the schedule at a moderate level of exercise vigor.

Whether the intensity level is determined by using the Karvonen formula or chart with predicted maximal heart rates, the intensity of exercise conditioning program should be carefully supervised by competent instructors. Each prescriptive method is effective in improving cardiorespiratory functions. A note of caution is indicated when using heart rate monitoring procedures such as 220 minus age formulas. Due to considerable variability in maximum heart rate at any age, norm tables may underpredict training heart rate by 10 to 15 beats/min^{-1}.[22]

Another means of expressing intensity of exercise is through the MET system. A *MET** is a categorization of activities relevant to their metabolic cost. The metabolic cost at rest is one MET; two METs are two times the resting level; three METs are three times the value at rest; and so on. The resting energy cost is measured in kilocalories (Kcal/min.) and represents a standard for evaluation and prescription of exercise loads, ranging from low to high intensities. The procedure entails reference to a table of values,

*One MET equals 3.5 milliliters of oxygen per kilogram of body weight per minute.

which delineate given activities in caloric costs and METs derived from calculated equations. For example, badminton play expends from 5 to 11 Kcal/min. and 4 to 9 METs; recreational bicycling uses 3.7 to 10 Kcal/min. and 3 to 8 METs.[23] The actual MET value varies depending upon the vigor of play, skill level of the participant, and type of activity.

The following classifications of caloric costs and their respective METs are based upon exercising continuously for up to 60 minutes, for participants of average fitness:[24]

Calories per Min.	METs	Intensity
Less than 5	3.5 METs	Low
5 to 10	4–8 METs	Moderate
10 to 14	8–12 METs	Moderate to high
More than 14	12 METs	High

Low and moderate activities such as knitting and playing cards fall within the 1.5 to 2.0 METs range; darts, bowling, and shuffleboard from 2.0 to 2.5; and walking, hiking, and dancing from 2.0 to 6.0 METs.[25]

Direct measurement of metabolic energy cost is time-consuming and requires expensive laboratory equipment. However, approximations can be made from other predictive tests, relying on estimates from heart rate, rather than complex oxygen and carbon dioxide analysis. The MET system offers another scientific approach for prescribing and assessing exercise intensity.

Determining Heart Rate. Each participant should be instructed to take his or her own resting and exercise target heart rates. This procedure is accomplished by counting pulse rate, which is generally the same as the heart beat, at one of three body sites; (1) over the *radial* artery (thumb side of wrist); (2) over the *carotid* artery (along the esophagus in the neck); or (3) over the *temporal* artery (right side of temporal bone on the head). The pulsations felt by the tips of the first two fingers indicate a rhythmic expansion and contraction of the artery as shown in Figure 5.18.

The choice of sites depends upon the ease and prominence of the pulse throbs felt by the tester. Care should be taken counting pulse. When counting at the carotid site, a light, rather than heavy, contact should be exerted because excessive pressure may slow the heart rate and give an inaccurate count. The thumb should not be used to feel the count since the radial arterial branch, which is embedded in the skin and subcutaneous tissue of the thumb, may pulsate and give an erroneous count. Some people may not be able to feel the pulse at any of the above sites. In this case, measurement with a stethoscope must be used, as shown in Figure 4.13.

Typically, the heart rate begins to slow down quickly after exercise, so

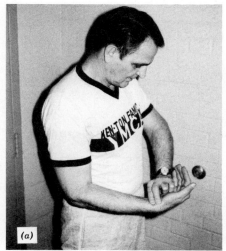

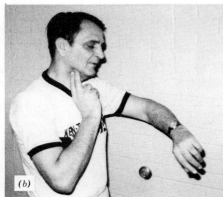

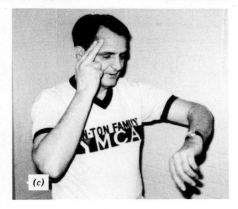

Figure 5.18 Counting pulse beats at the (a) wrist, (b) carotid, (c) temporal sites.

the pulse should be taken immediately after the cessation of activity. One method of estimating heart rate during training is to count the beats for 10 seconds, then multiply the rate by six to determine the pulse beat per minute. A clock or wristwatch with a sweep second hand can be used for timing. A stopwatch provides greater accuracy and should be used whenever possible. Some exercise leaders prefer a 15-second count multiplied by four. This procedure allows counting over a longer time period. Whatever method is used, the tester should count and calculate figures with care because a 5 to 10 percent error can occur with a faulty calculation.[26]

Each procedure requires some practice; however, the exerciser soon learns the signs and nuances of his or her pulse beat and can easily begin the count within five seconds after the exercise bout. Table 5.2 provides a 10- and 15-second conversion chart, which can be used for quick reference to determine heart rate beats per minute.

Duration of Activity. How long must an individual exercise to receive cardiovascular benefits? The answer may refer to one exercise session, or to a

Table 5.2   Conversion Chart for Transforming Heart Rate Counted for 10 or 15 Seconds to Beats per Minute

HEART RATE			
Beats per 10 Seconds	*Beats per Minute*	*Beats per 15 Seconds*	*Beats per Minute*
15	90	23	92
16	96	24	96
17	102	25	100
18	108	26	104
19	114	27	108
20	120	28	112
21	126	29	116
22	132	30	120
23	138	31	124
24	144	32	128
25	150	33	132
26	156	34	136
27	162	35	140
28	168	36	144
29	174	37	148
30	180	38	152
31	186	39	156
32	192	40	160
33	198	41	164
34	204	42	168
		43	172
		44	176
		45	180
		46	184
		47	188
		48	192
		49	196
		50	200
		51	204

Source: M. Pollock, J. H. Wilmore, and S. M. Fox III, *Health and Fitness through Physical Activity* (New York: John Wiley & Sons, 1978), p. 127. Reprinted by permission.

weekly or monthly time frame. People vary in their medical and dynamic fitness levels; thus, a single rule or format is inappropriate. In order to bring about significant changes in cardiovascular fitness, an exercise session must range from a minimum of 20 to 30 minutes per period, at the level of intensity prescribed for the exerciser's fitness status.

Deconditioned persons in their 60s and 70s can start an aerobic regimen of walking geared to raising the heart rate to 40 percent of maximum. This threshold, for a minimum of 15 minutes, can initiate improvement in cardiorespiratory fitness when performed at least three times per week over a period of six weeks. It should be remembered that this level of work should be gradually increased to the 60 percent level, and for some individuals to 75 percent of maximum heart rate as cardiovascular fitness status improves.

Big muscle activity, such as walking, bicycling, jogging, swimming, and rhythmic exercises, are advised for cardiovascular improvement as opposed to static or isometric forms of activity. All exercise programs that exceed intensity of raising the heart rate of 100 beats per minute should conform to the following sequence: (1) warm-up and stretching; (2) core of activity raising heart rate to 100 to 120 beats per minute; followed by (3) cool-down and relaxing movements. Figures 5.19 and 5.20 illustrate a sample rhythmic exercise routine coordinated with music and designed to stimulate the cardiovascular system not to exceed 120 beats per minute.

Frequency of Activity. The appropriate number of exercise sessions per week is contingent upon the fitness status of the participant. The American College of Sports Medicine recommends a range from three to five days per week depending upon the functional capacity of the individual.[27] Low-stress activities such as walking may be done daily, whereas moderate to vigorous intensity level workouts, such as jogging, bicycling, or swimming, can be performed every other day or three times per week.

It is important to apply the concept of regularity to frequency; that is, fitness workouts must be done with consistency throughout the year. Sporadic bouts of exercise, such as weekend walking, jogging, or swimming, may have negative rather than positive cardiovascular effects, and should be discouraged. Deconditioning occurs much faster than conditioning—in fact, twice as fast as getting in shape. Thus, if the exerciser misses one workout session, the loss of the conditioning effect is equal to two periods of exercising.

It is important to recognize that people vary in their desires, motor skills, and sport preferences; therefore, flexibility from a minimum of three to five days per week throughout the year is a key exercise frequency concept applicable for most people. For a few elite senior athletes preparing for sport competition, daily practice may be appropriate.

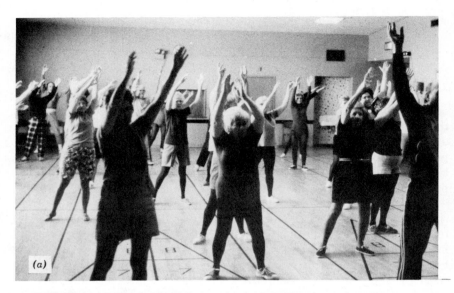

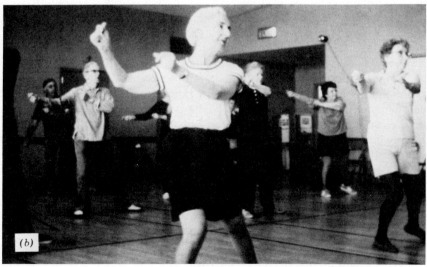

Figure 5.19 Rhythmic exercises: (a) warm-up; (b) cardiovascular core; (c) stretching and cool-down.

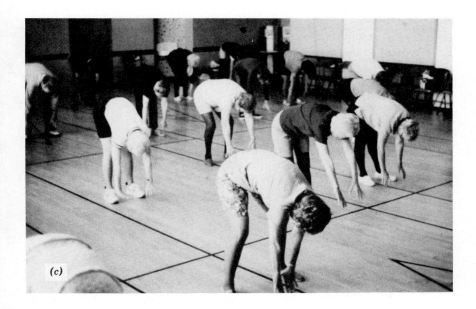

(c)

Progression Rate. The usual progression stages in an exercise activity program geared to aerobic fitness are: (1) the beginning training or conditioning stage, (2) the improvement stage, and (3) the maintenance stage. The rate for each person varies, depending upon his or her specific goals and capabilities. Stationary bicycling, walking, and jogging are common modes of exercise where quantitative rates of progress can be determined using the heart rate monitoring method.

In any progression of cardiorespiratory endurance training, the overriding factor must be safety because the risk of musculoskeletal injury and cardiac dysrhythmias increase as the person becomes older. The principles of conditioning, improvement, and maintenance for the senior adult are similar to the sequence applicable to younger persons, except that training and adaptation for each phase take place over a longer period of time. For example, a 25-year-old can make significant training improvement over a period of 4 weeks, but the typical sedentary 60-year-old may require a range of 6 to 20 weeks depending upon starting health and fitness status.

Improvement in aerobic capacity or the ability of the body to use oxygen (Vo_2 max) is directly related to mode, frequency, intensity, and duration of training. These fitness factors, described earlier, determine the amount of improvement in conditioning, ranging from 5 to 25 percent.[28] There is no list of magic exercises; hundreds of calisthenics and motor skills exist that will

Figure 5.20 Rhythmic exercises for older persons.

I.   *"SUMMER WIND"/ROGER WILLIAMS/STANDING POSITION*   2:45 min.

    A.   Head flexion and head extension—Bring chin to chest, raise head, slowly extend head backwards.

    B.   Keeping shoulders still, turn head sidewards left, face center, turn head sidewards right.

    C.   Drop left ear to left shoulder, face center, drop right ear to right shoulder.

    D.   Look over left shoulder, face center, drop ear to right shoulder.

    E.   Stretch sidewards left with left arm and left leg, come back to center, stretch sidewards right with right arm and right leg.

    F.   Stretch straight ahead with left arm and left leg, stretch straight forward with right arm and right leg.

    G.   End with shoulder rolls.

II.   *"MOON RIVER"/LAWRENCE WELK/CHAIR EXERCISE*

    A.   Inhale raising arms overhead.

    B.   Intermingle fingers and stretch palms to ceiling.

    C.   Exhale returning arms to sides. Do 4 times.

    D.   Legs apart, bring head to left knee while reaching to left ankle with hands. Return to center and repeat on right side. Slide hands down left and right leg while bending between legs. Repeat twice more.

    E.   Arms outstretched at sides, touch left hand to right foot. Come back to center and repeat, touching right hand to left foot. Do 4 times in all.

    F.   Have both arms outstretched on right side of body. Stretch arms out in front of body, over to left side, and swing arms up over head, repeating sequence again.

III.   *CHAIR EXERCISE/"LOVE POLLUTION"/EPIC*   3:09 min.

    A.   Clap hands while keeping toes on floor and hitting heels on floor.

    B.   Slap thighs keeping heels on floor and tapping toes to floor.

    C.   Make fists with both hands. Fling hands forward stretching fingers apart.

    D.   Shake hands shoulder height.

    E.   Leg walks—alternate legs as in a flutter kick.

    F.   Scissors—alternate crossing right leg over left and left over right.

    G.   Bring right knee to chest with help from hands. Bring left knee to chest with help from hands.

    H.   Reach forward between legs and do crawl stroke. Stress a nice reach and try to lift arms alternately.

    I.   Touch hands to top of shoulders. Extend arms sidewards. Do 4 times. Touch hands to top of shoulders. Extend arms overhead. Do 4 times.

IV.   *"LET'S ALL CHANT"/MICHAEL SAGER BAND CHAIR EXERCISE/ FRISBEES (2 EACH)*   3:07 min.

    A.   Hit Frisbees on floor 4 times, overhead 4 times. Repeat.

    B.   Hit Frisbees together and reach side to side—first right then left.

C. Reach forward with Frisbees in swimming fashion arm over arm.
D. Hit foot with Frisbee—first right then left foot.
E. Holding Frisbees in each hand—wave Frisbees at your friends.
F. Put Frisbee on head, move side to side trying to keep Frisbee on head.
G. Stand up keeping Frisbee on head. Sit down keeping Frisbee on head. NO hands allowed.
H. Stand up holding Frisbees in each hand. Swing Frisbees back and forward.
I. Hit foot with Frisbee. Hit seat with Frisbee.
J. Hit Frisbee on floor and overhead again.

V. *"CAN'T SMILE WITHOUT YOU"/BARRY MANILOW* 3:13 min.
A. Holding wand over head, bend side to side.
B. Holding wand over head bend left, up, center, up, right, up, back and up. Repeat.
C. Walk fingers down wands first with right hand and then left hand. Walk finger up at same time.
D. Cross wand in front of body. Cross in other direction. Holding wand in vertical position, wring as you would a dishrag.
E. Holding wand horizontally, lift alternate knees to wand.
F. Extend wand overhead, bring to center of body, then to floor. Repeat.
G. Bending knees half way, circle wand in front of body, holding wand in horizontal position. Keep back straight.
H. Place wand behind neck, bend side to side.

Source: Developed by Joan Magin, Fitness Specialist, Tonawanda Senior Center, Tonawanda, New York.

stimulate and condition the physiological endurance mechanisms of the body. However, the American College of Sports Medicine does set forth standards for the developing and maintaining of fitness in healthy adults that can be useful in designing programs for the healthy senior adult. These recommendations include the following general guidelines:

1. *Frequency:* 3 to 5 days per week.
2. *Intensity* of training: 60 to 90 percent* of maximum heart rate.
3. *Duration:* 15 to 60 minutes of continuous aerobic activity, depending upon intensity.
4. *Mode of activity:* Any activity that uses the large muscle groups, e.g., running-jogging, walking-hiking, swimming, skating, bicycling, rowing, crosscountry skiing, rope skipping, and various endurance game activities.[29]

*This intensity level applies to a broad range of young and middle-aged adults and should be lower (from 40 to 75 percent) for older persons.

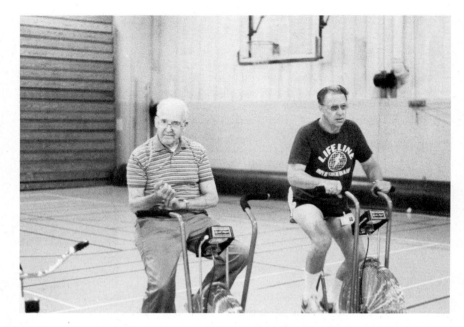

Figure 5.21 Quantitative rate of progress can be measured using bike ergometer.

The above guidelines are broad and must be modified to meet the individual capabilities of the senior adult. Intensity and duration must be carefully prescribed, usually at lower levels than for middle-aged and younger adults. Frequency of exercise is most important in terms of developing and maintaining endurance. Irrespective of age, activity consistency of at least three times per week is necessary before adequate changes in heart-lung endurance functions will occur.

Modified Walking Program. In some cases, for those men and women who are grossly overfat, or who exhibit limiting orthopedic conditions such as arthritis or muscle-joint problems, but can walk without pain or discomfort, a pulse rate monitoring modified walking program is appropriate. Table 5.3 illustrates a sequential and gradual progression of increasing intensity and duration of big muscle exercise, beginning with Level I, one mile in 20 minutes, to Level III, one mile in 14 minutes, gradually increasing the distance from one to four miles.

This walking program uses a self-monitoring heart rate system. The participants monitor their own heart rate and keep individual progress

Table 5.3 Modified Walking Program for Adult Fitness

Level I Mile Walk Program			Level II Mile Walk Program			Level III Mile Walk Program		
Pace: ¼ mile in 5 min. 1 mile in 20 min.			Pace: ¼ mile in 4 min. 1 mile in 16 min.			Pace: ¼ mile in 3½ min. 1 mile in 14 min.		
Exercise Period[a]	Miles	Min.	Exercise Period[a]	Miles	Min.	Exercise Period[a]	Miles	Min.
1	1	20	1	1	16	1	1	14
2	1¼	25	2	1¼	20	2	1¼	17½
3	1½	30	3	1½	24	3	1½	21
4	1¾	35	4	1¾	28	4	1¾	24½
5	2	40	5	2	32	5	2	28
6	2¼	45	6	2¼	36	6	2¼	31½
7	2½	50	7	2½	40	7	2½	35
8	2¾	55	8	2¾	44	8	2¾	38½
9	3	60	9	3	48	9	3	42
						10	3¼	45½
						11	3½	49
						12	3¾	52½
						13	4	56

Directions

1. Warm up with slow and easy walking. Do rhythmic loosening-up exercises.
2. Stride out the designated distance at the suggested time schedule.
3. Stop and monitor your pulse rate at the beginning, half-way point, and end of workout for 10 seconds.
4. Keep your pace to approximately 120 heart rate level per minute (20 monitored beats in a 10-second period).
5. Definitely keep your pulse rate below 132 beats per minute (22 in 10 seconds). Never surpass twice your normal beating heart.
6. Slow down your pace or stop and rest when winded, fatigued, or pulse rate is too rapid.
[a]7. Increase the distance walked a ¼ mile each exercise period in the recommended time only if your monitored heart rate and body fatigue warrant the change. Otherwise, stay at the same intensity level.
8. Keep a careful daily record of your accomplishments on the "Walking Fitness Progress Chart."
9. Additional distances may be added if advisable.

Source: R. E. Wear, "Conditioning Exercise Program for Normal Older Persons," in R. Harris and L. J. Frankel, eds., *Guide to Fitness after Fifty* (New York: Plenum Press, 1977), pp. 260–261. Reprinted by permission).

charts, which are kept on file with the fitness specialist. Dr. Robert Wear of the University of New Hampshire applies a progression program of modified walk, fast and slow walk, and adult jog walk protocols.[30] Each program is structured so that the intensity and duration is gradually increased. Tables 5.4 and 5.5 present instructions for these programs. Again, as with the modified walk program, exercise training heart rate is carefully monitored and evaluated before the senior moves up to the next level.

The progression sequence begins with simple walking at a comfortable pace, gradually increasing the distance and rate of walking and jogging up to a 20-minute period using the basic 220 minus age heart rate training formula. Once the maintenance stage has been reached (as determined jointly by the physician and fitness specialist), the participant can explore active games such as racquetball, extended jogging distance, tennis, and badminton where greater exercise stimulation may be found. The exercise activities selected should be aerobic and rhythmic, using the large muscle groups, not isometric, when pursuing gains in cardiorespiratory efficiency. It is important that fitness maintenance, once achieved, must be practiced consistently

Table 5.4 Instructions for the Adult Fast and Slow Walk and Adult Jog-Walk Fitness Programs

1. Carefully monitor your pulse rate for 10 seconds immediately after jogging at approximately the second, eighth and 15th minute periods of your workout.

    a. Locate your pulse at the carotid artery of the neck (one inch below the jaw level) or at the radial artery on the thumb side of the lower wrist immediately after fast walking.

    b. Stop your movement and count your pulse beats for 10 seconds using a wrist or stop watch. Multiply this heart rate by six to determine your approximate heart rate for one minute at this intensity or work.

    c. Record this rate in the appropriate space on the chart.

2. Continue your fast and slow walking program for 15 to 20 minutes. Slow down your pace if your monitored pulse rate is above your training heart rate.

3. Stop your workout and immediately contact your instructor if you have difficulty in breathing, chest tightness, dizziness, or loss of coordination.

4. Progress to the next exercise intensity prescription level only when your recorded three pulse rates for one day's workout are below your training level and with approval of your instructor.

5. Your workout has been too intensive if your pulse rate has not returned to 120 beats per minute or lower within three minutes following your last fast-walking session.

Source: R. E. Wear, "Conditioning Exercise Program," p. 265. Reprinted by permission.

Table 5.5   Adult Jog-Walk Fitness Program

Name _____   Address _____
Age Maximum Heart Rate _____   Training Heart Rate _____
Average Resting Heart Rate _____   Body Weight _____

DATE _____
PRESCRIPTION _____
H.R. 2nd min. _____
H.R. 8th min. _____
H.R. 15th min. _____

Exercise Prescriptions for Jog-Walking Program

Intensity Level	Minutes		Intensity Level	Minutes	
Special	Jog ¼	Walk 1	E.	Jog 1½	Walk ¼
A	Jog ½	Walk 1	F.	Jog 1¾	Walk ¼
B	Jog ¾	Walk ¾	G.	Jog 2	Walk ¼
C	Jog 1	Walk ½	H.	Jog 2–20	Walk ¼
D	Jog 1¼	Walk ¼			

Total time of interval training workout: 15–20 minutes. Cooling off period: minimum of 5 minutes. Slow walk. Easy rhythmic exercises and static stretching.

Source: R. E. Wear, "Conditioning Exercise Programs," p. 264. Reprinted by permission.

209

and regularly for a minimum of three times per week throughout life, since exercise benefits cannot be stored.

Enhancing Balance and Equilibrium

The anthropometric and kinesiologic changes and principles of balance and equilibrium were presented with considerable detail in Chapters 3 and 4. This section deals with activities that help to sustain normal balance skills and retard the decline of those mechanisms that control this fitness component.

Improving Upright Dynamic Balance Skills. Beam walking activities with variations in body positions and modifications in beam sizes and shapes offer a wide variety of interesting maneuvers that stimulate and sharpen the sensory and neuromuscular mechanisms which control such movements as walking, bending, turning, and skipping, all of which fall into the category of upright dynamic balance. The following activities are designed to enhance this particular balance skill:

1. Beam walking: use variable widths and lengths. Start with a 12-inch width, gradually decreasing width to 2 inches. Beams may vary in length from 10 to 20 feet. Place several beams in zig-zag arrangement (see Figure 4.18). Emphasize use of vision—focus eyes at the end of beam. Place weight primarily on the ball of each foot to stimulate sensory nerve ending on soles of feet.
2. Walk the low beam in a variety of body positions: arms raised sideward to shoulder length (allows for easier balancing), or arms placed behind the back. Walk to the center of beam, crouch, turn, and return to starting position. Walk backwards (slowly) on the beam. Walk to center, pick up a small object, continue to end of beam. Practice tandem beam walking with arms placed on shoulders of lead walks.

Balance beams should be approximately four inches from the floor. Lengths and widths may vary to allow progressive challenges as the participants improve their skill level. Senior adults should learn to assist and "spot" each other as they walk the beam in various positions. Figure 5.22 shows a low-cost improvised beam that can be made from easily obtained materials, with little, if any, special manual training.

Improving Upright Static Balance Skills. Activities such as those shown in Figure 5.23 are common household tasks that require proficiency in upright static balance. Reaching up and keeping the center of gravity over the feet raises the gravity center slightly higher over the pelvis and, therefore, re-

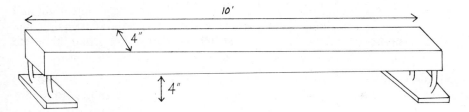

Figure 5.22 Low balance beam.

quires greater control to avoid falling. The following exercises stimulate and foster better upright stationary balance:

1. Stand on one foot: arms extended sideward, arms placed on hips.
2. From standing position: slowly lean forward, backward, sideward with hands on hips. Changing postures, shift the center of gravity and line of gravity inside and outside the body.

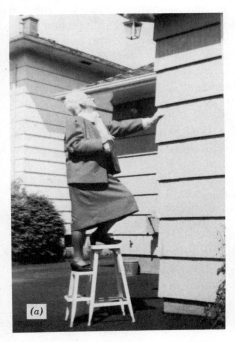
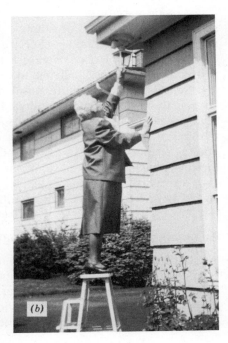

Figure 5.23 Maintaining upright stationary balance—an everyday living need.

3. From standing position: slowly move arms overhead, left, right and extend arm sideward to shoulder height. These movements change the height of the center of gravity within the body and stimulate balance adjustment mechanisms to maintain balance control.

Improving Inverted Static Balance Skills. Although upright, static, and dynamic balance postures are more common in everyday activities of senior adults, occasions arise where inverted balance skill is necessary. For example, bending forward from a sitting position to tie a shoe requires a "head-down, hips-up" posture, with an adjustment in head orientation that can cause loss of static balance and a fall. Figure 5.24 shows a simple exercise that helps to acclimate the exerciser to a head-down, hips-up inverted static balance sensation.

Inverted Dynamic Balance. Although of relevance to youth, this balance category has little value to the older adult (see Chapter 4). Sensations of moving upside down can be simulated by a surface dive in water, with the body directed to the bottom. In aquatic terms, this is a "porpoise dive." Exercises and activities that entail moving in the inverted position on land are too hazardous and should be avoided by the typical senior adult.

A wide variety of activities that involve holding and moving balance skills can be designed. For example, various standing and sitting chair exercises can be incorporated in exercise routines that require upright static and dynamic motions. Hoops, wands, Frisbees, and step benches can be used to add variety, fun, and challenge to balance activities.

Seniors who possess the desire and capability should be encouraged to participate in active sports and games such as bowling, shuffleboard, and diving, where balance requirements are part of the motor skill. One activity that appeals to most people is dance. Dancing, whether square, social, or ethnic, not only enhances agility and neuromuscular coordination, but also improves balance and kinesthetic acuity.

Appendix A contains a sample group of exercises and motor skills designed to improve balance and equilibrium.

Enhancing Body Composition and Build

As stated earlier, one of the major purposes of a senior adult fitness program is to enhance the physique and maintain reasonable control of adipose tissue. Essentially, improving muscular strength and flexibility and engaging in cardiorespiratory endurance activities influence body composition, subsequently altering the human physique when coordinated with proper nutrition.

One of the most variable tissue constituents of the body is adipose

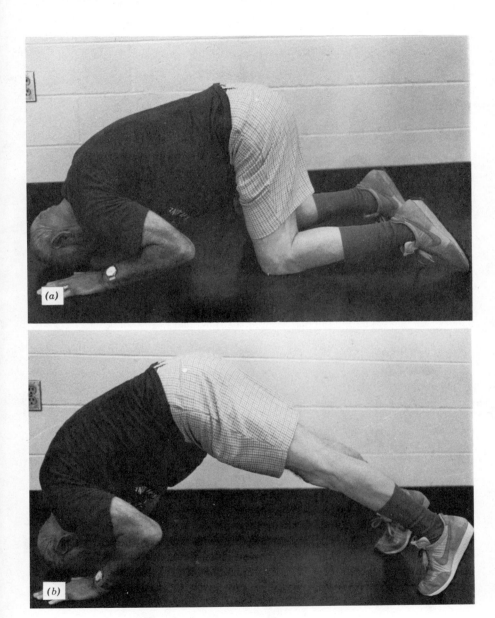

Figure 5.24 Improving inverted stationary balance skill.

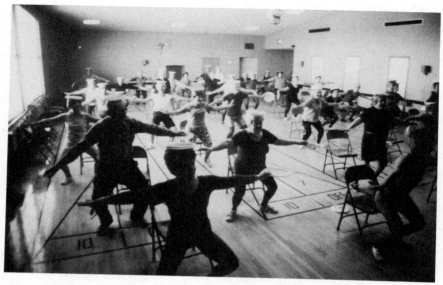

Figure 5.25 Seniors having fun balancing Frisbees on their heads.

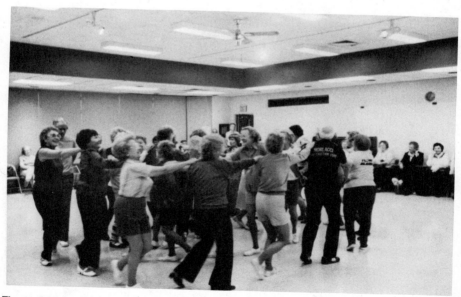

Figure 5.26 Improving upright dynamic balance through circle dancing.

tissue. Extreme obesity is reflected by an endomorphic appearance. By contrast, extreme leanness projects an emaciated and weak physique. Body fat normally tends to increase with age with some decline in later years. Muscle tissue tends to continue its decline throughout life. Extremes in leanness or adipose are inadvisable conditions, and a sensible approach to body composition strikes a balance between these two conditions.

Muscular Tone and Physique. Muscle tone is the quality of tension affecting muscles at rest. Actually, tone reflects the degree of muscle softness. Firmness of muscular tissue stems from two sources, neurogenic and myogenic. Neurogenic tone comes from a constant state of nerve impulse transmission to the muscle fibers which keeps the muscle in a partial state of contraction. Myogenic tone pertains to the degree of muscular firmness developed through exercise.

Each of these types of tone affects posture maintenance mechanisms. Adequate neurogenic tone depends upon a healthy nervous system and provides the basic blueprint for maintaining postural tonus, whereas myogenic tone serves to develop optimum levels of muscle hypertrophy as opposed to flaccidity and softness.

Participation in activities that abide by the basic overload and specificity of training principles enhance myogenic tone, and subsequently improve stability in maintaining upright posture by reducing excessive postural sway—a common condition among persons past 80.[31]

In the design of a program where improved posture is sought by the participant, calisthenic-type exercises that firm up the pectorals, abdominals, pelvic/hip region, shoulder blades, and extensor muscles of the upper back are recommended. Light weight loading, using any one of the exercise systems described in Chapter 4 is appropriate for developing high levels of myogenic tone. Appendix A contains a sample set of exercises designed to improve postural tone and physique.

Summary

Fitness programs should be designed within the boundaries of medical and dynamic fitness capabilities of the senior adult, emphasizing self-improvement, rather than attainment of fitness levels based upon population norms.

Four different target populations can be identified: (1) well-aging, (2) limited ambulatory and wheel chair, (3) frail elderly, and (4) bed patients. This chapter has presented guidelines for the design and conduct of programs for the noninstitutionalized well-aging.

Organized fitness programs are offered in assorted settings, from multipurpose senior centers to commercial health spas and fitness centers. Five important concepts apply to all programs pursuing excellence irrespective of organizational type: (1) program philosophy and goals, (2) personnel management, (3) budget and finance, (4) facilities and equipment, and (5) program evaluation and assessment.

Qualified professional staff are essential. The caliber of professional leadership, budgetary allowances, and availability of equipment and facilities also greatly affect the scope and quality of fitness programs.

The chapter next focused on the purposes, functions, and content of senior centers and similar organizations in considerable detail. Most centers conduct a wide variety of physical, social, recreational, and intellectual activities. Although senior centers provide excellent services in social and recreational areas, improvement is needed in the area of professional fitness leadership and programming.

The content of fitness programs of senior adults was then discussed, with appropriate guidelines and principles offered. Fitness elements of muscular strength and endurance, flexibility, cardiovascular-respiratory efficiency, balance and equilibrium, and body composition and build were described with illustrations of appropriate activities. The need for medical clearance and such diagnostic procedures as stress testing were emphasized.

Considerable detail was provided on the development of cardiorespiratory efficiency as a central fitness goal since this trait is related to cardiovascular disease, the leading killer of adults in our society. The following components of cardiorespiratory fitness were explained and applied to an exercise regimen; (1) type of activity, (2) intensity of exercise, (3) duration of workout, (4) frequency of participation, and (5) progression rate.

Flexibility, balance and equilibrium activities were then presented with specific suggestions for the enhancement of these fitness components. Finally, exercises focused upon improving body composition and build, stressing the development of myogenic tone, were explained, with ways and means of developing and maintaining postural efficiency indicated.

REFERENCES

1. U.S. Bureau of the Census, Department of Commerce, "Demographic Aspects of Aging and Older Populations in the United States," Current Population Reports: Special Studies, Series P. 22, no. 59 (May 1976), p. 1; and John Piscopo, "Indications and Contraindications of Exercise and Activity for Older Persons," *Journal of Physical Education and Recreation* 50, no. 9 (1979): 31–34.
2. *Catalogue of Programs and Services for the Aging* (Williamsville, N.Y.: Town of Amherst Multipurpose Senior Center, 1981–1982).
3. American College of Sports Medicine, *Guidelines for Graded Exercise Testing and Exercise Prescription,* 2d ed. (Philadelphia: Lea & Febiger, 1980), pp. 73–115.

4. Max Kaplan, *Leisure: Lifestyle and Lifespan* (Philadelphia: W. B. Saunders, 1979), pp. 102–105.
5. Committee on Aging of the American Alliance for Health, Physical Education, Recreation and Dance, "General Guidelines for Exercise Programs for Older Persons (age 50 and Older)," *The Easterner,* EDA-AAHPER, vol. 7, no. 1 (January 1982): 8.
6. Betty Van der Smissen, "Legal Aspects of Adult Fitness Programs," *Journal of Health, Physical Education and Recreation* 45, no. 2 (1974): 54–56.
7. C. W. Thompson, *A Manual for Structural Kinesiology,* 8th ed. (St. Louis: C. V. Mosby, 1981), pp. 59–62.
8. John E. Beaulieu, "Developing a Stretching Program," *The Physician and Sportsmedicine* 9, no. 11 (1980): 59–65.
9. Herbert A. de Vries, *Physiology of Exercise,* 3d ed. (Dubuque, Ia.: Wm. C. Brown, 1980), Chapter 21.
10. S. M. Walker, "Delay of Twitch Relaxation Induced by Stress and Stress Relaxation," *Journal of Applied Physiology* 16 (1961): 801–806.
11. Mercedes Lesser, "The Effects of Rhythmic Exercise on the Range of Motion in Old Adults," *Journal of American Corrective Therapy* 32, no. 1 (1978): 118–122.
12. Herman Kabat, "Proprioceptive Facilitation in Therapeutic Exercise," in S. Licht, ed., *Therapeutic Exercise,* 2d ed. (Baltimore: Waverly Press, 1965), pp. 327–343.
13. Charles B. Corbin and Larry Noble, "Flexibility," *Journal of Physical Education and Recreation* 51, no. 6 (1980): 23–24, 57–60.
14. G. S. Thomas et al., *Exercise and Health* (Cambridge, Mass: Gunn & Hais, Publishers, 1981) p. 78.
15. American College of Sports Medicine, *Guidelines,* pp. 36–37.
16. Ibid.
17. M. K. Karvonen, K. Kentala, and O. Muslala, "The Effects of Training Heart Rate," *Annals Medicinae Experimentalis et Biologiae Fenniae* 35, (1957): 307–315.
18. Herbert A. de Vries, "Exercise Intensity Threshold for Improvement of Cardiovascular-Respiratory Function in Older Men," *Geriatrics* 26 (April 1971) 94–101.
19. Ibid., p. 101.
20. Gene M. Adams and Herbert A. deVries, "Physiological Effects of a Training Regimen upon Women Aged 52 to 70," *Journal of Gerontology* 28, no. 1 (1973): 50–55.
21. Herbert A. deVries, "Physiology of Exercise and Aging," in D. S. Woodruff and J. E. Birren, eds., *Aging: Scientific and Social Issues* (New York: Van Nostrand, 1975), pp. 257–277.
22. E. L. Smith and C. Gilligan, "Physical Activity Prescription for the Older Adult," *The Physician and Sportsmedicine* 11, no. 8 (1983): 94.
23. M. L. Pollock, J. H. Wilmore, and S. M. Fox III, *Exercise in Health and Disease: Evaluation and for Prevention and Rehabilitation* (Philadelphia: W. B. Saunders, 1984), p. 258–259.
24. Ibid., p. 257.

25. Smith and Gilligan, "Physical Activity Prescription," p. 100.
26. M. L. Pollock, J. H. Wilmore, S. M. Fox III, *Health and Fitness through Physical Activity*. (New York: John Wiley & Sons, 1978), p. 125.
27. American College of Sports Medicine, "Position Statement on Recommended Quantity and Quality of Exercise for Developing and Maintaining Fitness in Healthy Adults," *Medicine and Science in Sports* 10, no. 3 (1978): vii-viii.
28. Ibid., p. vii.
29. Ibid.
30. Robert E. Wear, "Conditioning Exercise Programs for Normal Older Persons," in R. Harris and L. J. Frankel, eds., *Guide to Fitness after Fifty* (New York: Plenum Press, 1977), pp. 253–270.
31. Betty R. Hasselkus and Georgia M. Shambs, "Aging and Postural Sway in Women," *Journal of Gerontology* 30 (1975): 661–667.

6

Special Health and
Fitness Problems
Among Older Adults:
Program Implications

INTRODUCTION

Adaptation of activities to suit the capacity, ability, safety, and interests of the older adult is a key concept that should be applied to all programs serving those from the well-aging to the bed patient. Each population group requires some form of adjustment and accommodation in the rules of the game, sport, or activity, or modification in the environment surrounding the participant. Little change is necessary for the "super old" of the well-aging segment. As pointed out in Chapter 4, senior athletes participating in Master's tournaments continue to compete in sprint and distance races, tennis, bowling, archery, and discus events. The major adjustment required for this group is equalization of extreme age levels; that is, older persons should not be pitted against youth—a modification that respects the normal biological changes that occur with the aging process.

At the extreme end of the spectrum, elderly bed patients must be closely guided with regard to type and method of movement. For this group, physical activity of any sort is confined to one site, and exercises are performed in the prone, supine, or sitting position.

ADAPTATION GUIDELINES

Whether the instructor is working with the elite senior athlete or the bed patient, the following guidelines are recommended when adapting physical activities to senior adults:

1. Adjust the activity according to *medical status* of the senior determined by his or her physician.
2. Modify or alter the activity within the senior's motor *capacity* and *ability*.
3. Modify environmental surroundings *facilities* and *equipment* to ensure the *safety* of the participant.
4. Adapt activities according to *needs and interests* of the senior adult; foster and encourage skill development that is *personally satisfying* to the individual; explain the beneficial health effects of selected activities through participation.

Games and motor activities can be modified for one person or for the entire group. The changes or adjustments, of course, depend upon the condition of the participant. For example, the older diabetic with a lower-leg amputation can sit on the pool deck and participate in an enjoyable circle ball throw and catch game while other seniors are in waist-deep water.

Game and equipment elements also can be modified to accommodate sensory age changes. For example, dimming eyesight and the preponderance of bi/trifocal lenses make it difficult for seniors to see and track shuttlecocks in badminton. Decorating the birds with brightly colored ribbons, as shown in Figure 6.1, helps participants to see fast-moving objects and facilitates success in game play. This approach has been successfully used with senior citizens engaged in fitness programs, some of whom have not played the game for over 50 years.[1] The intensity of competition can be adjusted by shifting rules to allow for doubles and trio players on each side. This lessens the energy demands of the game and generates enthusiasm and motor skill achievement within the capacity of the players. Other badminton modifications with specific directions and adjustments are presented in Appendix .

Adaptations in the Conduct of Physical Activities

The conduct of physical activities and use of equipment should be flexible enough to allow individual adaptive changes within a group. The following accommodations are recommended for typical senior citizens participating in a group setting:

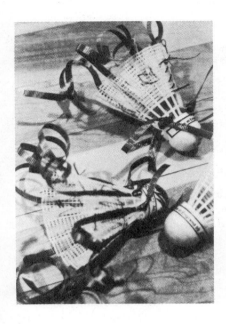

Figure 6.1 Using badminton shuttle-cocks decorated with bright colors allows better tracking of a fast-moving object. (Courtesy of Dorothy Chrisman, *Body Recall*, Inc., Box 412, Berea, Ky.)

1. *Slow the pace of movement;* that is, walk, fast-walk, or jog instead of running.
2. *Deemphasize speed of movement* as a major element in the game or activity.
3. *Allow enough time for repetition of movement* when introducing new motor skills.
4. *Use chairs* for alternating standing, sitting, and balanced movements.
5. *Allow frequent rest periods* between physical activity bouts.
6. *Stress participation,* rather than perfection of motor skills.
7. *Conduct rhythmic exercises with music in sitting position,* using small, lightweight equipment, such as wands and Frisbees.
8. *Use light weights with numerous repetitions* rather than heavy weights with fewer repetitions when exercising.
9. *Customize activities* that will ameliorate a specific health condition of the participant; for example, indicate swimming rather than weight-bearing land exercises in some arthritic cases.

Each person should be allowed to move at his or her own pace, and in a comfortable way. Fun in movement, at the individual's free tempo, without trying to keep up with other class members, should be emphasized.

ADAPTATIONS AND MOTOR SKILL CLASSIFICATIONS

Many sports and games in the vast array of motor activities reflect common characteristics according to their motion pattern. Such terms as *discrete and continuous skills* and *open and closed skills* represent categories used by motor learning specialists and kinesiologists to describe a given sport, game, or activity. This taxonomy method of identifying and describing appropriate motor activities for older adults with adaptations in the conduct of the game will be used in this text.

Discrete and Continuous Motor Skills

One way in which motor skills can be identified is through movement flow. Certain activities begin and end with a definite effort. For example, the senior adult tossing a ring at an upturned chair is performing a single action with three parts: initial, execution, and ending phases (see Figure 6.2).

Such activities as dart throwing, hitting a soft ball, diving, kicking, throwing, catching, calisthenic and gymnastic moves, free throw in basketball, and a net shot in badminton are examples of *discrete skills*—each task has a fixed beginning and end. Other motor skills do not abruptly end, but continue in a series over a long period of time and are repetitive in nature. Activities such as walking, skipping, jogging, running, bicycling, swimming, rowing, and skating are *continuous skills* (see Figure 6.3).

Discrete and continuous skill types affect retention of motor performance. Such activities as swimming and skating are retained indefinitely once the skill is learned well. Skill retention applies most directly to serial or continuous-type activities.

On the other hand, discrete skills are not remembered well unless practice is sustained throughout life. The identification of motor skills as discrete or continuous types have implications for the teaching of motor activities to older adults. For example, such skills as swimming, bicycling, and skating are easily recalled after long periods of practice abstinence, particularly in those sports that are self-paced and do not require acute qualities of speed and reaction time. It is not unusual to put on a pair of skates and move around the rink after 30 years of absolute nonparticipation in the sport. Since continuous skills are serial, repetitive, and habit-forming, they are most resistant to "forgetting." Such information about the participant's sports background can be useful in establishing initial prescriptive physical activities, and can help personalize fitness goals.

Closed and Open Skills

Another way of labeling motor activities is by environmental situations. Those skills in which the critical cues for successful performance are fixed or

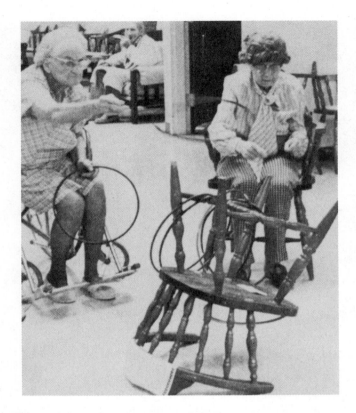

Figure 6.2 Ring toss—a discrete skill requires practice to maintain proficiency. (From S. Risso and C. R. Mayo, "Games and Kids Could Be the Key," *Journal of Physical Education, Recreation and Dance* 50, no. 7 (1979): 34–35. Used with permission.)

static in one position are called *closed skills*. For example, bowling and shuffleboard are closed motor skills because the requirements of the action depend upon the correct movements of the performer without concern of a changing environment. These activities are usually self-paced and performed in a stable setting when consistency of response is necessary for success. Accuracy is a component that is accented in closed skills—a motor trait that older persons tend to retain, which suggests at least one reason why bowling is a popular sport among senior citizens.

Closed skills, particularly those of low-intensity and repetitive skill movement characteristics, are appropriate for the nonathletic senior citizen. These motor skills are usually classified as individual sports, and skill improvement is readily enhanced with correct repetitive practice.

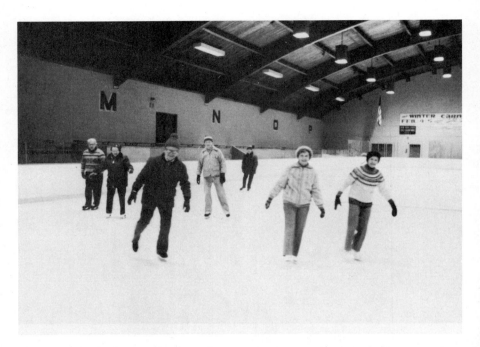

Figure 6.3 Skating—a continuous skill that is retained well into old age.

Skills performed in an environmental setting that is constantly changing are termed *open skills*. Two-person and team sports such as badminton, tennis, volleyball, and basketball are open skills. Open skills are conducted in an environment that is subject to unpredictable changes which require internal and external motor adjustments by the participant. Thus, proficiency in open skills requires considerable flexibility and versatility of movement response patterns. For example, whether an offensive smash or a strategic net shot is used in badminton may depend upon the opponent's court position at a particular moment in game play.

The principal difference between open and closed skills lies in response pattern. Open skills are very rarely duplicated in the same manner, whereas closed skills, because of their conduct in a calculable environment, can be repeated in the same way. Thus, consistency of response, applying correct mechanical principles, is the major concern of a closed skill participant. Flexibility, with varied and multiple motor responses, which are more complicated, is associated with open skills and requires greater athletic ability by the senior adult.

For some older people, participation in open skills may be contrain-

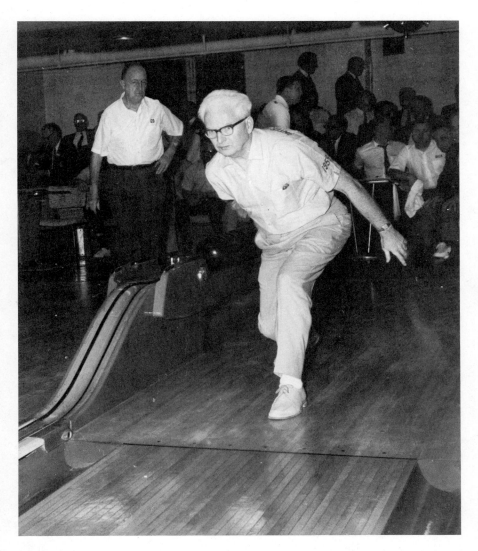

Figure 6.4 Bowling—a closed motor skill that stresses accuracy, and a popular choice of older adults. (Courtesy of Marvin Smith.)

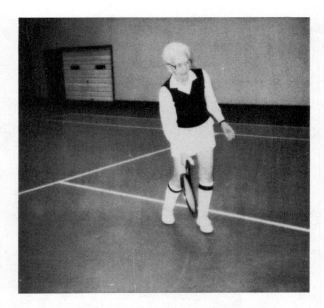

Figure 6.5 Tennis—an open motor skill, and a popular sport among older persons. (Courtesy of Bea Massman, undefeated city doubles champion for 15 years, Buffalo, N.Y.)

dicated, particularly when speed of movement, reaction time, and sudden changes are necessary parts of the game, as in handball, racquetball, tennis, and similar sports. On the other hand, the rule of individual differences prevails—older persons are a diverse group in health-fitness status, and those who have the capacity, ability, and desire for a given sport should be encouraged to participate and enjoy its benefits when supervised under competent leadership. Table 6.1 lists physical activities and indicates appropriate adaptations for the typical older adult.

The decision to select a discrete, continuous, closed, or open skill depends principally upon the participant's capacity (health and fitness level), ability (sport skill level), and interest (desire) in addition to the direct fitness goals sought. A wide variety of activities should be offered in an organized program to meet the needs of the participants, ranging from basic locomotion skills (walking, stepping, turning, bending) to free-time activities of gardening, sports, traveling, and handicrafts.

INSTITUTIONALLY BASED AND SPECIAL SETTING POPULATIONS

Older citizens who reside in institutional and special settings include: limited ambulatory and wheelchair adults, the frail elderly, and bedfast patients (see

Table 5.1 for population descriptions). These individuals reside in a variety of settings, such as extended-care facilities, intermediate-care facilities, and homes for the aged. Although many people in each category live independently at home or with relatives, the discussion here focuses primarily on settings where organized health-fitness programs are conducted under the supervision of an activity director or fitness specialist. Table 6.2 shows several important characteristics of residents in institutions and special settings.

Fitness Activities for Older Persons with Limited Capacities and Abilities

The health benefits of physical activity are not exclusive to the well-elderly; the frail and feeble, including bedfast patients, can improve their fitness and sense of well-being by participating in appropriate exercise directed by competent personnel. Most activities can be adapted and modified to provide mild low-stress-type physical stimulation that can improve the heart, circulatory, flexibility, and muscular functions of the older sedentary and deconditioned person.

The central effort of a fitness program for older adults with physical limitations is to increase their mobility so that they gain the means of "going places and doing things" to enrich the quality of their lives and become more self-sufficient and less dependent on others. The following section offers several activities and adaptations of sports and games designed to enhance fitness, mobility, and movement efficiency of the institutionally based and residents in special aggregate housing settings.

Limited Ambulatory and Wheelchair Elderly. This group of elderly, although ambulatory, needs the assistance of a cane or walker; or moves from one point to another in a wheelchair (see Table 5.1). Unless medically contraindicated, the goal is to instill the physical stamina and motor coordination through an appropriate and planned system of exercise and activities that will allow the chairbound individual to move from the wheelchair level to self-propulsion without assistance, or to let the cane and walker user discard the walking appliance. Thus, activities and related modalities that enhance the personal locomotion (walking, stepping, turning, bending, etc.) of the senior should be part of prescriptive programming. These include exercises that improve stretching, strength, and tone qualities of muscles; heart, blood flow, and lung action; and psychomotor control. These specific fitness parameters need attention and development in order for the limited ambulatory participant to realize locomotion freedom. As stated earlier, some activities may be medically contraindicated. for example, if the senior is afflicted with

Table 6.1 Physical Activities and Adaptations for Older Adults

Skill*	Type	Intensity Level	Fitness Components	Adaptations
Throwing	Discrete	Low	Hand-eye coordination	Use underhand throw instead of overhand; soft ball instead of hard ball; rolling ball along floor or table
Walking/Jogging	Continuous	Low to vigorous	Mobility, circulorespiratory	Slow walking to vigorous jog; progressive increase in pace and distance from ¼ to 3 miles; heart rate not to exceed 120 beats per minute
Swimming	Continuous	Low to high	Flexibility, circulorespiratory relaxation	Walking across pool; side stroke leg kicking; aquacizes; blowing bubbles; assisted prone and back floats
Horseshoes	Discrete	Low	Hand-eye coordination, balance	Use rubberized horseshoes; shorten target distance
Bowling	Discrete	Low	Hand-eye coordination balance, flexibility	Standing to sitting; shorten distance from foul line to pins; bright colors for pins; lightweight ball
Ice-skating	Continuous	Low to high	Balance, agility, circulorespiratory	Regulate tempo with music; skate with partners holding hands
Bicycling	Continuous	Moderate to high	Balance, agility, circulorespiratory	Use three-wheel bike; avoid up and down grade paths; increase pedal rate and distance gradually; tandem bike (21-inch wheel); large seats

Activity	Type	Intensity	Skills/Benefits	Modifications
Darts	Discrete	Low	Accuracy, hand-eye coordination	Shorten target distance; use bright colors for target areas
Bocci	Discrete	Low	Accuracy, flexibility, circulorespiratory, hand-eye coordination	None
Badminton	Discrete	Moderate to vigorous	Accuracy, flexibility, circulorespiratory, hand-eye coordination	Doubles and trio play; brightly colored shuttlecocks; use ribbons for shuttlecocks (see Appendix J)
Archery	Discrete	Moderate	Accuracy, shoulder girdle strength, hand-eye coordination	Use lightweight bow; shorten target distance
Bait/Fly Casting	Discrete	Low	Relaxation	None; chairs may be used, if standing over long periods
Golf	Discrete	Low to moderate	Coordination, relaxation, balance	Play nine holes; use electric golf carts; use miniature putting golf courses; play on level courses
Racquetball	Discrete	Vigorous	Circulorespiratory, coordination	Play doubles; shorten game score
Table Tennis	Discrete	Moderate	Coordination, balance, agility	Play doubles; lower table for wheelchair players
Tennis	Discrete	Moderate to vigorous	Coordination, agility, hand-eye coordination	Play doubles; reduce court size; use lightweight rackets

(*Continued*)

Table 6.1 Continued

Skill*	Type	Intensity Level	Fitness Components	Adaptations
Curling	Discrete	Moderate to vigorous, depending upon position	Accuracy, coordination, circulorespiratory, depending upon position	Use lighter brooms, stones; reduce rink distance
Horseback Riding	Continuous	Moderate to vigorous	Coordination, agility, balance	Depends upon skill level of participant; avoid racing at high speeds
Billiards	Discrete	Moderate	Accuracy, balance, hand-eye coordination	None
Softball	Discrete	Moderate	Coordination, agility, accuracy	Use plastic bats; shorten distance between bases and home plate; omit called balls and strikes; designated base runners for those unable to run
Fishing	Discrete	Low to moderate	Relaxation, agility, balance	Fishing from chairs; avoid walking in stream fishing
Paddle Ball	Discrete	Vigorous	Circulorespiratory	Play doubles; reduce winning score
Dance	Continuous	Moderate to vigorous	Balance, coordination, agility, circulorespiratory	Slow tempo with appropriate music; use social, folk, square, and ethnic dances; sitting and standing positions

Activity		Intensity	Components	Modifications
Hiking	Continuous	Moderate	Circulorespiratory, endurance, mobility	Start with short hikes; increase distance gradually; avoid unsafe and hazardous hiking trails; hike in groups with experienced leader
Croquet	Discrete	Low to moderate	Accuracy, hand-eye coordination, balance	Use brightly colored, larger wickets; reduce court size
Track Events	Continuous	Vigorous	Circulorespiratory, mobility, agility, balance	Shorten distance; widen running lanes
Volleyball	Discrete	Moderate	Coordination, agility, balance	Lower net height; allow ball to bounce on floor once before it is hit; allow server greater number of "tries" on service; use beach balls or plastic balls
Rollerskating	Continuous	Moderate to vigorous	Coordination, agility, balance, circulorespiratory	Use music to establish tempo; partner skating
Skiing	Continuous	Moderate to vigorous	Circulorespiratory, endurance, balance, agility, coordination	Modify (shorten) distance, slope, and type of terrain
Snowshoeing	Continuous	Moderate to vigorous	Circulorespiratory, endurance, balance, agility, coordination	Modify distance and terrain; use poles for balance

*Skill may be open or closed depending upon whether the participant is playing in a fixed environment or involved in competitive play with one or more players.

Table 6.2 Institutionally Based and Special Settings

Type	Population	Sponsorship	General Functions
Extended-Care Facility (SNF-Nursing Home)	Average age, 82; predominantly female; usually admitted for one of following causes: mental problems, incontinence, lack of mobility; length of stay—usually two years; chronic diseases, such as cardiovascular, arthritic, and orthopedic disorders prevalent; include limited ambulatory and wheelchair, frail, and bedfast patients; includes about 5 percent of elderly over 65; usually widows, white, and alone; mental illness is the most common disability; less than half can walk	Private; city, state, or federally sponsored; about 65 percent operate for profit	Skilled nursing facility, staffed by registered nurses, physicians, and other health specialists, such as: speech pathologist, occupational therapist, physical therapist, and activity director, prepared to perform specialized functions such as tube feeding, alleviation of incontinence, and other procedures under the orders of the attending physician; caters to persons who need round-the-clock nursing care and services
Intermediate-Care Facility (ICF)	Over age 65; accommodates limited ambulatory and frail elderly and bedfast patients who are convalescing; sometimes called a Health-Related Facility	Private; city or state sponsorship	Provides technical services under direction of licensed practical nurse; M.D. on call for conference and consultation; administers injections, medications injections, medications for individuals in a stabilized medical condition
Day-Care Facility (DCF)	Ambulatory and not incontinent elderly; group can administer their own	City, county, or state with funding from a variety of sources including public	Provides a variety of health-related services for maintenance of health-fitness,

232

	Population	Sponsorship	Services/Function
	elderly; individuals usually have some type of ailment or physical disability that needs attention during the day, but can live at home; this group is usually restricted in participating in normal everyday activities for a variety of reasons and need the support and services of day-care personnel		grams, social and activity events, transportation to and from home; emphasizes health restoration and rehabilitation; staffed by health team of physicians, physical therapists, occupational therapists, social workers, nursing personnel, and activity coordinators; attempts to keep people at home, and out of nursing home
Homes for the Aged (licensed and nonlicensed)	Usually ambulatory, over 65; may enter by preference or necessity; group may range from well-elderly to frail; person may seek group living situation; residents may keep outside contacts in community; some facilities may house small numbers up to 10 with other settings having as many as several hundred: usually such residents have few family ties and less likely to have a spouse	Private, church affiliated, fraternal organizations, founded by a variety of sources: city, state, federal, and charitable organizations; licensed dwellings must conform to care requirements of state and federal funding agencies	Provides intermediate care with supervision and help with everyday tasks of dressing, eating, medications; some provide continuing care as older person moves from self-sufficiency to possible total dependency; provides social and recreational services, physical activities, spiritual and religious programs; arranges transportation to doctor's office, shopping occasions; therapeutic recreation programs are usually provided; atmosphere of residential setting, rather than institution caring for the ill, prevails

swollen, inflamed and painful joints, movement of any kind may aggravate the condition and worsen its state.

The instructor should prescribe within the medical capabilities of the exerciser—this requires close articulation and communication with the senior's physician. Such conditions as circulatory disease, fractures due to osteoporosis, neurological impairments, vision and hearing losses, arthritic diseases, and general muscle flaccidity are common among adults past 65, and more prevalent among the limited ambulatory and wheelchair group.

Music and Rhythm Applications. Generally, musical accompaniment should be used in most exercise sessions. Music serves to reduce boredom, helps to maintain tempo, and actually can alter the mood of the exerciser, ranging from an exciting "Saturday Night Fever" state of a disco beat to a relaxing waltz time. Music, when correctly used, tends to integrate the emotional and mental aspects of the senior adult, reinforcing the holistic mind/body concept approach to presenting activities.

Music provides a stimulus for movement, and in some cases can help to reduce the trauma of pain that sometimes parallels exercise. For example, Palmer reports the positive effects of music in maintaining finger flexibility and prevention of severe contraction among wheelchair patients who usually sit with arms folded and clenched fists, even though it is frequently painful to stretch out the arthritic fingers.[2] Hearing a lively tune such as a German drinking song encourages the residents to clap along. For residents with more ambulatory power and greater movement functions, marching and dancing can be used to enhance locomotion skills and positive social behavior.

Although music has general application in bringing about positive changes in mood, motivation, and mental states of the older person, in some cases, this modality may be undesirable. A small portion of the adult population suffer from a condition called "musicogenic epilepsy" in which music of certain frequency triggers a particular brain wave pattern that causes epileptic seizures.[3] Seniors manifesting this condition should be excluded from music sessions.

In other cases, persons cannot distinguish between high and low tones and may not enjoy a melody. These individuals are tone-deaf. The instructor should be alert to individuals (although small in number) who for medical or emotional reasons do not respond to any kind of music. Such persons should not be pressured to participate in music sessions. The purpose of musical accompaniment is to stimulate and motivate the senior adult for greater physical movement.

The premise that elderly people prefer sedative tunes to stimulating music, and old music over current popular selections, is a common miscon-

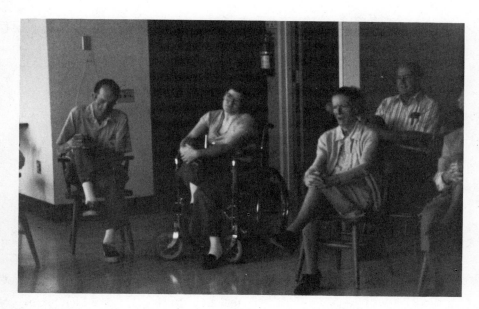

Figure 6.6 Using music and adapting activities to the capabilities of limited ambulatory persons. (Courtesy of the Episcopal Church Home, Buffalo, N.Y.)

ception. A revealing study by Gibbons about musical preferences involved 60 elderly persons, from various residential settings, between the ages of 65 to 95 years.[4] Musical selections representative of popular music in each 10-year period from 1900 through 1976 were played with a mix of stimulative and sedative music from each period decided by a panel of music experts. Table 6.3 shows selected music types with song titles used in the study.

The results of this study indicated that elderly persons strongly preferred popular music of their young adult years (20 to 30) to popular music of later life periods, and they elected stimulation to sedative music that was popular in all life periods. Thus it may be erroneous to assume that any old popular tune can be successfully used to elicit successful activity and behavioral responses. Musical accompaniment should be carefully selected to represent compositions of the participant's young adult years and to contain stimulating rhythm as well as serene and tranquil tempos.

The following guidelines are recommended for creating a positive experience for music activity participants:

1. Avoid extremely loud, rock-type music.
2. Use a variety of music from 1900s, 1920s, 1930s, and 1940s to stimulate past and familiar experiences.

Table 6.3 Song Types and Sequence by Life Periods

	Song Titles		
Type	65–75 Years	76–85 Years	86–95 Years
1. Sed.	Sentimental Journey	I'm Sorry[a]	Moonlight Bay
2. Stim.	You're 16, You're Beautiful and You're Mine[a]	If You Knew Susie	Over There
3. Sed.	Roses Are Red[a]	Moonlight and Roses	I'm Sorry[a]
4. Stim.	Deep in the Heart of Texas	The Lion Sleeps Tonight[a]	My Little Margie
5. Sed.	I Only Have Eyes for You	Roses Are Red[a]	Roses Are Red[a]
6. Stim.	Raindrops Keep Falling on My Head[a]	Baby Face	Sixteen Tons[a]
7. Sed.	Mandy[a]	Always	Always
8. Stim.	Marzidoats	Raindrops Keep Falling on My Head[a]	The Lion Sleeps Tonight[a]
9. Sed.	Over the Rainbow	The Way We Were[a]	Mandy[a]
10. Stim.	The Lion Sleeps Tonight[a]	I've Got Rhythm	Darktown Strutters Ball
11. Sed.	I'm Sorry[a]	Girl of My Dreams	Let Me Call You Sweetheart
12. Stim.	I've Got Rhythm	You're 16, You're Beautiful, and You're Mine[a]	You're 16, You're Beautiful, and You're Mine[a]
13. Sed.	I'm in the Mood for Love	Mandy[a]	The Way We Were[a]
14. Stim.	Sixteen Tons[a]	My Little Margie	Raindrops Keep Falling on My Head[a]
15. Sed.	The Way We Were[a]	I'm in the Mood for Love	I'm Always Chasing Rainbows
16. Stim.	You Are My Sunshine	Sixteen Tons[a]	Alexander's Ragtime Band

[a] Songs that were popular after 1950.

Source: A. C. Gibbons, "Popular Music Preferences of Elderly People," *Journal of Music Therapy* 14, no. 4 (1977) 184. Used with permission.

3. Carefully select music that evokes the desired tempo and rhythmic beat.
4. Encourage creative body movement of the participant—allow freedom of expression.
5. Use a varied collection of music, including melodic contemporary selections.
6. Use music that will arouse such movements as hand tapping, clapping for opening sessions of activity. End class with relaxing and melodic mood music for easy stretching.
7. Use familiar songs to promote discussion and shared experiences that stimulate group social interactions.
8. Use a good balance of slow, moderate, and relaxing music to parallel exercise and movement intensity.
9. Consider the participant's past experiences, ethnicity, religious preferences, and background in the selection of musical contents to enhance personal identity.
10. Avoid music in certain pathological cases of brain damage or emotional disturbance, or with individuals who are oversensitive to noise.

Older adults with limited ambulatory capacities usually occupy intermediate health care and day-care facilities. Many others are homebound and live at home with family or relatives. These individuals are semi-incapacitated with assorted mobility dysfunctions and other chronic disorders, but do not have serious psychological problems. Modifying and adapting games and sport activities according to the individual's medical and dynamic status is central in designing a program for this group.

Many activities indicated in Table 6.1 can be used depending upon the specific condition of the participant. For example, wheelchair relays, toss games with bean bags, soft balls, horseshoes, and group exercises help the senior adult to maintain necessary levels of fitness for self-transportation tasks essential for satisfying everyday living needs. Activities that mildly stretch muscles and improve joint flexibility and muscle strength should be emphasized. Supervised swimming activities are highly recommended.

Frail Elderly and Bed Patients. Frail elderly and bed patients, within the context of this discussion, are those individuals with significant deficiencies in ambulatory ability but without serious constrictions of incontinence and psychological problems (see Table 5.1). The members of this group may or may not be in an institutional setting, but they do require daily routine care and attention. It is recognized that multiple approaches and needs, such as speech training, occupational training, and social worker liaisons may be involved in the daily care of the frail elderly. The discussion here focuses upon practices and management dealing primarily with physical modalities and procedures that can sustain and improve the physical fitness components, such as strength, flexibility, and motor coordination necessary for everyday tasks.

The primary goal is to sustain and improve the individual's functional movement ability. Before activity prescription is implemented, each frail and bedfast adult must be evaluated by a physician to determine his or her medical and dynamic fitness status. Exercise and activity procedures must be guided by the organic condition of the participant. For example, if Mrs. Smith has had a stroke resulting in impaired motor ability on one side of the body (hemiplegia), physical exercise designed to prevent secondary disabilities will usually be instituted early. Exercises that mobilize joints either passively or actively to prevent muscle contracture and joint deformity, pressure sores, and muscle atrophy should be started as early as medically allowed.

Exercise classifications for frail and bed patients, according to type and intensity are as follows:

1. Passive Motion
2. Assistive-Active
3. Active
4. Active-Resistive

Passive motion is of the massage type, whereby joint movements of the patient are made without any assistance on his or her part. The therapist or fitness specialist kneads, strokes, and manipulates muscles and soft tissues for the purpose of preventing contracture of joints, muscles, and connective structures. Such procedures are essential in averting further tissue deterioration and secondary complications resulting in greater flaccidity and incapacitation. Operators should remember that massage is not a substitute for exercise in regaining muscle function, but principally serves as a means of sustaining blood circulation, lessening pain and stiffness, and retarding the development of pressure sores.

Assistive-active exercise is appropriate for those individuals who possess some voluntary movement ability, but need assistance in moving a joint through its range because of weakness and debilitation. Muscles usually possess nerve system innervation, but lack the power of lifting or moving a limb or body part. Great care is needed on the part of the exercise instructor to understand the anatomy and kinesiology of body joints when assisting the participant through various flexion, extension, lateral, and rotation movements. For example, elbow and knee joints do not possess significant lateral or rotation motions, so forced sideward and rotary movements can injure these hinge-type joints. Assistance may also be provided by a counterweight or the buoyant medium of water in watercizes. Aquatic activities offer the individual with muscle weakness help by buoying body parts.

Active-exercise requires muscle strength and motor coordination to move a limb or total body through joint ranges against gravity. Games, daily living skills, and assorted movements done without external assistance are examples of this category.

Active-resistive exercise entails resistance to movement, in addition to the normal weight or motion of a limb or body part. For example, flexing the elbow joint with a five-pound weight in hand is a typical active-resistive exercise. These several exercise classifications clearly indicate progression modes extending from nonmovement of massage to procedures requiring considerable strength typified by resistive-active protocols.

Certain frail and bedfast patients may not be able to partake beyond the massage state, whereas others can often exercise with weights and machines that provide graded resistance. The exercise type and intensity used depend upon the diagnosis and prognosis set forth by the older adult's physician. Appendix A contains a set of exercises designed to meet the needs of the frail elderly capable of some movement.

COMMON HEALTH PROBLEMS: FITNESS AND PROGRAM IMPLICATIONS

Earlier, it was stressed that normal aging and maturation are not synonymous with disease and pathology. Certain hearing (presbycusis) and vision deficits (presbyopia) are quite normal and age-related, and should not be confused with disease states. The acuity of these sensory receptors declines, which mean that activity modalities and environment must be adapted to accommodate changes. Other conditions such as arthritis and osteoporosis have unknown causes. Nevertheless, such problems are universal among the elderly and pose significant mobility predicaments involving the musculoskeletal system. Such health problems as obesity, diabetes, cardiovascular and neurological syndromes, respiratory diseases, and various orthopedic disorders also affect the quality and quantity of mobility and locomotion of many senior adults.

Certain conditions may emerge from pathogenic causes, others result from normal biological changes that accompany the aging process. Yet most conditions can at least be ameliorated through appropriate movement and activity protocols. The following section presents an overview of health problems commonly found among the elderly with a focus on maintaining desirable fitness and functional locomotion levels with due consideration to the limiting constraints imposed upon the senior adult.

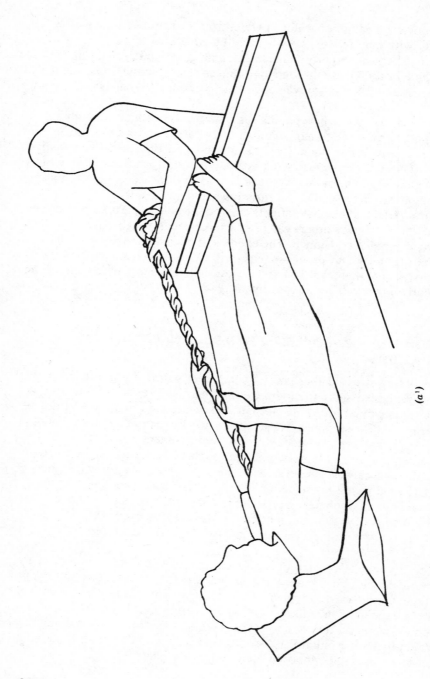

Figure 6.7 Exercises for the bedfast: (a1) assistive-active; (a2) assistive-active; (b) active-type exercise.

(a^1)

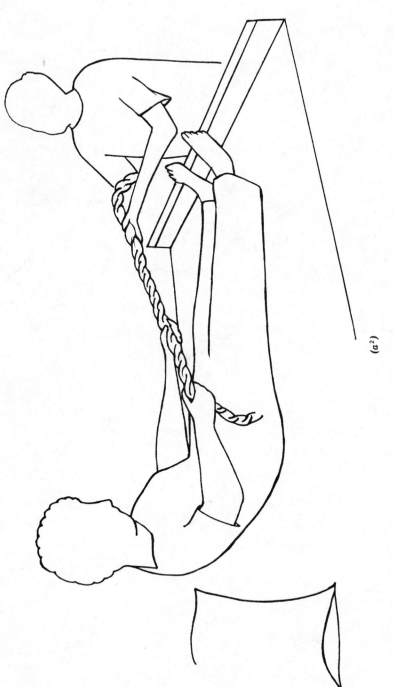

(a^2)

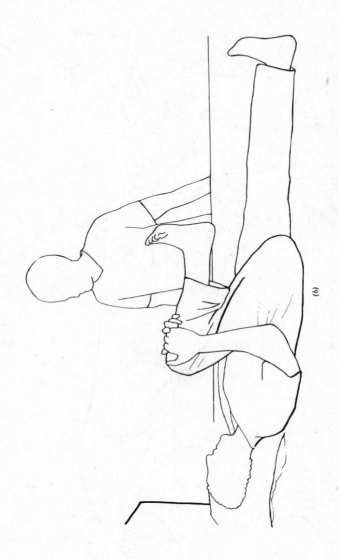

(b)

Arthritis

Arthritic diseases are manifold. Over 100 different arthritic conditions affect bones, joints, and connective tissue and impede the body's ability to move. these musculoskeletal diseases include gout, scleroderma, ankylosing spondylitis, bursitis, synovitis, rheumatoid arthritis, and osteoarthritis. Rheumatoid arthritis and osteoarthritis are two types common among older adults.

Rheumatoid Arthritis (RA). This type of arthritis is usually highly inflammatory to the joint and surrounding tissues resulting in marked pain, swelling, deformity, and movement impairment, depending upon the degree of severity. Since this kind of arthritis is systemic, it may invade more than one joint. Other characteristics of the disease include coldness and tingling of hands and feet and painful bouts of stiffness in the morning.

RA attacks more females than males, in a ratio of about three to one. It can strike at any age, but it seems to have a predilection for middle-aged and older persons. Table 6.4 shows the prevalence of RA in adults from 18 to 79 years of age. A steady rate increase in both sexes occurs from young adulthood to old age with a clear frequency of this disease among women over men, particularly in the 65 to 74 age group. RA rises dramatically with age among women.

The specific causes of RA are unknown. It somehow disrupts the body's antibody immune system, causing continuing inflammation in synovial membrane, which plays a major role in joint damage. The joints of the hands are

Table 6.4   Prevalence of Rheumatoid Arthritis in Adults by Sex and Age, United States, 1960–62*

	Both Sexes	*Men*	*Women*
	Rate Per 100 Adults		
Total, 18–79 years	3.2	1.7	4.6
18–24 years	0.3	0.2	0.3
25–34 years	0.3	—	0.6
35–44 years	1.3	0.5	2.1
45–54 years	3.0	1.5	4.4
55–64 years	6.3	4.2	8.3
65–74 years	9.2	3.1	14.1
75–79 years	18.8	14.1	23.5

*Although data are based upon 1960–62 figures, unpublished data from the National Center for Health Statistics indicate a similar pattern in 1981 of increased incidence from ages 17 to 65 + in the United States.

Source: National Center for Health Statistics, "Rheumatoid Arthritis in Adults, U.S., 1960–62," *Vital and Health Statistics,* series II, no. 7. Washington.

first affected, then the wrist, knee, shoulder, and hip. The cervical spine may also be involved in the early onset of the disease.[5]

The devastating results of the disease, particularly among widowed women, can be critical. For the elderly person with disabled hands, cooking and performing other everyday living tasks may become increasingly difficult. Thus it is not uncommon to find the rheumatoid person extremely thin with muscle atrophy and varying degress of osteoporosis. In its extreme manifestation of immobility, solitude, loneliness, and loss of human dignity can stalk the victim of this crippling disease.

Management Concepts. The severity and level of the RA directs its course of management. When pain is present with inflammation, rest and medication with steroids or aspirin are usually the principal modes of providing relief. This insidious disease tends to worsen with immobilization; therefore, appropriate exercise—passive, assistive-active, or active—is important for the prevention of joint contraction, muscle atrophy, and progressive bone loss.

Individuals with mild forms of RA may practice active and resistive forms of exercise, but those with severe conditions should not proceed beyond assistive exercise forms without pain. Therefore, exercise modes must be based upon capacity of joint range of motion and manual muscle evaluation before a program of movement is initiated. Noteworthy objectives of the fitness specialist should be to: (1) sustain and restore joint range, mobility, and locomotion; (2) prevent deformity of joints and limbs; (3) improve physical functioning and performance; and (4) relieve pain. These objectives can be accomplished by applying the correct mode of activity, tailored to the capacity and ability of the participant, ranging from passive to active-resistive exercise forms.

Finger and wrist extension applying light resistance, as shown in Figure 6.9, is especially effective for individuals who have difficulty with finger and hand maneuvers. Movements may start with 10 repetitions and gradually extend to 30 in a progressive stretching and resistive manner. Such movements can increase finger and wrist joint ranges, as well as help to maintain muscular strength of the forearm. Figure 6.10 shows an active-type exercise designed to improve joint range of motion of the hip through flexion movements of the thigh on the trunk. Exercises for the cervical spine (the first seven vertebrae), moving slowly left and right, forward and backward, and sideward, left and right, are shown in Figure 6.11.

Appendix A contains sample exercises specifically directed toward increasing joint range of motion of body parts and limbs affected by RA. Rheumatoid arthritis manifests itself in various stages from mild disturbances of function to severe body deformity. In some acute cases, complete bed rest to reduce inflammation may be prescribed. Relief of pain should be

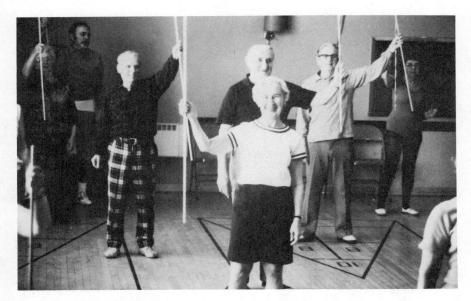

Figure 6.8 Active form of exercise for arthritis using a wand.

the foremost objective when this is the case. Physical suffering is usually alleviated by heat application of various types including hot packs, short wave diathermy, infrared lamps and paraffin wax. Each of these modalities provides palliative relief—not cure. The prudent fitness specialist or therapist should strive to break the vicious cycle of muscle atrophy and disuse, incapacitation, and enfeebling physical performance through individualized exercise prescription.

Osteoarthritis. This condition is commonly known as "wear and tear" arthritis because of its slow, noninflammatory degenerative effect upon joint cartilage, accompanied by bone and cartilage thickening or overgrowth. The disease primarily affects people over 40. The symptoms usually include increasing pain and stiffness.

Osteoarthritis is the most common form of arthritis, and it is estimated that 40.5 million Americans are touched to some degree by the disease.[6] Males and females are equally affected; however, more males have osteoarthritis in the younger group than in the 45-year-old age group, and more females are affected in the over-55 group.[7]

The cause of osteoarthritis is unknown, although factors associated with its incidence include obesity, genetics, and mechanical trauma to body joints. Obesity places undue stress on the weight-bearing joints, yet some

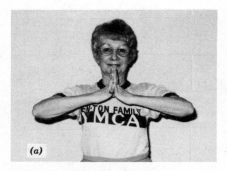

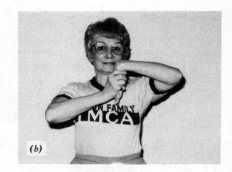

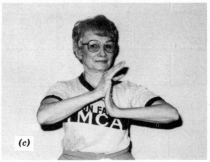

Figure 6.9 Active-resistive exercise for the fingers and hand.

studies do not find any particular prevalence of osteoarthritis among obese individuals.[8] Even though population studies show increased arthritis among obese individuals, the specific role of obesity in osteoarthritis remains uncertain. The mechanical trauma to joints found among athletes in football, baseball, and similar activities has led to the notion that overloading breaks down the integrity of the joint cartilage and triggers the biochemical processes that lead to structural changes that cause osteoarthritis. Genetics may also play a role; however, this is an irreversible factor about which little, if anything, can be done, at least for the present.

Until definite answers are found about a specific cause of osteoarthritis, the following rules will help to minimize the distress of the disease: (1) maintain moderate weight levels (avoid lean or obese states), (2) avoid undue trauma to joints, (3) eat well-balanced nutritious meals, and (4) exercise regularly.

Management Concepts. The management of osteoarthritis involves a multi-modality approach depending upon the severity of the disease and individual needs. The primary goals of therapeutic care in the control of osteoarthritis

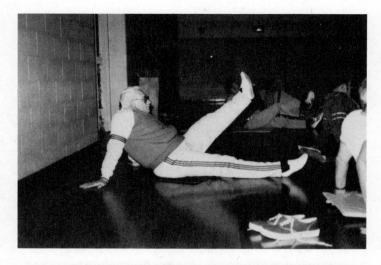

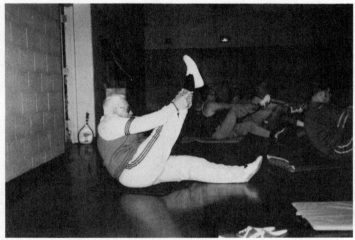

Figure 6.10 Increasing hip joint range of motion—flexion of the thigh.

are: (1) relief of pain, (2) maintenance and improvement of joint range of motion, and (3) delaying of further damage to joints.

When pain is present, relief may be gained by such drugs as aspirin, Butazolidin, and Motrin (nonsteroidal anti-inflammatory drugs). In some cases, cortisone (steroid) is used; the administration of this steroid must be under close supervision of the physician because of its probable side effects.

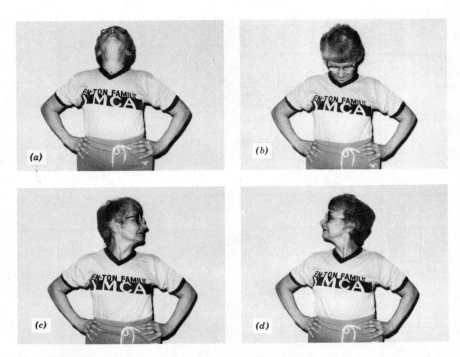

Figure 6.11 Active exercises for the cervical spine: (a) extension; (b) flexion; (c) rotation—left; (d) rotation—right.

Nonmedicinal forms of treatment entail rest, heat application, and exercise. Surgical procedures may be indicated for advanced cases; however, this discussion focuses upon noninvasive forms of treatment that fall within the domain of the fitness specialist and therapist.

Application of heat, such as hot packs, hot baths, and heat lamps, helps to soothe muscles—to relax and lessen spasm. Whirlpool baths also help to loosen stiff joints and decrease pain. Exercise prescription may follow heat treatments after pain is relieved. Care must be taken to preserve the supportive cartilage, ligaments, tendons, and muscles surrounding the afflicted joint. Because osteoarthritis is a local disorder, not a systemic condition, the disease affects one joint and is not necessarily transferred to another articulation.

The joints most commonly involved in osteoarthritis are the distal (last) joints of the fingers. Small bony growths called *osteophytes* develop, resulting in finger enlargement (Heberden's nodes) shown in Figure 6.12.

Other common sites of osteoarthritis are the joints of the hips, knees,

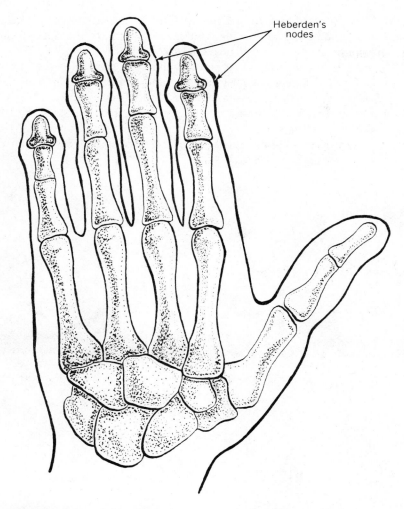

Figure 6.12 Osteoarthritis of the hand.

and spine. An understanding of joint motion is essential before prescriptive exercise can be applied. For example, finger and knee joints are essentially hinge-type structures with principal movements of flexion and extension; thus, directing motion in a rotary fashion, which is not a major movement of this articulation, may further damage the tissues. On the other hand, the hip is a ball-and-socket joint, and is capable of moving in all planes, which means that exercises involving flexion, extension, abduction, adduction, and rotation may be used for this particular joint.[9] Several exercises directed toward maintaining and improving troublesome joints of the hands, knees, hips, and spine are shown in Figure 6.13.

The course of exercises must be individually designed for each person, keeping in mind physical capacity, ability, and degree of osteoarthritic severity. Some individuals in the acute stage of the disease may need bed rest without movement, while others may begin at the passive stage with heat modalities. The ultimate goal is to pursue a path whereby the individual moves in a progressive fashion from passive to active-restive activities

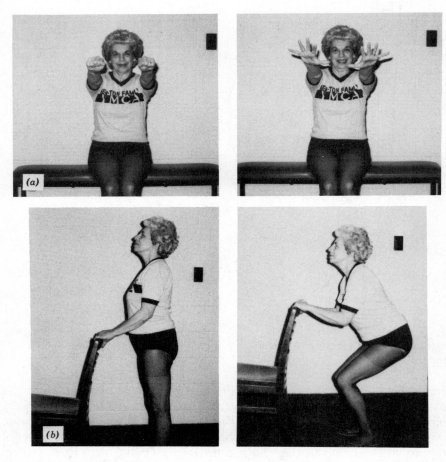

Figure 6.13 (a) Finger stretching; (b) Knee bend (half); (c1) Hip flexion; (c2) Hip extension; (c3) Hip abduction; (d) "Cat stretch" for the spine; (e) Low back stretch.

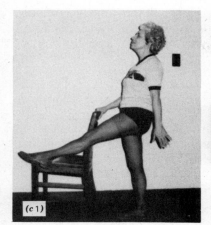

(c1)

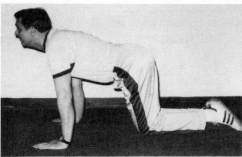

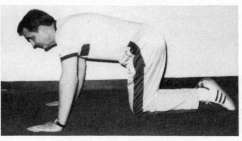

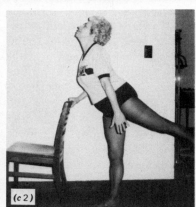

(c2)

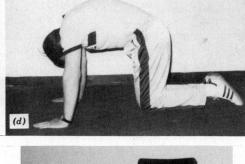

(d)

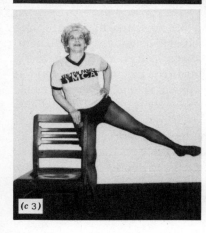

(c3)

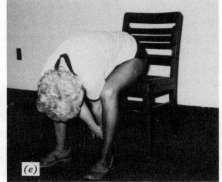

(e)

within structural and functional limits. At the present time, medical science has not found a cure for this form of arthritis. However, a proper balance of rest and prescriptive exercise can restore and maintain adequate levels of functional mobility.

Osteoporosis

As pointed out in Chapter 3, falls are a leading cause of death of persons over 65. Elderly women are particularly vulnerable to tripping and stumbling, which result not only from loss of balance and muscular strength, but also from a decrease in bone mass.

Fractures resulting from falls rise dramatically among older women. In the United States, women over 45 incur one million fractures yearly; and hip injuries in elderly females quadruple in every decade past 50.[10] Vertebral, wrist, and femoral neck fractures occur with increasing frequency in post-menopausal women. The question thus arises, How are these fractures related to osteoporosis? The common bond between these conditions is found in shrinkage of bone which results in decreased structural strength to withstand the compression, tensile, and trauma stresses placed upon various parts of the skeleton. The sources of these stresses range from simple sneezing, which can crack osteoporotic ribs, to stepping off a street curb, which can result in a break of the femur neck. Although we do not know the specific cause of osteoporosis, such factors as genetics, hormones, nutrition, and physical inactivity contribute to bone decrements. It is generally recognized that the management of osteoporosis entails supplemental dosages of calcium and Vitamin D, and, in some cases (prescribed by a physician), estrogen or fluoride treatment. However, regular physical activity and muscular exertion significantly retard the rate of bone loss and resorption.

Management through Physical Activity. Bonelike muscular tissue atrophies when subjected to continuous disuse or placed in a weightless environment. This phenomenon has been demonstrated by measuring bone loss of elderly patients in nursing homes and of the astronauts in the Gemini IV, V, and VII space flights.[11] For example, Smith et al. studied 51 nursing home female patients over a 36-month period.[12] These researchers found that patients who participated in light to mild exercises designed around sitting in a chair (i.e., sideward leg spread, leg walk, running in place, arm cross, and sideward bend), for a 30-minute session three times per week, actually showed an increase of 4.2 percent in bone mass, whereas, the nonexercise (control) group lost 2.5 percent. Aloia measured bone mass in 17 postmenopausal women, half of whom exercised for one year, and found significant bone mass gains among the exercising group.[13]

Thus evidence supports the hypothesis that physical exercise slows involutional bone loss. It is also clear that the positive effect of exercise upon bone strength is similar among young and old. Such a position confirms Wolff's classic law (established in 1892) which postulates that bone adapts and architecturally changes its structure when subjected to mechanical forces and stress.[14] The cellular changes that occur when strain and stress are applied to bone are unclear; however, one theory advocates that mechanical stress stimulates bone cell growth by piezoelectricity (electricity produced by mechanical pressure).

Muscular contraction, with or without resistance, and the pull of gravity provide the principal forces that stimulate bone growth. Although we know that physical activity vitalizes bone accretion, we do not know the exact type and degree of prescriptive exercise regimen that can maximize its benefits. For example, will swimming offer more protection from bone loss than walking or jogging? Will light-weight resistance exercises produce greater bone benefits than calisthenics without weights? Will three-pound resistive loads stimulate greater adaptive changes than one pound stresses? Although exact quantitative data with reference to type and degree of exercise intensity are lacking, it seems reasonable to suggest regimens that apply the basic principle of Wolff's law within the physical capacity and ability of the older person.

Figure 6.14 shows several recommended exercises for the vertebral column, forearm, wrist, and hip joints, the common fracture sites among older persons. Literally dozens of exercises can be used to stimulate bone accretion. The exercises shown in Figure 6.14 illustrate movements that specifically focus upon vulnerable bones.

Other forms of activity can be used whereby the pull of the muscle tendons creating mechanical stress on the origins and insertions of bone stimulate osteoblastic (cell) development. Walking and bicycling are well suited for strengthening bones of the hip, thigh, and lower legs. Arm exercises, using light weights ranging from three-quarters of a pound to five pounds, provide bone cell stimulation of the shoulders, upper chest, and upper back regions. For the adults with arthritic ailments, swimming offers a beneficial activity without placing undue stress on body joints. Adaptation of activities to fit the capacity of the participant is central for success when designing a fitness regimen for the osteoporotic person.

Sensory Deficits and Activity Principles

In some cases, besides general adaptations of the activity, equipment, and environment, special adaptations must be considered when the older adult is limited by impaired vision and hearing.

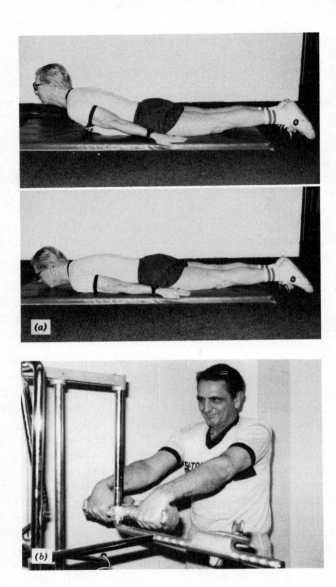

Figure 6.14 (a) Extending the thoracic spine; (b) wrist flexion; (c) wrist extension; (d) hip extension.

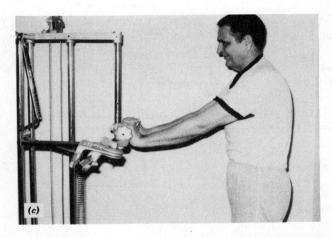

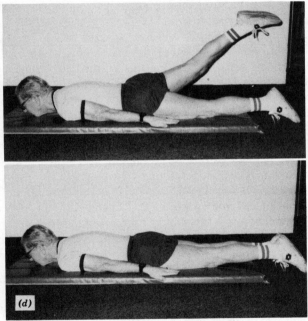

The degree of adaptation depends upon the severity of loss. Through our eyes and ears, we relate to the environment. Therefore, when, for example, a person is unable to see faces and places, or hear voices and music, missing out on the dozens of mundane activities that keep the individual in touch with the world, psychological disturbances of varying degree are inescapable—unless opportunities are provided to allow accommodations for the visually and hearing impaired to fulfill their physical, social, and emotional needs. The next section deals with several program designs for adults with limited sensory functions.

Vision Impairment. If we compare vision loss with hearing impairment, perhaps most of us would prefer deafness over blindness in an absolute sense. Vision is often considered the most important of the two senses. Yet, persons with hearing deficits tend to withdraw from the social milieu more quickly, thus initiating the vicious cycle of noncommunication, isolation, and depression. We do live in a visual world, which means that much of what we feel and learn comes from visual images, especially in the case of older adults. Peppers studied the leisure patterns of 206 retirees in several mid-Western communities and found that watching TV and reading were the most popular leisure activities among this group.[15] It should be noted that each of these pastimes require little physical effort, and is usually performed by one person. Sedentary-isolate experiences represent the antithesis of the activity-social way of life, and when pursued exclusively without a balance of physical activities hasten atrophy of the human machine.

What are some of the changes that make vision less effective? Table 6.5 indicates the significant alterations that can affect the way we perform everyday recreational or living activities.

It can be seen from Table 6.5 that visual acuity is affected to varying degrees by anatomical and physiological changes of the eye itself and of related neural mechanisms. It should be recognized that other ophthalmological defects such as detached retina, tumors, or conjunctivitis may also result in acuity, color and light adaptation problems.*

Practical considerations. The quality and quantity of illumination required for older persons vary depending upon the severity of the loss and the nature of the activity. Generally, older persons need more light for most tasks, yet too much light can cause glare. When colors are not clearly distinguished, elderly people may find it difficult to determine the placement of objects because of some loss in depth perception. As pointed out in Chapter 3, this

---

*See Edward Elkowitz, *Geriatric Medicine for the Primary Care Practitioner* (New York: Springer Publishing, 1981), for detailed information about these conditions.

Table 6.5 Common Vision Changes Past 50

Condition	Anatomical/Physiological Alteration	Visual Effect
Presbyopia	Loss of lens, elasticity, and power of accommodation	Inability to focus clearly on close work, such as fine print or numbers; farsightedness; lens usually well accommodated to distance vision
Myopia	Excessive curvature of the cornea or thickness of lens	Incorrect focus of light rays in front of the retina, resulting in a distorted image, reduced acuity for distance objects, nearsightedness
Astigmatism	Irregular curvature of cornea	Error in light refraction distorts image on the retina, reduces acuity
Cataract	Cloudiness of lens, common among diabetics	Light rays unable to pass through the lens to the retina; progressive loss of vision due to coverage of the pupil
Glaucoma	Elevated fluid pressure within the eye; usually accompanied by farsightedness	Loss of vision, halos, nausea, may have some pain; can result in blindness
Light Sensitivity Thresholds	Pupil size diminishes with age	Poor vision in dark or at night; eye needs more light in dark rooms, especially for close work
Glare	Increasing thickness of the lens (see Chapter 3)	Sensitivity to excess light; poor contrast and acuity of objects
Dark Adaptation	Errors in retinal function, yellowing of lens, and other central nervous system deficiencies (see chapter 3)	More time required when changing vision tasks from dark to light and vice versa
Color Discrimination	Deficiencies in retinal receptors that discriminate colors, usually between colors with short wave lengths, such as blues, blue-greens, and violets (see Chapter 3)	Cannot always distinguish among colors; reds, oranges, and yellows best for color perception among the elderly

change makes it more difficult for the older person to engage in daily living tasks, such as walking up and down stairs.

Program suggestions. Accommodations for persons with limited vision can be made by adjusting the activity itself to fit the visual needs of the participant, and by modifying the equipment and facilities surrounding the involved action. Several suggestions are presented in the next section about typical fitness activities appropriate for older persons. Rather than detailed motor and sport skill descriptions, modifications of techniques and adjustments of selected activities that can be transferred from one skill to another with minor changes are offered.

Group Games and Sports. Games, and their variations, such as volleyball, softball, circle ball, wallball, kickball, and parachute play are found in senior settings. Each requires a ball or piece of equipment and a relatively large playing area; thus attention needs to be directed to the type ball used and action arena. Volleyball represents an open-type skill (see Table 6.1), of moderate exercise exertion; however, because game play constantly involves unpredictable movement patterns, rules should be modified to allow

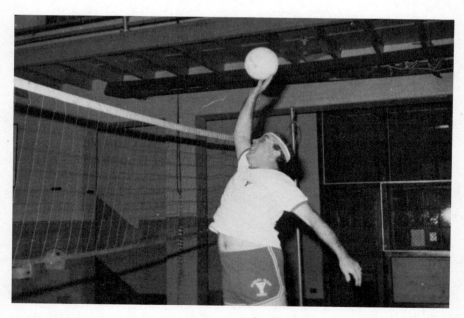

Figure 6.15 Volleyball—an excellent activity for developing hand-eye coordination and team spirit.

more time for response in serving and hitting the ball. Using large, brightly colored (red), light balls, such as beachballs, is preferred. The floor and walls should be of contrasting colors. The game itself should be changed to allow one-bounce floor rebound before it is hit, allowing players more time to "see" the ball. The playing area should be well-lighted with minimum glare.

Parachute play is another group activity that can be played with 20 or more seniors. The parachute should be about 22 feet wide in a bright color for clear visual contrast with the floor. Nylon fabric with contrasting end-lining material from the chute itself is recommended so that the hand grasp site can be easily seen.

Individual and Two-Person Sports. These fitness activities range from mild forms of energy expenditures such as bocci and horseshoes to the vigorous exercise activities of jogging and paddleball. The visual adjustments depend upon the equipment used and the playing area. The general rules which apply to all motor activities are: increase illumination (avoiding glare); use bright, contrasting colors—particularly on floors and walls; and allow more time by slowing the pace of the game so that participants can see the visual clues before a movement is performed. For example, using brightly painted bleach bottles with nerf balls on top that can be easily seen and knocked off with a shuffleboard cue and puck is one activity successfully used by an activity director of a resident home for the elderly.[16]

Whether participants are engaged in team or dual sports, protective glasses should be worn by those who use corrective lens. Glasses should be sturdy enough to withstand the impact of a ball or piece of equipment in the event of an accidental hit (see Chapter 8).

Aquatic Activities. Visual requirements for swimming activities are not as acute as those for physical activities on land. It is recommended that persons wear their glasses for exercise activities performed on the deck area; however, spectacles should be removed while swimming because of the probability of losing them in the turbulence of the water. Actually, vision becomes obscured when glasses are wet, making them a hindrance rather than a visual aid. Seniors should wear eye goggles to keep irritating chlorinated water out of the eyes. Wearing aquatic goggles (the type used by competitive swimmers) also improves vision when the head is underwater and helps to maintain confidence of participants with weak swimming skills.

Many pools are poorly illuminated. Although some natatoriums are equipped for 50-foot candles overhead lighting, we recommend 100-foot candles with a greater concentration over the end walls. Indoor pool windows on the side walls should be tinted to reduce glare and reflection off the surface of water. Water clarity should be such that the bottom and end line

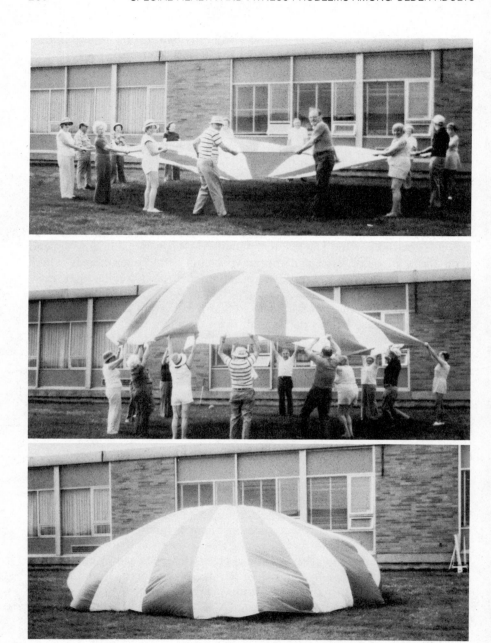

Figure 6.16 Parachute play—an excellent group activity for developing strength of shoulders, arms, and hands.

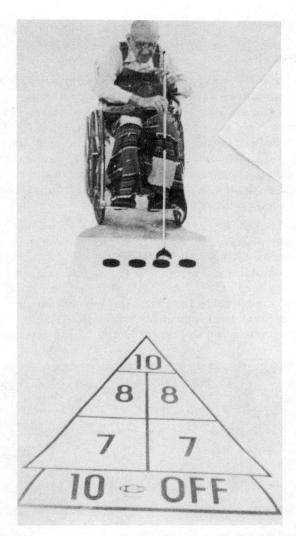

Figure 6.17 Shuffleboard—a suitable activity for wheelchair elderly. (From Risso and Mayo, "Games and Kids," p. 34. Used with permission.)

markings can be clearly seen while standing at midpoint on either side of the pool deck. (Chapter 8 contains a detailed presentation on swimming pool facilities and equipment.)

Rhythm Activities. Rhythmic activities, through various dance modes from square to social ballroom types, provide an opportunity to reinforce the senior's kinesthetic sense by stimulating the nerve receptors in the muscles and skin, particularly of the hands and feet (see Chapter 5). Touch and physical contact become more important and more meaningful as vision acuity decreases. In some cases, when individuals are severely limited by vision approaching blindness, activities that offer touch, physical contact, and less space-orientation with more verbal instructions using clearly accented music accompaniment are recommended.[17]

Hearing Impairments. The ear as an internal control mechanism in maintaining balance was discussed in Chapter 3; the focus here is on an equally important function of this sensory organ—hearing. Hearing loss is more prevalent among older persons than is visual deficiencies. Too often, this sensory loss has been perceived as merely one of life's minor annoyances, but, in fact, psychiatrists and gerontologists agree that significant hearing impairment can cause serious mental dysfunctions because it both interferes with verbal communication and breeds inertia for the development of isola-

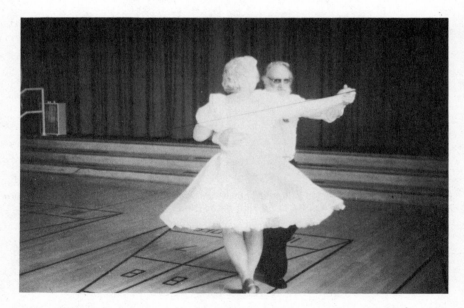

Figure 6.18 Dancing increases keenness of touch receptors as vision acuity decreases.

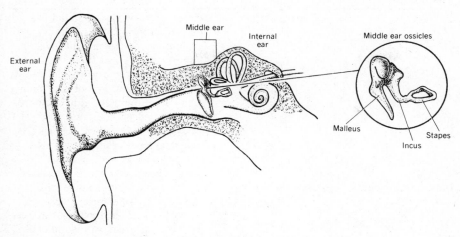

Figure 6.19 External, middle, and internal ear.

tion and depression. Helen Keller once said that "deafness is even more isolating than blindness."

The human ear is a fragile and intricate structure; fortunately, the hard bony structure of the skull provides some protection. Figure 6.19 shows the principal components of the external, middle, and internal ear.

Although hearing loss occurs at all ages and results from many causes including infections, genetic factors, and traumatic lesions, this discussion is confined to common conditions associated with persons past 50. Hearing losses usually are classified into three types: (1) conductive, a form of mechanical obstruction or damage to the outer or middle ear causing the blockage of sound waves through the ear passages; (2) sensorineural, damage to the inner ear mechanisms or brain causing erroneous or complete lack of sound perception; and (3) mixed, a combination of conductive and sensorineural losses. Table 6.6 lists several types of hearing impairments associated with aging.

Hearing losses also may result from other causes not shown in Table 6.6. Certain infections, such as *otitis externa* and *otitis media,* are usually cured quickly with appropriate medications; other problems, such as *acoustic neuromas* (tumors), can present a serious threat to hearing and to life itself, however, they may be successfully treated with early discovery. Most hearing losses are not threats to longevity, but they do create, in some cases, a serious emotional handicap by isolating the older adult from society at a time when the support of family and friends are needed.

Nature of Sound. What we hear as sounds are actually vibrations of the air, moving like the ripples caused by throwing a stone into a pond. These

Table 6.6 Common Hearing Disorders among the Elderly

Condition	Type	Characteristics
Presbycusis	Sensorineural	Varying degrees of high sound frequencies loss; problems in discriminating consonants like *p* as in *pain*, *s* as in *score*, *sh* as in *should* (only parts of these words are heard); most common type of loss among aging adult population; usually progressive, but does not cause total deafness; involves both ears; hearing aids, in certain types of frequency loss, may help restore some hearing; "words heard as a jumble of sounds"
Impacted Cerumen (Ear Wax)	Conductive	Soft wax-like secretion in outer canal, causes partial or complete blockage of sound to middle and internal ear; hearing restored when wax is removed
Otosclerosis	Conductive	Bony growth on parts of the bone capsule between middle and internal ear resulting in fixation of the *stapes;* probably genetically caused; appears to affect more women than men; usually can be corrected by modern methods of microsurgery
Noise Deafness	Sensorineural	Nerve deafness; damage to nerve hair cells within the inner ear; loss of hearing to varying degrees; may be caused by high levels of city noise and industrial noise; damage generally irreversible
Menière's Disease	Sensorineural	Disturbance of fluid in inner ear; common in middle-aged women and beyond; persistent ringing (tinnitus) accompanied by balance problems and vertigo; treated with variety of medications, such as diuretics and antihistamines
Ototoxicity	Sensorineural	Cumulative effect of certain medicines leading to hearing loss, such as aspirin (when overused), diuretics, and certain tranquilizers and other medications; may also result in dizziness and some loss of balance; not uncommon among elderly who consume aspirin for arthritis and diuretics for heart/circulatory problems

vibrations have two central characteristics: pitch and loudness. *Pitch* (or frequency) is the wave length, determined by the cycles or vibrations per second (cps). Since sound travels at an even speed in a particular medium, the closer the waves are together (shorter wave lengths), the more frequently the waves will strike the ear drum. From the top of one wave to the top of the next is considered one cycle; hence, the frequency or number of vibrations per second is often referred to as cycles per second. The greater the frequency (short wave lengths), the higher the pitch. The human ear can perceive frequencies from 16 to 30,000 cps. As a general rule, perception of high frequencies are best in early childhood, with a gradual decrease throughout life, so that the normal adult may have difficulty with anything over 10,000 or 12,000 CPS.[18]

Presbycusis, a common hearing loss among older adults, affects the individual's ability to hear higher-pitched sounds. Figure 6.20 shows an audiogram of typical presbycusis with principal losses in higher frequencies.

Loudness refers to the intensity of sound. It represents the height of the sound wave, and is expressed in decibels (db). A decibel is a relative measure of sound intensity. A sharp gain in loudness occurs with each decibel increase. Specifically, each increment of 10 db indicates a tenfold increase in

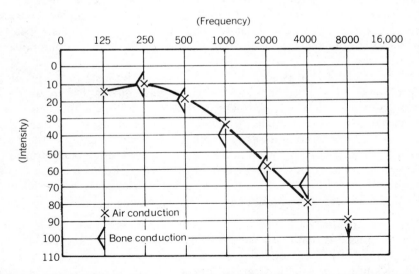

Figure 6.20 Audiogram of typical presbycusis. (From D. Myers et al., "Otologic Diagnosis and Treatment of Deafness," copyright © 1970 CIBA Pharmaceutical Co., Division of CIBA-GEIGY Corp. Reprinted with permission from *Clinical Symposia*, illus. by Frank H. Netter, M.D., all rights reserved.)

Table 6.7   Decibel Ratings

Normal breathing	10 decibels
Leaves rustling in the breeze	20 decibels
Whisper	30 decibels
Quiet restaurant	50 decibels
Normal speech	60 decibels
Busy traffic	70 decibels
Niagara Falls	90 decibels
Subway	100 decibels
Pneumatic riveter	130 decibels
Jet takeoff (discomfort)	140 decibels

Source: R. N. Butler and M. L. Lewis, *Aging and Mental Health* (St. Louis, Mo.: C. V. Mosby Co., (1982), p. 139. Used with permission.

sound intensity; thus, a sound of 10 db is ten times as intense as one db. Table 6.7 shows examples of noises with increasing decibel levels.

Practical Considerations. The first consideration in dealing with hearing loss is to understand the nature and effects of the auditory deficiency. It is obvious that merely amplifying sound or speaking louder may not help the individual with sensorineural loss. In fact, lowering the pitch of the voice and talking more slowly when speaking to persons with presbycusis help the listener to better discriminate the different sounds of words. Persons affected by conductive loss such as that found in otosclerosis can benefit by an increase in the db level or loudness threshold. Certain individuals appear to hear better in noisy places; others find it difficult when background noise is present.

Hearing decrement is specific to the cause of the loss; that is, seniors with conductive loss need approaches to assistance modes that are different than do persons with sensorineural problems. Thus a reliable medical evaluation is required, by a physician who specializes in diseases of the ear. The diagnosis and rehabilitation process should be shared, using a team approach to include the physician and all allied health personnel involved in senior program activities. The professional worker should be alert to the following hearing loss clues, ready to refer the individual to a physician as quickly as possible when an impairment is suspected:

1. Prefers the TV a little louder than anyone else in the room.
2. Complains that others are slurring words or mumbling.
3. Habitually turns one side of his head toward the speaker.
4. Continually asks persons to repeat phrases or words.
5. Complains of ringing in the ears or other head noises.
6. Has trouble hearing at church, movies, etc.
7. Finds it difficult to locate the source of sounds.

Program Suggestions. A keen awareness by the health professional to the type and extent of individual hearing impairment within any group provides direction in the design and conduct of activities. Generally, persons with slight or moderate loss (e.g., 30 to 40 db) need little or no program adaptation of fitness activities, unless the inner ear balance mechanism is affected. Most of the conversational intensity range falls between the 40 to 60 db levels; however, persons with slight or moderate losses may miss whispers or some ordinary conversation, particularly when the listener is beyond a distance of three feet.

Visual aids such as slides, films, and blackboards should be extensively used because most hearing-impaired persons automatically learn to depend upon vision for directions and explanations of activities. When planning activities, groups should be arranged so that both the instructor and the clear display of visual materials may be seen easily. Hearing-impaired individuals also are sensitive to gestures and movements by the instructor. Any hand motions and facial expressions are quickly noted and interpreted by the participant. Male instructors should be cognizant of the hindering effect of beards or moustaches, which tend to obscure the mouth, possibly interfering with a participant's ability to read lips.

When rhythmic or musical accompaniment is used, careful attention should be given to the pitch and volume. Usually, persons with presbycusis respond to and enjoy tones in the lower frequency since the higher-pitched sounds cannot be heard. Volume too often is set to accommodate normal hearing, even more of an annoyance to hard-of-hearing persons.

In team game action, some hazards may exist for the auditory impaired since they are unable to respond quickly to typical sound signals. In these instances, colored flags should be used or horns of sufficient intensity so that warnings and other game action changes can be perceived. Signals such as dimming the lights rather than using a whistle can be used in some cases where stop and go actions are required.

All activities listed in Table 6.1 may be learned and enjoyed by hearing-impaired persons. In team games, those participants without hearing deficits should be alerted to sign and color signals. This approach adds a safety measure to the activity and enlists cooperation from all team members.

Individual and two-person sports, such as bowling, tennis, badminton, horseshoes, and bocci can be played without any major changes. The manner of keeping score should be visual, and scores should be recorded so that the game can progress without the embarrassment of depending upon auditory signals.

Swimming and pool activities, in some cases, may be contraindicated when the participant has a medical or balance problem, such as Menière's syndrome or other dysfunctions in balance mechanism. Water temperature should be about 82 degrees with the deck temperature approximately 10 degrees higher than that of the water. Extreme cold water (less than 60 degrees) should be avoided, as stimulation of the labyrinth of the ear by low temperatures can produce *coloric labyrinthitis* (inflammation of internal ear) with vertigo, loss of balance, and nausea.[19] However, most older persons with presbycusis or conductive loss can partake in most aquatic activities without restrictions.

Rhythm and dance activities need to be selected carefully since movement response depends upon hearing the sound and beat of the music. When introducing social and folk dancing, playing the record or tape first helps the participant to determine the beat. The instructor should participate with the group since members can profit by watching the action to complement hearing reception.

Group leaders should be sensitive to the reactions and responses of hearing-impaired persons. Demonstration is especially important and more meaningful than lengthy explanations of the activity. It is not unusual for hearing-impaired individuals to show lack of attention or interest—because they are not hearing and understanding what is happening.

The following suggestions are useful when presenting activities to hearing impaired persons:

1. Determine type and extent of hearing loss of individual members, and adapt the presentation and activity to accommodate the loss; e.g., speak in lower tones when the problem is presbycusis.

2. Accent demonstration of activities rather than detailed verbal explanation.

3. Face the hearing-impaired person directly and speak on the same level with him or her whenever possible.

4. Avoid talking or providing directions from another room.

5. Use an efficient sound system that can control pitch as well as volume.

6. Use blackboards, slides, charts, audiocassettes, and pictures to reinforce verbal explanations.

7. Avoid introducing new activities when the participant is tired; hearing and understanding diminish with fatigue.

8. Avoid smoking, chewing, or eating when presenting activities since these interfere with clear enunciation.

9. Avoid games and activities that depend upon whispered signals. Use color or hand/body signs.

10. Use percussion instruments, metronomes, music with definite beat and cadence to maximize auditory cues.

OTHER HEALTH-FITNESS RELATED ELEMENTS

While movement and exercise are crucial to the maintenance of fitness and well-being of older adults, nutrition, Kegel exercises, and obesity also are important elements in the health-fitness of the senior adult.

Nutrition and Aging

We know that proper foods are essential at all ages from the pediatric set to the very old. We also know that undernutrition (too little of essential foods) can cause certain diseases at each age level, and that overnutrition (too much of the essential foods) can result in serious health dysfunctions. While a vast literature exists on the importance of nutrition and health, the discussion here is focused upon selected factors and problems about nutriments that affect the elderly with particular reference to maintaining an active lifestyle.

Two general types of factors affect the nutrition status of the elderly: external and internal, external factors include social influences, economic forces, and life style; internal factors entail the anatomical and physiological changes within the body that influence the quantity and quality of what we eat.

The external factor of living alone applies to about one-third of all people over 65; apathy and isolation contribute to reduced food intake, as well as do irrational eating habits. Widows tend to select foods that do not require much preparation and thus become vulnerable to poor nourishment. The sheer economic reality of elderly widows, some of whom subsist on $4000 per year, means some must choose between rent/fuel and food supply because of continued inflation—and food reduction usually takes preference.

Older persons also tend to become sedentary. Thus creeping weight gain occurs more rapidly, and to a greater degree, unless the person's nutritional pattern is modified.

The internal factors of physiological changes, as with other biological parameters, exhibit great heterogeneity. For example, some older people need less calorie intake because of sedentary living and low metabolic rates, while others require more to satisfy the energy requirements resulting from a continuing vigorous exercise and activity lifestyle.

Certain elderly develop diabetes, which results in the inability of the pancreas to manufacture insulin. Such dysfunctions require a specific kind of nutrition control, based on an ascertainment of the carbohydrate needs of the body in conjunction with the individual's activity and medication protocols.

Although older adults show similar physiological decrements, their nutritional needs may be quite different from each other, depending upon their individual environmental lifestyle and physiological status.

Calories. Most authorities recommend lower caloric intake at advanced ages. However, as we have previously stressed, essential calories depend upon the particular energy requirement of the individual. Nevertheless, the following recommended allowances of the Food and Nutrition Board of the National Academy of Sciences may serve as a working guide for individuals free of metabolic or chronic diseases:[20]

Energy (k cal)

	Men*	Women**
Age 51–75	2400	1800
Over 75	2050	1600

*Average height 70 in., 154 lbs.
**Average height 64 in., 120 lbs.

The above allowances are merely guidelines and should not be considered as absolute. The genetic makeup, energy needs, and medical status of the individual may alter his or her caloric needs to a considerable degree.

Protein. There is general agreement that a high protein diet, particularly at levels exceeding recommended dietary allowances (56 gms/day for men; 44 gms/day for women) of the Food and Nutrition Board of the Academy of Sciences, causes urinary calcium excretion. It is further hypothesized that the hypercalciuria (excess calcium in urine) increases the risk of osteoporosis.[21] We know that men and women lose bone mass as part of normal aging, women more so than men. Thus it appears prudent to refrain from exceeding the RDA allowance of protein because of its link with the absorptive mechanism of calcium and osteoporotic bone development.

Fat. Saturated and unsaturated fats are high in calories and generally make up about 40 percent of the American diet. Such foods as butter, margarine, and fat spreads are examples of saturated fats; fish oils and vegetable oils are classified as unsaturated fats. Unless the individual is a competitive endurance runner or an extremely high energy consumer, the older person should maintain a maximum level of about 30 percent fat in the total daily calories. Research has shown that diets high in saturated fats contain cholesterol, a powerful predictor of coronary artery disease for some individuals. Since the basal metabolic rate generally declines, along with activity levels with maturity, a prudent dietary course of moderation in fat content and the substitution of unsaturated fats for saturated fats usually satisfies the energy and nutrition requirements of most older people.

Carbohydrates. A relatively large percentage of the energy necessary for muscular effort is derived from the breakdown of muscle and liver carbohydrate stores (glycogen). Some marathon athletes who participate in endurance events that last for one hour or more ingest high-carbohydrate foods through a dietary regimen called *carbohydrate loading*. The intent is to increase glycogen to muscle stores and allow the athlete to perform longer before exhaustion. Although this procedure is acceptable for young competitors, it is unwise for the older athlete because of possible disturbances to the cardiac functions that may result from disruption of normal metabolic processes.[22]

Carbohydrates are consumed in the form of simple sugars and complex forms. The complex types are broken down into components that can be used by the body, such as starch; those components that are not used are passed through the gastrointestinal tract and excreted. The latter group is classified as fiber. Simple sugars are a source of carbohydrates, but contain low-bulk calories and should be taken in moderation.

The starches found in potatoes or grains such as wheat, corn, and rice, if unrefined or enriched, contain other essential nutrients including vitamins, minerals, and fiber. The fiber acts as a bulking medium and promotes efficient movement of the stool through the lower intestines. This can help to prevent or reduce the stress of flatulence and constipation, a common complaint of the elderly. About 55 percent of the older adult's daily calories should come from carbohydrates, primarily from unrefined starches, whole grain, or enriched flour; the diet should also be high in fiber content (see Table 6.8).

Calcium and Phosphorus. The requirement for calcium is affected by age, sex, hormonal status, absorption efficiency, and physical exercise—all factors that vary according to the individual. However, varying degrees of calcium loss and the consequences of osteopenia and osteoporosis appear with persistent regularity among older persons, particularly in women. Research is not conclusive as to whether negative calcium balance is due to the lack of quantitative intake or malfunctions in the metabolic absorptive process. The role of phosphorus appears to be controversial. Some investigators report that high phosphorus should be reduced, while other researchers indicate that this mineral does not negatively influence calcium utilization in humans.[23] Although the mechanism of calcium loss in adults is not clearly known, and phosphorus is found in abundance in the U.S. diet of meats, poultry, and fish, some reduction in the average diet of this mineral would still be within adequate RDA levels. Calcium consumption, however, should be increased to about 1000 mg/day (see Table 6.8).

Iron. The transport and metabolism of iron generally slows with age, past maturity. Many older individuals secrete less hydrochloric acid than do

Table 6.8   Nutrient Recommendations for the Elderly

Nutrient	Men	Women
Calories	2300/day	2000/day
Protein	56 gms/day	45 gms/day
Fat	25–30% of total daily calories (64–76 gms/day)	25–30% of total daily calories (55–66 gms/day)
Carbohydrates	55–60% of total daily calories (310–345 gms/day)	55–60% of total daily calories (275–300 gms/day)
Fiber	Increase to approximately 10 grams	Increase to approximately 10 grams
Vitamins	Increase B_{12} to greater than 3 mcg	Increase B_{12} to greater than 3 mcg
Calcium	1000 mg/day	1000 mg/day
Phosphorus	Reduce	Reduce
Iron	18–40 mg/day	18–40 mg/day

M. Winick, ed., *Nutrition and Health* 1, no. 6 (1979): 3. Used with permission.

younger people. This transport reduction has been linked with iron-deficiency anemia. This condition is accompanied with symptoms of weakness, pallor, and breathlessness. It is not unusual to find nutritional anemia among older persons who survive on a diet of milk, crackers, tea, and toast. In fact, a survey of a scientifically chosen random sample of persons aged one through 74 years showed that persons over 60 had nutritional deficiencies of iron as well as of vitamin A, C, and calcium.[24] Such foods as liver, fortified cereals (low-sugar type), lima beans, and lean meat are good sources of iron. Intake of 18 to 40 mg/day of iron are advised (see Table 6.8).

Vitamins. Vitamins do not contain calories, but they do control vital chemical reactions within the body in relationship to the food consumed. For example, vitamin B_{12} is necessary for the utilization of ingested iron; vitamin D is associated with the metabolism of calcium necessary for healthy bones; and vitamin C is important for forming connective tissue and promoting wound healing, as well as in the absorption of iron.

Vitamins that are especially important to older persons are vitamin D and B_{12}. These vitamins are associated with bone integrity and iron metabolism. Research dealing with the effects of aging of the utilization of vitamins and minerals is sparse. Based upon the present evidence, we can say that intake of large doses of vitamins not only is a waste of money, but usually provides no unique nutritional benefit and may even lead to undesirable effects ranging from minor to serious body dysfunctions.[25]

The elderly with chronic or incurable diseases are especially vulnerable to the promises of food zealots. Such diseases as heart disease, arthritis, diabetes, and hypertension are frequent targets of megavitamin promoters. Although vitamin supplements may be indicated based upon individual needs (e.g., in cases of osteoporosis or nutritional anemia), for the normal individual vitamin enrichment should come directly from eating a variety of foods in accordance with his or her genetic and caloric energy requirements.

Obesity

As noted previously, a gain in weight generally occurs with advancing age up to the middle 50, followed by decline. Hazards associated with obesity, all of which are well documented, include hypertension, diabetes, and skeletal trauma. Each of these conditions indirectly affects longevity.

Obesity is a complex phenomenon involving the interaction of heredity, nutrition, and lifestyle. Some experts hold the view that mild to moderate levels of adiposity may not be deleterious to longevity, some even arguing that moderate obesity may have a positive relationship with longevity.[26] Research studies have yet to reveal what these health benefits may be. Nevertheless, enough solid evidence does exist to verify that gross over-weight due to excess adipose tissue is hazardous for the following reasons:

1. Merely carrying excess weight can injure joints and their surrounding tissues—e.g., tendons, cartilages, and ligaments.
2. Postive relationships exist between higher levels of obesity and coronary heart disease, hypertension, and diabetes.
3. Physical endurance performance level is reduced, and fatigue occurs sooner in obese individuals.
4. Increased levels of obesity result in elevated plasma cholesterol.
5. Increased levels of obesity foster hypokinetic disease (disuse syndrome), and subsequently, muscle weakness and atrophy.
6. Excess adipose tissue accumulation around the chest and diaphram interferes with respiratory efficiency.
7. Obese individuals are more vulnerable to serious injury due to accidental falls since excess fat prevents quick movements to adjust balance errors.
8. Obesity is associated with gallbladder, digestive, and kidney diseases.
9. Obesity places undue strain upon arthritic joints.
10. Excess adipose around the abdominal area increases stress on spinal discs and facilitates likelihood of low back pain.
11. Obesity is associated with disturbed body image and lower self-esteem.

This list does not include all of the health consequences of obesity, but it does offer a persuasive rationale for keeping adipose levels within normal limits.

Program Considerations. Most adults are increasingly interested in maintaining their health and well-being as they approach the middle adult and late maturity cycles. Any approach to correcting obesity must consider the element of motivation. Success in weight reduction programs is unlikely unless interest, drive, and incentive are present. This means that fitness specialists need to individualize a prescriptive program based upon the senior's organic capacity and ability, personality, and temperament. For example, if Mrs. Brown is primarily interested in losing adipose tissue because she wants to "look better," the sage fitness specialist will design a program of activities that will both condition her postural muscles and include aerobic-type activities that burn up calories.

Another senior adult may be mainly interested in reducing his or her exposure risk to a cerebrovascular accident or stroke. Suggesting activities that focus upon improving cardiac function and peripheral vascular circulation can serve to motivate that person to pursue an exercise course. The point here is to recognize that motivation among individuals differs, and that generally most people will respond positively to a program when the prescription satisfies their personal needs and desires.

A prescriptive agenda for dealing with overweight involves three segments: (1) providing an understanding of obesity and its effects on health-fitness; (2) nutrition counseling; and (3) implementing program activities. The first component should include basic facts about the biological, psychological, and sociological ramifications of obesity. Suitable topics could include: (1) obesity and overweight—differences and similarities; (2) nutrition and fatness; (3) diets—facts and fallacies; (4) specific nutrients for the older adult; (5) practical methods of assessing obesity; (6) high- and low-calorie foods; (7) energy expenditure and exercise; and (8) exercise—conceptions and misconceptions.

Nutrition counseling should be given during the same period as the cognitive information and physical activity segments. This part of the program can be done in small seminar groups of six to eight persons or on a one-on-one basis. The purpose is to deal with what the obese person is eating and to modify his or her dining habits in terms of "what they do for you." Topics should be relevant to the interests of the participants. Such counseling provide an opportunity to give information on such subjects as: (1) balanced nutrition, (2) overnourished and undernourished individuals, (3) right and wrong foods for seniors, (4) high-energy foods, (5) low-calorie foods that provide essential nutrients, and (6) appetite and eating habits. Such topics are merely examples: lead topics and cues should be taken from the participants to ensure meaningful dialogue. Appendix F provides a sample nutrition profile form that can be used in conjunction with nutrition counseling.

The third component, implementation of program activities, includes measurement and assessment of base-line data on physique, such as height, weight, girths, and skinfolds (see Chapter 9), along with other basic physical fitness components. Assessment is followed by an individualized program of activities primarily aimed at burning up excess weight over an extended period of time (6 months), with a progressive loss of no more than two pounds per week. The type of activities can be varied, but two principles should be followed: (1) activity should be primarily aerobic in nature, and (2) intensity should be geared to the physical capacity and limitations of the participant. The following activities are particularly suited for overweight persons:

walking briskly	bowling
stationary bicycle	punching bag
swimming	volleyball
dancing	bocci
calisthenics	shuffleboard
table tennis	

Concurrently with aerobic activities, posture exercises can be introduced for those participants who are mainly interested in enchancing their appearance. The exercises suggested here focus on four body areas: (1) chest region, (2) abdomen and waist, (3) pelvic and gluteal regions, and (4) shoulder girdle.

1. *Pectoral stretching.* This exercise may be done ballistically or non-ballistically (e.g., controlled—not jerky movements), or deep stretching held for minimum of a 10-second count. The purpose of this exercise is to stretch the chest agonists while contracting the upper back antagonists (principally, rhomboids), and countering the kyphotic or round upper back effect by adducting the scapula. Ten to 20-second stretching bouts are recommended.

2. *Modified abdominal flexing.* This exercise is designed to prevent ptosis, or sagging abdominal wall. Trunk twisting sit-ups in varying positions may be performed depending upon the initial strength of the individual. Hyperextension of the lower back should be avoided during the sit-up movement. In certain cases, sit-ups may be started from the "jackknife" position, with the arms outstretched overhead. The individual will make the sit-up easier by swinging the

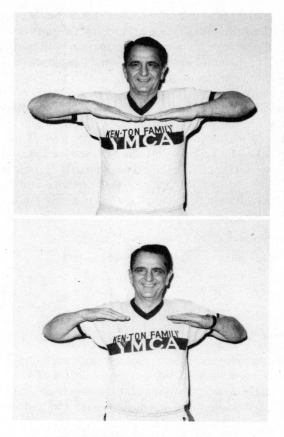

Figure 6.21 Pectoral stretching.

arms upward and legs downward. The downward momentum generated by the legs is transferred to the upper trunk, assisting the individual to the "up" position of the sit-up.

3. *Pelvic and gluteal strengthening.* The third area involves the hip area of the body namely, the gluteal maximus, medius, and minimus muscles. These muscle groups can be firmed and strengthened by (a) hopping on one leg, (b) running in place, or (c) vigorous backward extension of the leg, alternating left and right limbs. Jogging is also recommended, since this type of activity consumes calories and stimulates the cardiorespiratory system in addition to strengthening the pelvic and gluteal muscles.

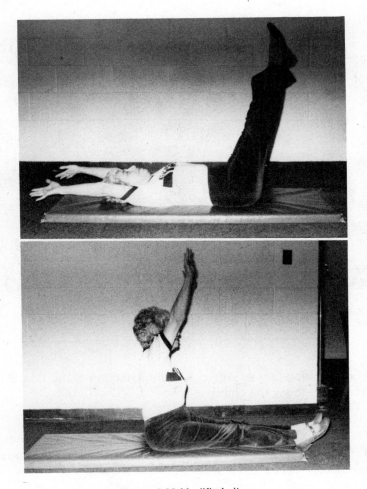

Figure 6.22 Modified sit-up.

4. *Agility exercise*. The calisthenic activity commonly known as the "squat thrust" or "burpee" can be modified by thrusting one leg at a time backward in an alternating manner, as shown in Figure 6.24. Body control and maneuverability are also enhanced along with agility. Speed should not be a concern in the performance of the exercise.

An ideal fitness program for the obese adult requires the cooperation of a physician, a fitness specialist, and a dietitian. Together, they can provide a

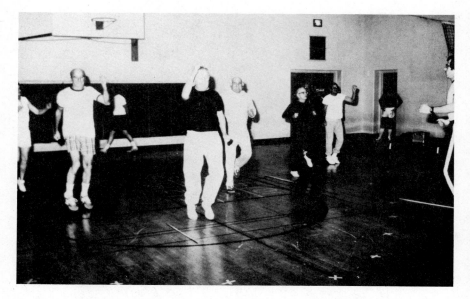

Figure 6.23 Strengthening pelvic and gluteal muscles while stimulating the cardiorespiratory system.

powerful combination for the prevention and reduction of this common nutritional problem among the elderly.

"Kegels"

Up to 63 percent of postmenopausal women may have a problem with urinary stress incontinence (lack of bladder control). The problem arises when the senior adult woman is unable to control bladder contractions, as the result of either neurogenic (neural) or myogenic (muscular) causes. Some women develop myogenic or muscular weakness of the pelvic floor musculature (peroneal muscles), a condition that may be caused by multiple childbirths resulting in damage to the muscles. In such cases, the bladder becomes distended and overfilled and the pelvic floor muscles are unable to sustain sufficient constriction; thus, urine control is lost. Loss of control may happen when the woman is laughing, coughing, or whenever the detrussor or "pushing down" muscle mechanism is involved.

Special exercises developed by Dr. Arnold Kegel can be of help in controlling myogenic urinary problems.[27] These exercises are designed to strengthen the *pubococcygeous* (or PC) muscle, which is a part of the pelvic

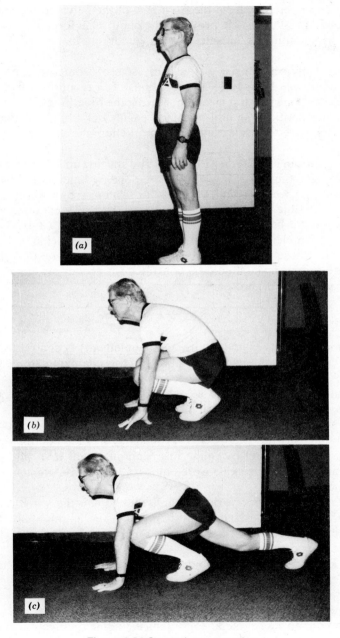

Figure 6.24 Squat thrust exercise.

muscle group stretching from the front part of the pelvis to the back part of the tailbone. The PC muscle provides the contractile force that controls the flow of urine—thus its muscle tone is important in maintaining urinary control.

Kegel exercises consist of five daily sets of isometric exercises, progressing over time from 10 to 30 repetitions. Ten repetitions five times per day should be done the first week, increasing the repetitions to 15 the second week. Five repetitions should be added each week until 30 repetitions are reached. Improved muscle tone and contraction should occur within two weeks.

A woman can identify her PC muscle by starting and stopping urine flow without moving the legs. Slow Kegels are done by holding or tightening the muscle for three seconds. Quick Kegels, or tightening and relaxing the PC as rapidly as possible, are also an effective method of conditioning. Natural breathing should be done while contracting, during both types of Kegels. While mild to moderate forms of incontinence due to muscular weakness can be helped by these special exercises, severe types may require surgery. In either case, a physician should be consulted for proper evaluation and prescriptive management protocol.

Summary

Adaptation of activities and environmental elements is central to the selection and conduct of older adult programs. In this chapter adaptive guidelines were presented emphasizing the need to adjust fitness activities to suit the individual capacity and ability of each participant. Flexibility in the conduct of games or sports to allow individual adjustments was emphasized.

The role of discrete and continuous skills as appropriate activities for older persons was then addressed. Proficiency in such continuous skills as skating, swimming, and bicycling may continue well into old age. Thirty discrete and continuous skills were enumerated with recommended adaptations for older adults.

The need for a wide variety of activities to suit the varied interests of participants was emphasized. Adult populations in institutionally based and special settings were described, with recommended exercise guidelines for limited ambulatory, wheelchair, and bedfast residents.

The discussion of music and rhythm in fitness programs emphasized their potential for facilitating interest and contributing to a positive mental and emotional outlook. Passive, assistive-active, active, and active-resistive types of exercises also were described.

Common musculoskeletal conditions including rheumatoid arthritis, osteoarthritis, and osteoporosis affect mobility and locomotion. Appropriate exercises to lessen the effects of these conditions were presented. Physical activity also enhances the development of bone mass in osteoporotic persons.

Sensory deficits in vision and hearing among older adults were explored. Analysis of vision and hearing losses revealed that auditory decrements beyond moderate levels can result in severe temperament and personality disturbances. Visual problems associated with persons past 50 were briefly described, with suggested adaptations in the conduct of activities. Program principles and guidelines to accommodate both visual and hearing-impaired persons were discussed.

Other health-fitness–related elements—nutrition, obesity, and incontinence—were introduced with a focus on their relationships to mobility and motor performance. External and internal factors were identified as causes of nutritional anomalies. Calories, protein, fats, carbohydrates, calcium, phosphorus, iron and vitamins were examined with particular attention to the nutritional needs of persons past 50.

Obesity was defined, analyzed and interpreted, and suggestions for developing a program for the purpose of maintaining weight control were offered.

Finally, the problem of urinary stress incontinence was explored. Special exercises (Kegels) for the purpose of toning and strengthening the peroneal muscles were explained.

REFERENCES

1. Dorothy Chrisman, "Badminton at 65 and Older," *Journal of Physical Education and Recreation* 50 (October 1979): 26–28.
2. Marian A. Palmer, "Music Therapy in a Comprehensive Program of Treatment and Rehabilitation for the Geriatric Resident," *Journal of Music Therapy* 14, no. 4 (1977): 190–197.
3. Ruth Bright, *Music in Geriatric Care* (London: Angus & Robertson, 1972), p. 52.
4. Alicia Clair Gibbons, "Popular Music Preferences of Elderly People," *Journal of Music Therapy* 14, no. 4 (1977): 180–189.
5. A. Fleming, J. M. Crown, and M. Corbett, "Incidence of Joint Involvement in Early Rheumatoid Arthritis," *Rheumatology and Rehabilitation* 15 (1976): 92–96.
6. National Commission on Arthritis and Related Diseases, National Institutes of Health, *The Arthritis Plan: Vol. I: Report to the Congress of the United States*, DHEW no. 76-1150 (April 1976): p. 102.
7. Robert W. Schrier, *Clinical Internal Medicine in the Aged* (Philadelphia: W. B. Saunders, 1982), p. 194.
8. P. Lee et al., "The Etiology and Pathogenesis of Osteoarthrosis: A Review," *Seminars in Arthritis and Rheumatism* 3(1974): 189–218.

9. John Piscopo and James A. Baley, *Kinesiology: the Science of Movement* (New York: John Wiley & Sons, 1981), Chapter 2.
10. Schrier, *Clinical Internal Medicine,* p. 182.
11. Everett L. Smith, "Exercise for Prevention of Osteoporosis: A Review," *The Physician and Sports Medicine* 10, no. 3 (1982): 72–83.
12. Everett L. Smith, W. Reddan, and P. E. Smith, "Physical Activity and Calcium Modalities for Bone Mineral Increase in Aged Women," *Medicine and Science in Sports and Exercise* 13, no. 1, (1981): 60–64.
13. John L. Aloia, "Exercise and Skeletal Health," *Journal of the American Geriatric Society* 29, no. 3 (1981): 104–106.
14. J. Wolff, *Das Gesetz der Transformation der Knocken* (Berlin: Aug. Hirschwald, 1892).
15. Larry G. Peppers, "Patterns of Leisure and Adjustment to Retirement," *The Gerontologist* 16, no. 5 (1976): 441–445.
16. Shirley Risso and Constance R. Mayo, "Games and Kids Could Be the Key," *Journal of Physical Education, Recreation, and Dance* 50, no. 7 (September 1979): 34–35.
17. Erna Caplow-Lindner, Leah Harpaz and Sonja Samberg, *Therapeutic Dance/Movement* (New York: Human Sciences Press, 1979), p. 68.
18. D. Myers et al., "Otologic Diagnosis and the Treatment of Deafness," *Clinical Symposia* 22, no. 2 (1970): 36.
19. Daniel Kuland, *The Injured Athlete* (Philadelphia: J. B. Lippincott, 1982), p. 241.
20. Food and Nutrition Board, *Recommended Dietary Allowances,* 9th rev. ed. (Washington, D.C.: National Academy of Sciences, National Research Council, 1980).
21. National Dairy Council, *Dairy Council Digest* "Diet and Bone Health," 53, no. 5 (September/October 1982): 25–30.
22. Kuland, *Injured Athlete,* p. 56.
23. Myron Winick, "Nutrition for the Elderly," *Nutrition and Health* 1, no. 6 (1979): 1–6, and National Dairy Council Digest, "Diet," p. 270.
24. *Anthropometric and Clinical Findings, Preliminary Findings of the First Health and Nutrition Examination Survey (HANES), U.S. 1971–1972,* DHEW Publication no. 75–1220 (Washington, D.C.; U.S. Government Printing Office, 1975).
25. National Dairy Council, "Nutrition Misinformation," *Dairy Digest* 52, no. 4 (July/August 1981): 19–23.
26. Reuben Andres, "Relationship of Obesity to Aging" (Paper delivered at Symposium on Aging, Multidisciplinary Center for the Study of Aging, State University of New York at Buffalo, 17 March 1977).
27. Arnold H. Kegel, "Genital Relaxation, Urinary Stress Incontinence and Sexual Dysfunction," in J. P. Greenhill, ed., *Office Gynecology* (Chicago: Yearbook Medical Publishers, 1965), Chapter 24.

CHAPTER 7

Drugs and the Elderly: Implications for Fitness Programs

UNDERSTANDING DRUGS IN GERONTOLOGY

The elderly constitute a population group that consumes a greater proportion of drugs in the United States than does any other age segment. It has been estimated that older persons ingest 25 percent of all prescribed medications even though they make up only about 11 percent of the population.[1] A report from the National Center for Health Statistics indicates that Americans spent $8 billion on prescription drugs in 1980.[2] These figures point out that drug use, particularly among the elderly, is a significant part of our daily lives. The consumer is barraged each day with drug claims extending from the relief of pain to complete cure.

The older members of the population, especially the very old (over 75), are particularly vulnerable to the numerous, sometimes dangerous, consequences of drug effects. However, informed and intelligent use of drugs and medications can be valuable in the prevention and amelioration of common problems that affect personal health-fitness. Our discussion will focus upon the common drugs and medications used by the elderly that are primarily associated with mobility and locomotion.

Before pursuing any discussion on drugs, a general knowledge about their content and characteristics is helpful. It is not our purpose to delve deeply into the biochemistry and pharmacology of drug composition, but rather to present an overview of the practical considerations of drug makeup, and of the course of drugs in altering body functions, particularly when combined with physical activity.

Dorland's Medical Dictionary defines a drug as: "Any chemical compound that may be used on or administered to humans and animals as an aid in the diagnosis, treatment of disease, or prevention of disease or other abnormal condition, for the relief of pain or suffering; or to control or improve any physiologic or pathologic condition."[3] This definition explicitly states that drugs are chemical substances administered for the enhancement of health; however, it should be noted that the alteration of physiologic function may also have deleterious results, in some cases, inducing *iatrogenic illness* (disorders resulting from treatment itself). For example, uncontrolled use of tranquilizers over a long period of time can damage brain cells and cause various organic brain disorders resulting in psychotic behavior patterns; extensive use of diuretics can lead to dehydration; and certain antiarthritic drugs can cause gastric dysfunctions.

Older persons, because of declining physiologic functions, reduced metabolic efficiency of the liver and kidneys, and increased tissue sensitivity, are vulnerable to acute drug reactions not usually found among young people. Also, standards for the use of most current therapeutic agents are set up through tests of young adults, and application of these same guidelines to the elderly is often hazardous.[4]

In addition, dimming vision and the gradual onset of presybyopia make it more difficult to select the right size, shape, and color from assorted pills, capsules, and containers at two-, six-, twelve-, or twenty-four-hour intervals. It is not unusual for older persons to ingest six or more different drugs each day.

Thus, the combination of individual variability, declining physiologic and cognitive functioning, and increased prevalence of disease and dysfunctions makes the risk of errors in prescription of type, mode, frequency, and dosage indeed probable. A better understanding of how a drug works and of its effect on body functions can help reduce the danger of drug toxicity.

Principles of Drug Application for Older Persons

It can be seen from our discussion that the effects of drugs depend upon the variables among individuals, and the environmental milieu of the individual, as well as conditions in the administration of the drug itself. The following principles should be followed as a safeguard for the older person when prescription drugs are indicated:

1. Special consideration must be paid to biological age as well as chronological age. In general, drugs tend to be absorbed more slowly and less efficiently with advancing anatomic and physio-

logic maturity. Drugs should be administered at low doses and then gradually raised if increased dosages are indicated.

2. All previous medications should be carefully reviewed before new drugs are prescribed.

3. Drug regimens should be as simple as possible to accommodate changing cognitive and sensory functions.

4. Written instructions on prescriptions should be clear and large enough for easy reading.

5. Consideration in drug frequency and dosage should be balanced with activity lifestyle; e.g., insulin absorption is affected by caloric expenditure (exercise), so prescription must consider energy consumption. That is, exercise lowers blood glucose levels. Exercise regimens should be coordinated and regulated with frequency and dosage of the drug to prevent hypoglycemic (low blood sugar) states.

6. Side effects of the drug must be considered, and the benefits of a drug should outweigh its adverse effects. This is especially important when more than one drug is taken simultaneously; e.g., dosage of blood thinners such as Coumadin must be monitored very carefully with any medication containing aspirin, since the combination of these two drugs can cause internal bleeding.

7. The effects of alcohol (also a drug) with other drugs must be considered; e.g., when alcohol is taken with barbiturates, tranquilizers, or antihistamines, nervous system depression and oversedation can result.

8. It must be emphasized to the patient that compliance with drug prescription regimen is necessary for maximum benefits; if certain drugs are taken at irregular frequencies, their advantages may be negated and may trigger adverse side effects.

9. Consideration should be given to possible allergic reactions to certain foods when a particular drug is taken.

10. Drugs should be administered only when necessary, and as few as possible should be consumed at any given time.

Drugs are important for the control of illness; however, complications may arise that can create severe dysfunctions and threats to health. Such chemical compounds alter body functions and must be carefully used. The next section deals with common drugs, with particular concern on how these medications affect mobility and performance of persons over 50.

Drugs and the Cardiovascular System

Cardiovascular disorders are the most common cause of death among the elderly; and those who reside in nursing homes receive more medications for heart-circulatory disorders and related diseases than for any other systemic ailment. Chapters 4 and 5 contain exercise prescription protocols for healthy persons. Our focus in this section is on individuals who use drugs for the management and control of heart and circulatory dysfunctions. Any exercise regimen that involves cardiac patients must require a valid informed consent of the exercise participant and physician approval before testing and activities are initiated (see Appendix E for sample forms).

Many of the pharmacologic agents commonly used by cardiac patients may be classified into the following categories: (1) antianginal, (2) antihypertension, (3) antiarrhythmic, (4) anticoagulant, and (5) digitalis. This listing is not a comprehensive index, but does provide a representative sample of drug agents dispensed to the elderly.

Antianginal Agents. Angina pectoris is evidenced by a sudden sensation ranging from mild pressure discomfort to a suffocating and crushing pain, which often radiates from the lower breastbone to the left shoulder, along the inside of the left arm. Such a state may develop when the heart does not receive the necessary oxygen supply to carry on its contraction-relaxation cycle. When the myocardium (heart muscle) is deprived of its oxygen-carrying blood supply, ischemia (blood flow obstruction) results and can precipitate angina pectoris.

Angina is usually of sudden onset and may strike without warning. It frequently follows physical exertion, strong emotional stress, or eating, however, some attacks occur without these conditions. Angina pectoris is symptomatic of long-standing coronary arterial disease.

The prime objective of therapeutic care is to restore the supply of oxygen to the heart. Two major approaches to treatment are modification of lifestyle and the use of drug therapy to decrease the oxygen demands of the heart. Such practices as eliminating cigarette smoking or participating in supervised exercise programs help to reduce blood pressure and heart rate, consequently decreasing the risk of angina pectoris episodes.

The primary drugs used for angina are nitroglycerin and beta-adrenergic blockers. *Nitroglycerin tablets* taken in sublingual form (under the tongue) decrease arterial resistance (through the dilation of blood vessels), thereby lowering blood pressure, which results in a decreased oxygen demand of the heart. The onset of vessel dilation and relief occurs within 20 to 30 seconds and lasts about 30 minutes. Occasionally, dizziness may accompany tablet ingestion because of the quick vasodilation and sudden drop in blood pressure.

Beta-adrenergic blocking agents are used for long-term drug therapy. These drugs work by decreasing myocardial oxygen consumption, causing a reduction in heart rate, blood pressure, and heart muscle contractibility.

Sometimes nitrates (nitroglycerin) and beta-adrenergic blocking agents are used in combination to control angina.

Antihypertensive Agents. High blood pressure is a common and powerful predictor of stroke and related coronary diseases. As indicated in Chapter 4, hypertension is a condition in which arterial blood pressure is consistently elevated. It is also associated with stiffness of the arteries. Figure 7.1 shows average blood pressures by age of men and women. As mentioned earlier, diastolic (lower figure) blood pressure tends to rise with age, but it stabilizes after 60 years of age (Figure 7.1). Systolic (upper figure) pressure continues to rise considerably in men and women after age 50. Although such elevations are common, care should be taken to detect and control inordinate rises because of their positive association with premature cardiovascular disease.

When drug therapy is necessary, *diuretics, vasodilators,* and *adrenergic blocking* agents affecting the central nervous system may be administered. A diuretic such as Lasix is useful if the body retains fluids. It assists the heart by removing the excess liquids. As with all drugs, frequency and dosage must be prescribed on an individualized basis. Too weak a dosage may not effectively reduce fluid and consequently will fail to decrease high blood pressure; on the other hand, too high a dose can cause body potassium loss, dizziness, and ataxia (loss of coordination), particularly when the elderly person is mixing diuretics with other drugs taken for diabetes and various forms of arthritis.

Vasodilators such as Minipress reduce blood pressure by directly relaxing the smooth muscles of the blood vessels. These drugs can cause adverse side effects, such as headache and rapid heart beat, and in some cases, can aggravate heart conditions. Thus they should be taken with care.

Reserpine and *Aldomet* also are commonly prescribed for hypertension. These drugs control the sympathetic (involuntary) nervous system by reducing heart rate and decreasing peripheral vascular resistance through their adrenergic blocking effect (inhibition of neural receptors and excitation responses to heart and blood vessels). Such drugs can result on *hypotension* (abnormally low blood pressure) because of their interference with sympathetic neural functions, and should be used conservatively.[5] Some elderly persons do have low blood pressure, and if antihypertensive drugs are mistakenly prescribed for such individuals, unstable behavior and movement may result.

Antiarrhythmic Agents. The heart beats constantly at an average rate of 72 beats per minute, circulating over 2000 gallons of blood each day. The sequence of blood flow through the heart is shown in Figure 7.3. The heart rate is regulated automatically by neurons emanating from the autonomic ner-

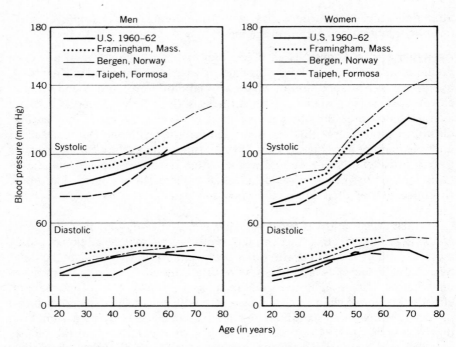

Figure 7.1 Mean blood pressure by age of men and women 18–79. (From L. E. Feinberg, "Hypertension in the Aged," in R. W. Schrier, ed., *Clinical Internal Medicine in the Aged.* [Philadelphia: W. B. Saunders, 1982], p. 67. Used with permission.)

vous system known as the *vagus* and *sympathetic* nerves. Stimulation of the vagus nerves to the heart slows down the rate whereas activation of the sympathetic nerves speeds up the rate.

Constant irregularity of heart beats is known as *arrhythmia.* The two most common types of arrhythmia are tachycardia (abnormally fast heart action) and bradycardia (abnormally slow heart action).

Persistent rapid heart beat can be controlled by such drugs as *Quinidine* and *Lidocaine,* which stimulate vagus nerves and lessen the heart rate. These drugs are eliminated by the body mainly through liver and kidney metabolism. Since approximately 35 percent decrease in total drug clearance is found in the elderly as compared with the younger population, lower doses of Quinidine and Lidocaine are advisable.[6] Quinidine may also cause tinnitus (ringing in the ears), dizziness, blurring of vision, headache, and diarrhea. Lidocaine is frequently used to treat certain types of arrhythmias during surgery. Drowsiness, dizziness, lethargy, and gastrointestinal disturbances are common side effects. Lidocaine is also an anesthetic agent. It has a

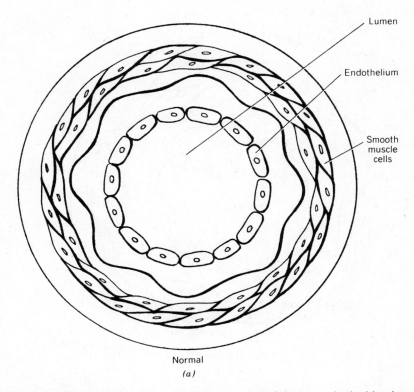

Figure 7.2 One cause of hypertension is the narrowing of the lumen in the blood vessels due to atherosclerosis and arteriosclerosis.

depressing effect on the nervous system and is effective in producing seda-tion; however, it must be used carefully because of its association with hypotension. Quinidine is generally used for long-term arrhythmias, whereas Lidocaine is prescribed for short-term and immediate treatment of tachycardia.

Anticoagulant Agents. Older persons are vulnerable to *thrombosis* (develop-ment of a blood clot obstructing a blood vessel or heart cavity), which may lead to an *embolism* (a roving blood clot). Thus, we often hear of blood clots in the brain (cerebral thrombosis) and the heart (coronary thrombosis). *Thrombophlebitis* is a troublesome clotting condition usually occurring in the legs whose principal danger is that clots may become dislodged and move to the lung where pulmonary embolism can result.

Anticoagulants are used to reduce normal clotting of the blood for the

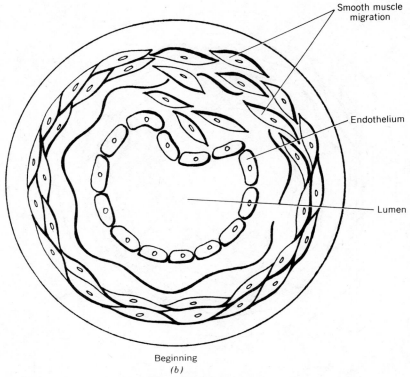

Beginning
(b)
Figure 7.2 (Continued)

purpose of treating stroke, heart disease, and phlebitis. *Heparin* and *Couma-din* are two common anticoagulants used to inhibit blood clotting. Heparin does not dissolve clots, but it does tend to prevent their extension.[7] Couma-din agents act slowly in preventing clot formation and are used for long-term therapy. Adverse effects include internal hemorrhage, which may be mani-fested by bleeding gums, blood in the urine or stool, and spontaneous bruises; thus, dosages must be diligently monitored.

Individuals using such drugs over an extended period of time need to be alert to small cuts because of their tendency for continued bleeding. Factors such as diet and other medications also can affect blood clotting time. Aspi-rin and anti-arthritic drugs increase the effects of anticoagulants. Therefore, such anti-inflammatory medications can be hazardous to individuals who are also on anticoagulants.

Digitalis. Digitalis therapy is used for cardiomyopathy (degenerative heart disease) and tachycardia. Compounds such as Digoxin and Digitoxin, which

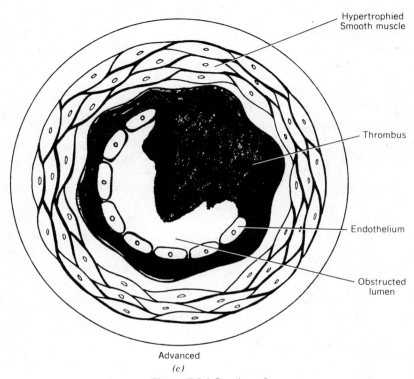

Advanced
(c)

Figure 7.2 (*Continued*)

are derived from plants, are digitalis preparations called *glycoside agents*. Diuretics such as Lasix, and Diuril are commonly used with digitalis, but in some cases when these are combined, a toxic reaction, such as *hypokalemia* (low potassium content in the blood), may result.

Digitalis stimulates the vagus nerves (nerves that lower the heart rate) and increases the strength of the heart beat while reducing its rate. Thus the blood supply to body tissues is improved. Older persons require lower dosages of Digoxin, as compared with young adults to attain therapeutic results.[8] A narrow line exists between positive therapeutic and dangerous dosage. Toxic reactions can be a consequence of inappropriate high Digoxin quantities.[9]

Digitalis preparations are cumulative; that is, they tend to build up in the body. Thus, their ingestion over a period of time can create problems, such as lack of appetite, nausea, weakness, dizziness, and mood disturbances. Digitalis dosages must be periodically monitored and evaluated to ensure the correct prescription and the prevention of adverse reactions

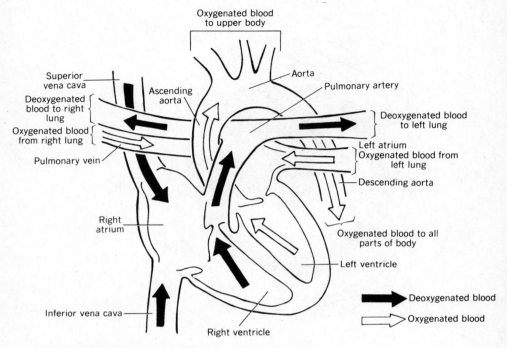

Figure 7.3 Sequence of blood flow through the heart.

when used over extended periods. Casual use of these medications can be risky and should be avoided.

Drugs and the Musculoskeletal System

A number of disorders affect the musculoskeletal system, ranging from simple muscle strains to severe rheumatoid arthritis. Our discussion focuses upon bone and joint medications commonly used by the elderly that affect mobility and locomotion. The universal problems involving bones and joints, which generally increase in severity from maturity to advanced age are generally related to such conditions as bursitis, tendinitis, rheumatoid arthritis, osteoarthritis, and osteoporosis. Each of these ailments limits movement and often generates such pain that physical activity is contra-indicated (at least temporarily) and drug intervention is necessary for the relief of aching, swelling, or inflammation.

Arthritis Medications. Two of the most common types of arthritis, rheumatoid and osteoarthritis, tend to be chronic, with the former, if allowed to progress, leading to joint destruction. Medications and therapeutic modalities offer pain relief (but not a cure) for RA, with some reduction of swelling and deformity. Since RA manifests itself at various levels of severity, a hierarchy of drug therapy from least to greatest toxicity potential is usually administered. The medication procedure begins with an analgesic, such as aspirin (acetylsalicylic acid), and progresses to steroids (corticosteroids), as shown Figure 7.4.

Aspirin is most frequently prescribed as an anti-inflammatory drug. It does reduce pain, and is one of the safest drugs available (when used correctly); however, as a treatment for arthritis it must be taken in large doses regularly, and even though it is considered a common household remedy, type and dose should be prescribed and monitored by a physician. For some people, high doses of aspirin can cause stomach irritation and tinnitus.

Indomethacin (Indocin) and *phenylbutazone* (Butazolidin) are newer anti-inflammatory agents that may relieve symptoms from rheumatoid arthritis, gout, and osteoarthritis. These drugs frequently help younger people with rheumatoid arthritis, but are fully effective in only a small proportion of aged arthritics.[10] Such drugs can be toxic and produce symptoms of headache, dizziness, and nausea. Caution should be observed in prescribing such drugs for individuals who have bleeding problems or cardiac adults on anticoagulants, because of their interference with the formation of blood platelets (which play a major role in blood coagulation). These anti-inflammatory drugs are used for short durations of about five days.

Some dermatologic reactions, such as hives, rash, and oral ulcers may also accompany the use of these drugs. All of these side effects warrant close medical supervision. *Ibuprofin* (Motrin) is rapidly absorbed after oral ingestion, and its side effects are similar to those of other arthritic drugs, although sometimes to a lesser degree.

Naproxen (Naprosyn), *sunlindac* (Clinoril), and *tolmetin* (Tolectin) are also used for rheumatoid and osteoarthritis with varying adverse side effects depending upon the individual's tolerance. These nonsteroids are useful in both long-term treatment and for acute flare-ups.

All of the above drugs work specifically to reduce inflammation, pain, and swelling. Each medication should be carefully supervised. Some individuals may find great arthritic relief, while others may experience such adverse effects that drug ingestion is intolerable.

Gold compounds are used primarily in the treatment of rheumatoid arthritis. Gold salts are usually administered by injection, and their benefits vary from person to person. Adverse side effects include skin rash and

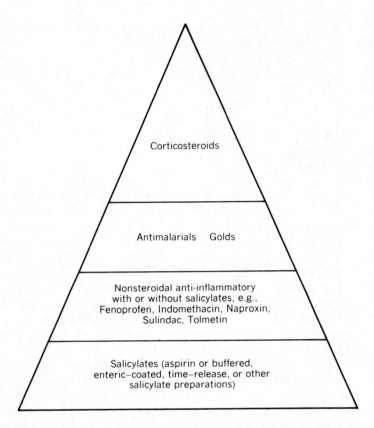

Figure 7.4 Pyramid of therapy for rheumatoid arthritis. (Adapted from E. P. Gall, "Analgesic and Anti-Inflammatory Agents," in K. A. Conrad and R. Bressler, eds., *Drug Therapy for the Elderly* [St. Louis, Mo.: C. V. Mosby, 1982], p. 227. Used with permission.)

irritations to the mucous membranes. Since the probability of toxicity increases with age, all dosages should be individually adjusted, starting with low amounts and increased gradually under careful supervision of a rheumatologist.

Antimalarials, which are derivatives of quinine, such as Atabrine, are used to treat rheumatoid arthritis (in addition to malaria). They are also used in the treatment of other joint and skin disorders. Toxicity levels among older persons can be low, with side effects that can impair vision or cause dizziness, headache, gastrointestinal disorders. Careful follow-up of antimalarial agents should be done to determine the positive benefit, if any, of the drug.

Corticosteroids, or steroid agents, are the most potent anti-inflammatory drugs available. They are also the most toxic, as shown in Figure 7.4. Therefore, their use is particularly discouraged for elderly persons with arthritis.[11] These powerful anti-inflammatory agents should be used only for specific reasons (functional incapacity) and monitored closely.

Such diseases as hypertension, diabetes, and osteoporosis are common among the elderly, and corticosteroids can aggravate these conditions. Steroids have also been implicated in the appearance of acute psychosis in persons of all ages; older adults may develop a chronic dementing syndrome as a result of these drugs.[12] Thus, when the use of steroids is being considered, the benefit/risk ratio should be weighed carefully.

Exercise, Diet, and Diabetes

Diabetes, a common disease of older people, can be controlled by *insulin*—a hormonal substance normally secreted by the pancreas, an organ located near the stomach. Diabetes is associated with obesity and impaired glucose tolerance. A careful balance of diet, insulin, and exercise must be maintained to avoid serious secondary medical problems, such as retinal damage and circulatory disorders.

Diabetes is recognized by the body's inability to use carbohydrates (starches and sugars) in the blood. The loss of the capability of metabolizing carbohydrates may affect people at any age; however, its effects can be more severe in older persons, leading to malnutrition, weakness, and greater susceptibility to infection.

The signs and symptoms of diabetes are: hyperglycemia (high blood sugar), sugar in the urine, frequent urination, increased thirst, craving for sweets, weakness, drowsiness, and, in its extreme state, coma. Fortunately, in many cases, older persons can control their glucose level through diets and exercise. These modalities help to lower blood glucose to tolerable levels; however, moderate to severe diabetics need carefully determined timed dosage regimens of oral hypoglycemic tablets or insulin injections.

Therapeutic Exercise. Two potential problems can develop among diabetics with respect to exercise and physical activity: the hyperglycemic effect and the hypoglycemic effect. *Hypo* results when there is a decrease in glucose in the blood, and *Hyper* occurs when too much glucose is deposited into the circulatory system.

Exercise has an insulin-like consequence; that is, it reduces the sugar content in the system. Thus, prolonged physical activity may cause hypoglycemia unless its intensity and frequency are regulated. It is important to remind the diabetic exercise participant that nourishment in the form of sugar, fruit juice, or some other digestible carbohydrate should be taken in the event of low blood sugar symptoms occur such as weakness, pallor, and mental confusion. On the other hand, not enough exercise and inadequate insulin intake create hyperglycemia, with similar symptoms of weakness, pallor, and, in some cases, unconsciousness.

Shephard believes that activity is a particularly valuable treatment for elderly diabetic patients since as many as 30 percent are unable to understand the simple components of a planned diet.[13] Physical activity consistently on a daily basis is important in the regulation of the body's energy demands.

Dr. Philip Felig of Yale University cautions that acute exercise can intensify hyperglycemia in a poorly regulated diabetic by exaggerating the normal increase in counterregulatory hormones produced through exercise.[14] He advocates careful control of insulin and suggests that diet is probably more important than exercise.

Exercise without control of insulin ingestion and diet can disturb metabolic regulatory mechanisms. Diabetic coma can occur when too much sugar and acetone appear in the blood. Insulin shock may be caused by an overdose of insulin, too much exercise, or too little carbohydrate food. The ultimate responsibility for maintaining correct balance of the modality triad rests with the participant.

Diet Control. Before insulin was discovered, diet and exercise were the only available modes of treating diabetes. Strict adherence to a prescribed diet, with each gram of food carefully weighed and recorded was required. Diet continues to be a principal method of treatment, but the scope and diversity of food allowed the diabetic is broader with recent discoveries of various drugs and expanded knowledge about the disease.

Since late-onset diabetes is a deficiency of carbohydrate metabolism, and because carbohydrates are primary sources of energy, the diabetic must control the amount of carbohydrates the body has to metabolize. Weight should be maintained within a moderate range, avoiding extreme leanness or fatness. Caloric needs recommended for adults by the Academy of Sciences are shown in Table 7.1.

Physically active diabetics require greater numbers of calories than inactive diabetics. Also, prolonged and vigorous types of exercise such as swimming, backpacking, cross-country skiing, and jogging decrease insulin dosage requirements.

It is advisable for older persons with diabetes to include a variety of nutritional foods in their diets, with emphasis upon fruits, vegetables, proteins, and vitamins and minerals. Carbohydrate intake must be carefully balanced with energy consumption. Such foods as sugars, pies, jellies, and

Table 7.1 Recommended Energy Intake for Adults

Age (years)	Energy Needs (with range) (kilocalories)
Males	
23–50	2700 (2300–3100)
51–75	2400 (2000–2800)
76+	2050 (1650–2450)
Females	
23–50	2000 (1600–2400)
51–75	1800 (1400–2200)
76+	1600 (1200–2000)

Source: Food and Nutrition Board, National Academy of Sciences, National Research Council, *Recommended Dietary Allowances,* 9th ed. (Washington, D.C.: 1980).

candies are forbidden. High-fat foods, such as meat, butter, bacon, and lard, should be avoided. Such foods may add to the complications of vascular diseases, which are not uncommon among older diabetics. Dietary management should be tailored to the level of physical activity practice and insulin dosage to compensate for the body's inability to manufacture this vital hormonal compound.

Drugs and Diabetes. As the pancreas grows older, the cells producing insulin frequently fail to yield sufficient insulin, thus causing diabetes. However, even though the prevalence of diabetes increases with age, most older individuals are not diabetic. This disorder of carbohydrate metabolism and impaired glucose tolerance is most likely genetically based since the disease appears to run in families.

The discovery of insulin by the Canadian physicians T. G. Banting and C. W. Best in 1922 allowed those afflicted with diabetes to extend their longevity to normal limits. Although diet continues to be a principal treatment of diabetes, the use of insulin permits the diabetic to eat more of a variety of foods than was allowed previously.

Insulin Therapy. Insulin is given by injection only. It cannot be taken orally because the drug is destroyed by the juices of the digestive process. Insulin is absorbed quickly and stimulates carbohydrate metabolism by facilitating the transport of glucose to the cells, especially sugar deposited in the muscles and fatty tissue.

It can be difficult for a person at any age to accept the fact that daily needle injections and a regulated diet are necessary for survival. Nevertheless, many persons adapt and continue to lead normal and happy lives.

The use of insulin by elderly persons requires careful monitoring. With older people, blood flow to the brain, which contains neural regulators of glucose concentrations (hypothalamus), is not as efficient as it is in young adults in keeping glucose within tolerable levels. Thus, the risk of insulin-induced hypoglycemia is higher in older persons. For this reason, blood glucose concentrations should be kept higher in elderly patients.[15]

Careful attention to foot care is especially important for the elderly diabetic because of the corresponding vascular problems that often accompany foot infections and injuries. In some cases, poor vision, arthritis, or memory problems mean that injections should be administered by another person. Such problems require decisions made in collaboration with family members, support staff and the physician.

Oral Antidiabetic Agents. Most diabetes discovered after 65 can be controlled with diet and oral medications known as *hypoglycemic agents.* These drugs are sulfonylureas commonly identified as Orinase, Diabenese, Dymelor, and Tolinase. Such nonhormonal synthetic drugs are chiefly used in the treatment of older diabetics. These medications are not usually recommended for young persons or severe cases of diabetes. A sulfonylurea tends to increase the release of endogenous insulin (originating within the pancreas), subsequently lowering the blood sugar level.

Orinase (tolbutamide) is widely used in the United States, and, when administered properly, it is helpful for the control of mild diabetes. Side effects may include dizziness, nausea, and other gastric disturbances. Aspirin, anticoagulants, and certain anti-inflammatory drugs increase the action of Orinase and the risk of a hypoglycemic reaction. Thus caution is advised when such drugs are taken concurrently.

Diabinese (chlorpropamide) is similar to Orinase; however, its duration of action is longer—up to 36 hours as compared to about 5 hours for Orinase. Because of strength and longer duration, it has a greater potential for causing hypoglycemia and should be carefully monitored, especially during early trial periods. Diabinese is occasionally associated with jaundice, and low blood sugar may appear among individuals who do not eat regularly or exercise without adequate caloric and nutritional intake. Care should also be taken when individuals are using tranquilizers, sedatives, and sleep-inducing drugs, as Diabinese increases the effect of sedatives and hypnotics by slowing their elimination from the body.

Dymelor (acetohexamide) is used in mild forms of adult diabetes. This drug also works to stimulate the secretion of insulin from the pancreas and has an effective action of up to 24 hours. In some cases, gastrointestinal disturbances, rash, and jaundice may appear as side effects. Individuals with allergic reactions or impaired liver or kidney function are advised not to take this drug. Elderly persons over 60 usually require smaller doses, and they should be carefully observed for signs of hypoglycemia, particularly if the compound is used over a long period of time.

Tolinase (tolazamide) has an effective action time of up to 16 hours. The action of this drug is similar to that of the other oral antidiabetic compounds, with possible side effects of low blood sugar, rash, and kidney and liver disorders. Tolinase may increase the effects of sedatives and other sleep-inducing drugs by slowing their elimination from the body. Alcohol should be taken with discretion when using this drug.

Oral hypoglycemic agents allow the patient to avoid hyperdermic injections. However, a regimen of drug oral intake requires persistent attention to correct dose and development of probable side effects. Since older persons are generally on different medications in addition, other health problems can arise. Regularity of diet, exercise, and drug use is essential in order to maximize the beneficial effects of oral sulfonylurea drugs.

Physically active adults particularly need to guard against hypoglycemia since exercise produces insulin's effect of lowering blood sugar. Each diabetic is different in terms of quality and magnitude of response. Careful records should be maintained with close coordination among the user, physician, and fitness specialist to ensure the health and safety of the older diabetic adult.

Drugs and the Mind

Like other illnesses, mental disorders become more prevalent with each passing decade after maturity. Adapting to multiple physical, psychological, and social changes creates tensions that place undue mental stresses upon the senior adult. Such events as loss of spouse, medical illness, retirement, and the onset of financial worries increase the probability of cognitive with psychotic ailments, from mild forms of memory loss to severe dementia.

In aging, the ability to cope with random stresses declines, as the energy resources to maintain homeostasis (biological equilibrium) diminish. For example, the self-reliant independent person with high self-esteem who becomes ill but attempts to fight the illness by denying its existence, may give up, after a few weeks of futility and withdraw, become dependent, and fall into greater depression.

The senior who can adjust or adapt to his or her decline in energy is best able to neutralize the stressors that interfere with the ability to successfully function within the environment. For example, a previously active and productive businessperson or homemaker, because of retirement, widowhood, or disability, may redirect energy in productive ways, such as involvement in church, community, or grandchildren. This pattern of living channels the retiree towards others and away from self, as well as allowing a healthy continuation of energy flow in a less demanding manner, commensurate with the normal age changes. Mind-affecting drug intervention enters the life of the elder citizen when natural coping mechanisms break down, with the possibility of serious psychological illness emerging.

Drugs and Depression. Short bouts of depression are common among the elderly and account for about 25 percent of suicides among the elderly.[16] White males in their 80s are at highest risk.

Depression is a condition of excessive emotional dejection and withdrawal characterized by sadness usually prolonged over an extended period of time. Factors that increase the perils of depression are poor health, divorce, loss of a spouse, loneliness, and alcoholism. Each of these states can breed isolation and poor physical fitness which hastens the course of serious depression. Staying active physically and mentally is perhaps the best preventive medicine against depression. This implies staying involved with family and friends and maintaining a lifestyle that includes correct nutrition and sensible physical exercise.

The major types of depression are grouped into *acute* and *chronic* categories. Acute depression is generally short-lived. It may follow the death of a loved one, last about six weeks, and be followed by reemergence into more normal behavioral responses. Chronic depressions can last for years. For example, the energetic executive who slows down after retirement has lost something of value to him—his position and status—and his slow-down is not the result of old age, but a depressive response.

Acute depression, as in the case of losing a loved one, can be quite normal and is amenable to treatment, whereas chronic depression is serious and far more difficult to remedy. Since depression is associated with personal and environmental losses in life, the elderly are vulnerable because this is a time of change and decline in physical stamina, income, death of spouse, living accommodations, etc.

The following characteristics are often signs of depression:

1. Change in sleep habits (insomnia).
2. Feelings of lack of worth—poor self-image.
3. Loss of appetite and weight.
4. Loss of libido.
5. Undue fatigue—tiredness without apparent cause.
6. Lack of concern about personal appearance.
7. Excessive alcohol use.
8. Self-blame and guilt complexes about past failures.
9. Distinct changes in mood, with sadness, apathy, and loneliness.

Mild forms of depression are often treated successfully by increasing support of understanding family and friends; however severe depression requires intervention by a physician, and medication depending upon the type and severity of the condition.

The following section deals with several major drugs used for depressive states. Two principal drug groups are used for depression: antidepressants, including tricyclics such as Tofranil, Elavil, Sinequan, and Norpramin, and monoamine oxidase inhibitors such as Marplan and Parnate; and antianxiety agents, such as, barbiturates (e.g., Phenobarbital), Librium, Valium, Mellaril, Thorazine, and Compazine. Table 7.2 presents salient features of each of these above drugs.

Tricyclic Antidepressants. These drugs produce a sedating effect with few side effects. Elavil, Tofranil, and Sinequan are common and fairly effective in treating depression. As is the case with all drugs administered to persons past 60, small doses should be given and carefully monitored by the physician until the individual's tolerance level is established. These drugs should be used cautiously, not administered casually when relief may be gained through human and moral support.

Antidepressants can cause a wide variety of side effects, such as dry mouth, blurred vision, loss of appetite, insomnia, and headache. Elavil should be used judiciously in the presence of cardiovascular disease because of probable induced hypotension and heart rhythm disruptions.

Monamine Oxidase Inhibitors (MOAI). This group of antidepressants was the first class of drugs used for depression; however, due to their many side effects and adverse effects in conjunction with foods and other drugs, usage has decreased. In certain cases they can cause blood pressure disturbances, such as hypotension, as well as insomnia, nausea, dizziness, urinary problems, and constipation. Because of their high toxic risk, MOAI should be used only in hospitalized patients where food and drug consumption are carefully regulated.

Antianxiety Agents. Anxiety is a common state of persons of all ages. It can be characterized as an unpleasant emotional state associated with feelings of apprehension and uncertainty. Such feelings can have real or imaginary causes. Real anxiety is precipitated when actual danger threatens the individual, whereas imaginary anxiety is caused by an illusory menace or distress. Although the causes of anxiety may be real or unreal, symptoms that follow this disorder are similar. All of us experience normal periodic anxiety; however, when the condition is excessive, that is prolonged over an extended time period, drug intervention may be indicated.

Life experiences that trigger anxiety are individualistic and greatly

Table 7.2 Principal Drugs Used for Depression

Drug	Type	Classification	Effect
Barbiturates, e.g., Phenobarbital	Antianxiety	Minor tranquilizer	Sedative; sleep-inducing
Valium	Antianxiety	Minor tranquilizer	Muscle relaxant; reduces tension; sedative
Librium	Antianxiety	Minor tranquilizer	Reduces fears and anxiety; used in simple and severe forms
Tofranil	Antidepressant	Tricyclic	Improves mood and relieves emotional depression
Elavil	Antidepressant	Tricyclic	Calming effect; drowsiness; mood improvement similar to Tofranil
Norpramin	Antidepressant	Tricyclic	Quick relief for psychogenic depression; effect similar to Tofranil and Elavil
Thorazine	Antipsychotic	Major tranquilizer	Restores emotional calm; relieves severe anxiety, unrest, and psychotic behavior
Mellaril	Antipsychotic	Major tranquilizer	Strong tranquilizer; effects similar to Thorazine
Compazine	Antipsychotic	Major tranquilizer	Strong tranquilizer; used for acute or chronic schizophrenia
Marplan	Antidepressant	Monoamine oxidase inhibitor	Used for moderate and severe depression; greater potential for side effects than tricyclic antidepressants; used in hospital setting
Parnate	Antidepressant	Monoamine oxidase inhibitor	Used for various depressive states; has many contraindications; used in hospital setting
Sinequan	Antidepressant	Tricyclic	Used for depressed and anxiety states; well tolerated by geriatric patients; improves mood and emotional disturbances

diversified. Anxiety can be aroused by small, inconsequential episodes, such as missing a bus, or by more serious events, such as loss of position, forced retirement, and illness. Whatever the cause, anxiety can produce multiple mental and physical disturbances including fast heart rate, increased blood pressure, nausea, vomiting, excessive perspiration, dilated pupils, diarrhea, insomnia, muscular tension, rapid breathing, and overactivity.

Equanil (meprobamate) is a mild tranquilizer that is widely available. Although this drug relieves temperate cases of anxiety, the danger of overdose is possible, particularly with older people. The elderly are highly susceptible to normal standard doses; and ingestion can cause lightheadedness, weakness, and confusion. This drug may impair alertness, mental judgment, and reaction time, and should not be taken when operating machinery or driving a vehicle.

Valium and Librium (benzodiazepines) are among the most common antianxiety tranquilizers for mild chronic tension. These drugs have been shown to be safer and more effective than barbiturates in the control of anxiety.[17] They often are prescribed as preoperative tranquilizers for those individuals who are particularly nervous and tense before surgery.

The sedating effects of benzodiazepines means they also serve as muscle relaxants. Although these agents are helpful in acute and chronic anxiety cases, their potential for misuse and abuse is high. Overdose can cause oversedation, dizziness, and undue postural hypotension. Other side effects of Valium and Librium include confusion, nausea, skin rashes, decreased libido, and hallucinations. Continued use can result in mental and physical dependence, and withdrawal from these drugs can entail severe adverse effects. Their sedative-hypnotic properties accumulate in the body, and multiple daily dosages are usually inappropriate for the elderly.[18]

The major tranquilizers, Thorazine, Mellaril, and Compazine are potent antipsychotic agents that should be used only when absolutely necessary because of undesirable side effects. Extreme pain or fear, combative and hostile actions, delirium, delusions, or hallucinations may warrant the use of these drugs. In some cases, the individual may feel "drugged" or "spaced out" after usage. Such agents have been known to produce tremors, body "plucking movements," drooling, confusion, and strange facial expressions. In addition, these agents can be particularly dangerous to the older person because they may cause falls, resulting in fractures of hip, skull, ribs, etc. The benefits of such drugs must be carefully weighed against their risk.

Barbiturates are used for sedation and anxiety states. Their hypnotic effects induce sleep. The high incidence of addiction and excessive drowsiness make them poor choices for older people. Moderate doses of barbiturates can produce results similar to alcohol intoxication: impaired speech, staggering, and disorientation.[19] Overdose of these drugs can result in death, and mixing with alcohol is dangerous since these drugs reinforce each other in sedation.

Drugs and Parkinson's Disease

Parkinsonism, also called paralysis agitans, is a disease of the nervous system. It is seen almost exclusively after the age of 65. The characteristic symptoms are hand tremors, small steps in walking, shaking head, and shuffling gait. The face usually lacks expression. All of these mannerisms can cause extreme embarrassment to the victim and further exacerbate a depressive state that may already rexist. Older persons normally have higher resting muscle electrical activity than younger persons; however, palsy patients have even higher rates.

The Parkinson's sufferer's intelligence usually is not affected, although mood swings and depression can occur. If mental deterioration does happen, it develops late and in severe stages of the disease. Parkinsonism results from too little dopamine (amino acid that provides an inhibiting effect in motor movement) and too much acetylcholine (cholinergic that exerts a facilitatory effect on motor movement); i.e., a biochemical imbalance in the brain which affects smooth motor movements.

Two important antiparkinsonian agents used are: dopaminergics (Levodopa), and anticholinergics (Artane and Symmetrel). Antihistamines (Benadryl) are also used, as these have some anticholinergic properties; however, they are not as effective as anticholinergics for most cases.[20]

The drugs used to relieve the symptoms work by replenishing dopamine with Levodopa and by blocking the cholinergic receptors with Artane or symmetral agents. Dopaminergics and anticholinergics may be used alone or in combination depending upon the severity of the disease and individual reactions. Although these drugs help to restore the biochemical balance of dopamine and acetylcholine, they afford only relief, not a cure.

In addition to drug therapy, exercise and rhythmic activities are essential for maintaining coordination, balance, and equilibrium, and muscle tone—all of which slowly deteriorate as the disease progresses. Several suggested activities are discussed in the final section of this chapter.

Although Levodopa dramatically relieves tremor and abnormally slow movements in some individuals, side effects of nausea and loss of appetite are not uncommon. Other adverse consequences include dizziness, cardiac arrhythmias, and emotional disturbances such as restlessness, anxiety, irritability, insomnia, and hallucinations. As with all drugs, the dosage of antiparkinsonian agents should start at the lowest effective level and be regularly adjusted according to the person's tolerance level. In addition, close scrutiny must be given other medications prescribed. For example,

Marplan and Parnate (MOAI) interfere with the metabolism of Dopamine, and may cause severe hypertension in conjunction with Levodopa. Careful prescription and monitoring are crucial.

Organic Brain Syndromes (OBS)

Organic brain syndromes refer to a group of mental diseases that impair brain function. OBS may be acute and reversible, or chronic and irreversible. The former type is usually associated with some physical illness or acute physiological disturbance. Cardiac, nutritional, and cerebrovascular disorders, together with alcohol and drug ingestion, account for most acute brain syndromes in the older group.[21] These disorders usually impair memory and intellectual functioning, including comprehension and judgment. Acute syndromes of short duration that are related to a particular physical ailment can be successfully treated with drugs and psychotherapy.

On the other hand, chronic syndromes are characterized by a slow and gradual onset of impaired memory and intellectual deterioration. Two of the most common conditions producing chronic brain syndromes in the aged are senile brain disease and arteriosclerotic brain disease (hardening of the arteries in the brain).

One of the most puzzling brain diseases, whose victims occupy up to 50 percent of nursing home beds, is Alzheimer's disease (AD). This form of dementia is also referred to as "presenile dementia" because it may strike individuals in their 50s. Diagnosis is difficult since symptoms of AD are also found among persons in states of depression.

However, when other forms of brain dysfunctions are excluded, AD is suspected in the presence of such signs as slow loss of memory, language disturbances, difficult in comprehension, and disorientation—all increasing in severity as the disease progresses.

Alzheimer's disease is anatomically characterized by loss of brain cells and neuronal degeneration. Senile plaques (patches of flat substances between neurons) and neurofibrillary tangles appear throughout the cortex of the brain. Thus AD is due primarily to tissue degeneration, but its cause remains unknown.

Drug therapy has been focused on: (1) compounds that attempt to improve brain function, and (2) substances that facilitate increased oxygen to the brain cells. *Hydergine,* a compound derived from ergot, has been used to increase biochemical neural transmission. Results have shown a modest improvement in alertness and confusion states.[22] A drug called *Lecithin* (a phosphatidyl choline used to increase cholinergic brain activity), has shown no statistical positive consequences. *Vasodilators* such as Papaverine, meant to increase blood flow—and theoretically improve oxygen supply to the brain—also have been tried in demented elderly without satisfactory results.[23]

The use of *hyperbaric oxygen* in elderly OBS patients was tested under the theory that brain cells in the cortex were not receiving enough oxygen. Jacobsen et al. treated OBS elderly patients afflicted with cognitive deficits using 90 minutes of 100 percent oxygen exposure twice daily for 15 consecutive days.[24] Her studies showed significant improvement in memory (short-term retention and recall) among patients with histories and symptoms of chronic OBS, a majority of whom had been in the hospital for many months. Edwards et al. also found cognitive improvement after using hyperbaric oxygen among a group of men and women outpatients who had exhibited memory lapses, some inability to attend to problems, and slight confusion regarding time and place.[25] On the other hand, other researchers have found hyperbaric oxygenation to be of no value.[26] These conflicting findings point out the individualistic characteristics of the disease and accent the need for further research about oxygen and its effects upon the brain.

Antipsychotic and sedative drugs used to suppress OBS symptoms must be employed with caution since these chemical compounds can cause toxic reactions and further mental deterioration. Overmedication often results in hospitalization for illnesses that are really drug side effects.

Greater attention must be directed toward natural means of stimulating brain function; i.e., by creating a living environment that keeps people out of bed, active, and in touch with reality. Physical and sensory stimulation of the remaining cognitive and emotional abilities of the individual should be accented. Such modalities as art, music, rhythmic activities, exercise, and movement therapy can sometimes help to counter further mental deterioration and the malaise of greater dependence.

Caffeine, Tobacco, and Alcohol

Each of these substances has one central common characteristic—potential addiction. However, all persons using these drugs will not become addicts. Addiction may develop slowly, depending upon the individualistic nature of the user and his or her surrounding environmental lifestyle. This discussion focuses upon the health-fitness concerns that particularly affect the older citizen.

Caffeine. The popular beverages coffee, tea, cocoa, and colas all contain caffeine, which acts as a powerful stimulant on the central nervous system. Caffeine is one of three *xanthine* drugs—the other two are *theophylline* and *theobromine*.

Does the ingestion of these beverages pose any health problems for senior adults? These stimulants have been linked with heart attacks, strokes, hypertension, anxiety, gastric disturbances, and a variety of other conditions, including cancer of the pancreas, breast, and bladder. The incidence of these health problems does increase with age, but whether caffeine is a major cause remains questionable. Perhaps the principal risk of the drug for older persons pertains to its effect of stimulating the vasomotor center in the medulla (lower part of the brain stem), which induces peripheral vasoconstriction and a rise in blood pressure, increase in heart rate, and disruption in heart rhythm.

Most people can tolerate moderate amounts of caffeine. However, in sensitive people and in others who consume excessive amounts of coffee and tea, caffeine can endanger cardiovascular functions and contribute to hypertension and cardiac arrhythmias. The approximate caffeine content of popular beverages is shown in Table 7.3.

Caffeine constricts the cerebral blood vessels and dilates peripheral vessel walls. However, the decreased peripheral vascular resistance is offset by an increase in heart rate and cardiac output induced by the drug's stimulation of the vasomotor center in the brain—thus resulting in a rise in blood pressure. Most people with high blood pressure or a tendency toward higher rates would be wise to avoid beverages containing caffeine; this means shunning regular coffee when systolic and diastolic pressure approaches 150 (systolic)/90 (diastolic).

Caffeine is related to anxiety and insomnia because it increases adrenalin, in addition to contributing to higher blood pressure and irregular heartbeat. Many older adults experience wakeful nights. A study of sleep patterns of older men and women, using electroencephalographic measurement methods, showed that older individuals exhibited more frequent and prolonged awakenings and shorter sleep stage periods than did younger peo-

Table 7.3   Approximate Caffeine Content of Popular Beverages

Beverage		*Caffeine*
Regular coffee	(average cup)	100–150 mg.
Instant coffee	(average cup)	80–100 mg.
Coffee-grain blends	(average cup)	14–37 mg.
Decaffeinated coffee	(average cup)	3–5 mg.
Tea	(average cup)	60–75 mg.
Regular cola	(6 ounces)	36 mg.
Diet cola	(6 ounces)	18 mg.
Cocoa	(6 ounces)	10 mg.

Source: The Essential Guide to Prescription Drugs (p. 103), Third Edition, by James W. Long, M.D. Copyright © 1982 by James W. Long. Reprinted by permission of Harper & Row, Publishers, Inc.

ple.[27] Caffeine adds to the dilemma by increasing nervousness, restlessness, and breathing rate, all of which reinforce wakefulness. Since caffeine is one of the xanthines, it is also classified as a diuretic, and, as such, can disturb sleep patterns of the elderly by causing frequent nocturnal urinary calls. Consuming caffeine beverages also often leads to dependence; when caffeine is cut out, withdrawal symptoms are evidenced by severe headaches and lethargy. Thus, although the drug enhances alertness, stimulates the brain and delays fatigue, these effects are hardly worth the risk of exacerbating high blood pressure, anxiety, sleeplessness, and arrhythmias—conditions that are common among the elderly.

Tobacco. The comprehensive U.S. Surgeon's Report on Smoking and Health released in 1979 firmly established the deleterious effects of smoking upon mortality and morbidity. The report documents the following links between cigarette smoking and death and disabling diseases:

MORTALITY

- Mortality increases with amount smoked. Two-pack-a-day male smokers have a mortality ratio two times that of nonsmokers.
- Overall mortality ratios are proportional to duration of cigarette smoking—the longer one smokes, the greater the risk of dying.
- Overall mortality ratios increase with the tar and nicotine content of the cigarette.
- Female dose-responses (quantity, age at initiation, duration of smoking, inhalation, tar and nicotine content) are the same as those for male cigarette smokers.

MORBIDITY

- Smoking cigarettes is a major risk factor for arteriosclerotic and peripheral vascular disease.
- Smoking increases the possibility of heart attack recurrence among survivors of myocardial infarction.
- Cigarette smoking increases appreciably the risk of peripheral vascular disease in diabetes mellitus.
- Smoking is causally related to coronary heart disease for men and women in the United States.
- Smoking is causally related to lung cancer in both men and women.
- Cigarette smoking is a significant causative factor in the development of cancer of the larynx in men and women.
- Adult cigarette smokers have respiratory symptoms more frequently than do nonsmokers (i.e., cough and sputum production increase with greater dosage of cigarettes).

- Cigarette smokers have a higher prevalence of chronic bronchitis emphysema than do nonsmokers, as well as an increased chance of dying from these diseases compared to nonsmokers.[28]

It is clear from this list that tobacco use, particularly cigarette smoking, represents a powerful menace to health. Yet despite the facts, and the warning "The Surgeon General Has Determined That Cigarette Smoking Is Dangerous to Your Health" on each pack of cigarettes, tobacco is still used by one out of three adults in the United States.[29]

Smoking is a complex act involving varied human physiological responses caused by the pharmacologic compounds found in tobacco and the psychosocial milieu surrounding the individual. Approximately 4000 compounds are found in cigarette smoke. Many of these compounds serve as pharmacological reinforcers and facilitate the establishment of the smoking habit. A pack-a-day smoker takes more than 50,000 puffs per year, and each puff delivers a risk assortment of chemicals into the lungs and bloodstream. Secondary smoking habit reinforcers include psychosocial ingredients, such as sight and smell of cigarettes, the milieu and ambience of a meal, a cup of coffee, or a cocktail—all of which bring pleasure to many people.

The nicotine, tar, and carbon monoxide found in tobacco have been identified as the compounds most harmful to health. *Nicotine* is a powerful stimulant on the nervous system. It also releases body chemicals such as catecholamines and epinephrine that cause increases in heart rate, blood pressure, arrhythmia, and vasoconstriction. The combined result of increasing heart rate and constriction of blood vessels is especially hazardous to older adults, many of whom already manifest higher blood pressure readings.

Tar is the sticky dark brown mass produced when the tobacco is burned. A chemical agent known as *polycyclic aromatic hydrocarbon* is generally blamed for a substantial portion of the carcinogenic activity of tar. The incidence of lung cancer, and of a host of chronic bronchial diseases, is significantly higher among smokers of cigarettes with elevated levels of tar content. Tar is an irritant to bronchial tissues and is one cause of the "smoker's cough" characterized by increased mucus, sputum, and congestion. Irritants affect the action of bronchial cilia responsible for expelling the mucus. Tar and other substances found in tobacco smoke first slow, then stop, ciliary action and eventually destroy the cilia, thus exposing the delicate membrane to possible tumor growth.

Older persons in general are more susceptible to lung infections such as bronchitis and pneumonia. Prevention of lung disability from chronic bronchitis and many other pulmonary diseases depend upon early detection and on cessation of smoking.

Carbon monoxide (CO) is the third substance that produces acute pharmacologic reactions upon the body. Carbon dioxide, which has 230 times the affinity of oxygen for hemoglobin, impairs the oxygen-carrying capacity of the blood, and can result in a condition called carboxyhemoglobinemia (union of CO with hemoglobin). Some evidence suggests that when CO is combined with nicotine, catecholamines (autonomic nervous system agents causing vasoconstriction of peripheral blood vessels) are released, enhancing the risk of cardiovascular disease.[30] Carbon monoxide has a depressive effect upon ventilation and the ability of the blood to use oxygen (a basic requirement for endurance-type activities).

Some evidence shows that low levels of CO in the blood are associated with impaired performance of psychomotor tasks when perception and reaction response to a stimuli is required in such skills as driving. However, it is unclear whether this factor is responsible alone, or only in combination with other variables such as fatigue and faulty vision and hearing.[31]

CO and other chemicals in tobacco clearly pollute the cardiovascular and pulmonary system. Therefore every person, irrespective of age, should be encouraged to avoid smoking.

Alcohol. A central consideration about alcohol and the elderly relates not to its use, but to its abuse. The temperate use of alcohol (no more than one or two drinks per day) probably presents no significant health risk to typical healthy senior adult (other than adding more calories to daily food intake). This is not to condone the use of alcohol, since the human organism can survive biologically and psychosocially very well without its consumption. The real perils lie in the potential risks of dependence and addiction, which, without question, shorten longevity and cause an endless list of cognitive and physical disorders.

Although the reasons why people drink are debatable, several possible explanations for excessive alcohol use among the elderly include:

- Boredom, habit, attendance at many cocktail parties.
- Loneliness, minimum contact with other people (family or friends).
- Loss of a spouse, relative, or close friend; stress; and daily strains of living.
- Financial exigencies and insecurity.
- Medical problems; relief of pain and discomfort.
- Loss of esteem and self-worth related to retirement.

This list is not exhaustive, but it does point out that some individuals, for biological or psychological reasons, resort to alcohol use as a coping mechanism for the relief of stress or to satisfy hedonistic wishes.

At the outset, it should be stated that alcoholism is less frequent among the elderly than among the young (although this may be partly due to the fact that many problem drinkers do not survive to old age). Those elderly who drink moderately are more socially active and perceive themselves as healthy individuals.[32] This perception probably can be attributed to the integration of drinking as part of an active social life, reflection of pleasure, and the ability to cope with the effects of alcohol. Heavy drinking is uncommon among men and women past 70.

The majority of those who abstain in late life stopped drinking after the age of 45.[33] Busse and Blazer reported the findings of drinking behavior patterns of 695 persons living in high-rise apartments, nursing homes, and domiciliary settings.[34] This investigation showed that among the 55-to-69 age group (young old), the rate of problem drinking was 22 percent; among individuals 70 years and older, 4 percent were problem cases. The older problem drinker was typically single, divorced or separated, socially inactive, underemployed, and male. These findings reinforce the premise that lonely and socially inactive individuals are vulnerable to alcohol abuse.

Alcohol is used in some nursing homes and other senior settings as a therapeutic agent. The values attributed to spirits such as wine and cocktails are associated with improving the social atmosphere, stimulating appetite, and relieving tension. However, such practices should be carefully weighed because of the diverse biological and psychological characteristics of older persons. Some elderly persons are vulnerable to alcohol dependence and addiction, while others may be under prescriptive psychotropic drugs or have alcoholic histories which demand absolute abstention. Activity directors in senior settings should provide alternate activities and programs to the daily or weekly "cocktail hour" in order to safeguard the health of high-risk seniors.

Although alcohol patterns range from taking an occasional drink at a ceremony or special event to chronic alcoholism, gradual steps do not necessarily follow in progressive order. Some individuals can maintain a pattern of infrequent drinking, while others do become dependent upon its use. The National Council on Alcoholism has set forth the following criteria for diagnosing alcoholism:

- Drinking a fifth of whiskey a day or its equivalent in wine or beer, for a 180-lb. person.
- Alcoholic blackouts.
- Withdrawal syndrome—gross tremor, hallucinosis, convulsions, or delirium tremens (DTs).
- Blood alcohol level about 150 mg/100 ml. without apparent intoxication.
- Continued drinking despite medical advice or family or job problems clearly caused by drinking.[35]

The majority of elderly persons use medications of one kind or another, such as the drugs for cardiovascular diseases, arthritis, diabetes, and depression discussed earlier in this chapter. The interaction of alcohol and certain drugs can produce serious consequences and sometimes death. For example, when taken with barbiturates, alcohol may cause a variety of neurological disturbances, such as dizziness, incoordination, loss of balance, staggering gait, and excessive drowsiness. Table 7.4 lists several common drugs used by older persons and their possible interactions with alcohol.

Many other drugs contain ingredients that may interact with alcohol and cause adverse effects. Aspirin taken in conjunction with alcohol can cause gastric irritation and metabolic and blood clotting disorders. The prudent senior adult should be aware of the effects of prescribed medications and their interactions with alcohol. Alcohol abuse can lead to serious forms of nutritional deficiencies and organic brain diseases; but when alcohol is used in moderation, without disqualifying medications, it may provide some positive therapeutic value.

IMPLICATIONS FOR FITNESS PROGRAMS

Drugs alter body functions. Thus the question arises, Should a senior adult partake in physical activity when under medication for cardiovascular disease, arthritis, diabetes mellitus, depression, or organic brain disorders? In

Table 7.4   Alcohol and Interactions with Other Drugs

Alcohol taken with	Possible Interactions
Barbiturates	Incoordination, dizziness, loss of balance, staggering gait, drowsiness and disorientation, and general oversedation; can be fatal
Tranquilizers	Increased sedative results of tranquilizer and intoxicating effects of alcohol
Antidepressants and Antianxiety Agents	Exaggerated effects of antidepressant and antianxiety agents; further depression of central nervous sytem and oversedation
Antidiabetic Agents	Interference with metabolism of insulin or oral antidiabetic agents, reducing their effectiveness and resulting in hypoglycemia
Anticoagulant Agents	Reduced metabolism of the anticoagulant, leading to increased blood thinning effect with danger of hemorrhage
Antihistamines	Oversedation and central nervous system depression
Antibiotics	Reduced anti-infective ability of the agent

most cases, the answer is a resounding yes. Movement and exercise are essential for all living organisms, and when used appropriately in accordance to the specific needs of the individual for specific purposes to improve or ameliorate a medical problem can hasten the healing process or retard the deteriorating effects of the many disorders affecting the elderly.

When the senior adult is taking one or more drugs, it is essential to regulate the type, intensity, duration, and frequency of activity. For example, individuals with diabetes must carefully balance each exercise variable with insulin or oral agents to avoid insulin shock. Persons taking anticoagulants such as Coumadin should avoid environmental conditions that present a danger of bruising tissues and activities that could cause injury and result in excessive bleeding. The next section deals with program suggestions with a focus upon drug medications commonly used by senior adults.

Fitness Activities and Cardiovascular Drug Therapy

Before any program of physical activity or exercise is pursued, program directors *must* have a properly completed informed consent form and physician approval form (similar to those shown in Figure 5.5 and Appendix D). Such release and approval forms are essential for the safety of the participant, as well as for the legal protection of those individuals involved in the conduct of the program. No persons under prescriptive drug treatment should be allowed to participate in exercise programs without their physicians' approval. In certain cases, individuals using cardiovascular disease medications should not engage in exercise programs. Those with such conditions as severe aortic stenosis, dangerous arrhythmias, or congestive heart conditions fall in this category. Thus, careful medical evaluation by the physician is crucial before establishing a program of exercise prescription.

Antianginal Drugs and Exercise. Nitrates such as nitroglycerin and beta-blocking agents may cause excessive drops in blood pressure. Such conditions can cause unexpected dizziness, lethargy, and fatigue. These symptoms also reflect inadequate blood flow (oxygen) to the brain. The alert fitness instructor should be aware of participants using these drugs and the possibility of fainting or dizziness spells. Prolonged standing, heavy exercise, and exertion should be avoided. Carefully determined progressive rates and intensity of exercise should be approved by the physician and monitored regularly. Exercise modes such as walk/jog and the stationary bicycle, using target exercise rates described earlier, provide an excellent way to regulate the intensity of the activity workload.

Antihypertensive Agents and Exercise. As indicated earlier, vasodilators and adrenergic blocking agents are used for the relief of hypertension. These drugs lower blood pressure by relaxing blood vessels, altering excitation responses to the heart, or relieving excess body fluid. Systematic exercise also tends to lower blood pressure; therefore, careful attention needs to be given to the intensity and duration of the exercising pattern to avoid abnormally lower blood pressure.

Adults under medications should follow carefully planned regimens using heart rate target exercise modes. Exercise routines should begin with a 5- to 10-minute warm-up and end with a similar cool-down phase to allow for natural and gradual blood pressure adjustments. Since isometric exercise tends to increase blood pressure more than do isotonic exercises, it is advisable for hypertensive individuals under medication to avoid static exercise and, instead, to engage in dynamic modes such as walking, jogging, bicycling, or swimming.

Antiarrhythmic Agents and Exercise. Individuals using antiarrhythmic drugs also must be constantly monitored. Exercise activity may be contraindicated depending upon the nature and severity of the dysfunction. Activity regimens should be meticulously prescribed with specific instructions regarding intensity and duration. Exercise involving isometric work is inadvisable because of its interference with blood flow and the probability of inducing serious ventricular arrhythmias or ischemia. Fitness specialists should be alert to the probable toxic side effects of Quinidine and Lidocaine, which include nausea, dizziness, headaches, and drowsiness.

Anticoagulant Agents and Exercise. These agents exhibit hemorrhage as a possible side effect. The risk of bleeding while on Heparin increases with age, particularly in women.[36] Mild exercises, accenting flexibility and muscle toning without heavy exertion, are preferred. Exercise and equipment areas should be free of obstructions and collision hazards that can cause bruising and skin cuts. Although seniors should be encouraged to participate in sport activities of their choice, individual activities such as walking, jogging, stationary bicycling, swimming, and bowling are recommended since these are less likely to result in falls and collisions.

Digitalis and Exercise. Any exercise regimen for adults using digitalis preparations must be specifically approved by the senior adult's physician since these agents are used for serious cardiomyopathy and certain types of arrhythmias. Vigorous and sustained physical exercise is contraindicated. Low-gear, mild forms of dynamic movement, such as walking and slow stretching movements to maintain sufficient levels of physical energy and mobility for daily living tasks and leisure activities, are advisable. Heavy weight lifting and static exercises should be avoided since these types of activities can exacerbate an already weakened heart. Digitalis, especially when combined with a diuretic, can produce side effects of nausea, low body potassium content, and, in some cases, mental confusion.

Fitness Activities and Arthritic Drugs

It was pointed out earlier that the principal goal of the various drugs used for osteoarthritis and rheumatoid arthritis is to relieve pain, swelling, and deformity. The toxic effects of arthritic drugs increase in progressive order (see Figure 7.4) from simple aspirin to corticosteroids. The steroids, such as cortisone, are powerful anti-inflammatory drugs that can bring about dramatic reduction of pain and inflammation; however, if taken in high daily doses over long periods of time, they can cause a variety of side effects including swollen ankles, weight gain, and gastrointestinal disturbances. These drugs can be particularly damaging when used in conjunction with hypertensive antidiabetic medications. The key to success with arthritis medications is to find a balanced mix of appropriate drugs, dosage, exercise, and rest.

The blend of these elements depends upon the individual's tolerance to a particular drug, the specific nature of the arthritic condition, and its severity. Chapter 6 contains specific protocols ranging from passive to active-resistive exercises; the activities that foster greater range of joint motion, such as static stretching and swimming, are advisable.

Fitness Activities and Antidiabetic Drugs

Diabetics can participate in most sports and physical activities unless other medical problems prohibit involvement. The proper mix of insulin, diet, and exercise is necessary to avoid the consequences of insulin shock or diabetic coma.

Special precautions with footwear and for the avoidance of sores or skin infections should be taken, particularly for those exercise participants who walk or jog daily. Most experienced diabetics do not always change their insulin doses with exercise but increase their food intake instead; however, the insulin-dependent diabetic who starts an exercise program should first decrease his or her insulin by 20 to 40 percent.[37]

Regular exercise, especially endurance-type activities such as walking, jogging, and swimming, reduce the need of insulin. Decreased daily doses of insulin should be administered one-half to 3 hours before extended exercise, using abdomen or arms as the preferred sites for injection since increased circulation in the exercised part may allow insulin to be absorbed too fast.[38]

Exercising diabetics also should consume foods that are high in carbohydrates and low in fat and protein. Any injury to tissues should be treated promptly as a safety measure against possible infection. In the event of insulin shock, the exerciser should be given sugar, in the form of sweet drinks or candy, and allowed to rest. These emergency procedures should be planned in advance and approved by the senior adult's doctor or the physician supervising the fitness program.

Fitness Activities and Mind Drugs

Physical activity and exercise have mind-healing effects. In addition to stimulating metabolic processes, exercise tones the heart, lung, and blood vessels to bring blood more efficiently to the muscles and brain. Exercise stimulates the production of chemicals in the body that give a sense of well-being and combat depression—one of which has been identified as endorphin (see Chapter 4).

It is obvious that drug therapy may be used when other natural means of therapy such as supportive counseling and various forms of psychotherapy fail to help mental problems. However, we know that physical activity relieves stress and anxiety, and some studies with younger populations have shown that jogging reduces depression. Fletcher reports on a study whereby 700 younger subjects were psychologically tested before and after a 10-week jogging, tennis, and mixed-exercise program.[39] Essentially, it was concluded that a rational, safe, and effective treatment for depression should include vigorous exercise to bring about and maintain optimal effective functioning.[40]

While such research does offer some evidence that exercise relieves depressive states, especially vigorous activity such as jogging, relatively few older men and women jog with intensity and duration equal to that of their younger peers. DeVries has conducted studies with older male and female adults from the ages of 52 to 70, comparing the effects of a commonly used tranquilizer (meprobamate) and moderate exercise upon muscular tension.[41] Using electromyographical procedures in assessing muscle tension, he found that a 15-minute walk at a moderate rate (sufficient to raise heart rate to 100 beats per minute) was effective in bringing about a tranquilizer effect greater than that of meprobamate.

Some questions arise with regard to the intensity, duration, and frequency of exercise as a therapeutic modality. At the present time, we cannot answer these questions precisely because of the individualistic psyche make-up of people. It appears that moderate exercise of an aerobic nature, such as walking, jogging, biking, swimming, etc., can induce a feeling of well-being and create a natural buffer against depression without the hazards of side effects caused by antidepressant drugs.

Fitness Activities and Caffeine, Tobacco, and Alcohol

What effect does caffeine have upon exercise and sports performance? It has been noted that caffeine, an activating drug found in popular beverages, is capable of raising catechol levels in the blood and stimulating action of the nervous system, skeletal muscles, kidneys, respiratory rate and depth, and possibly the adrenal glands.[42] Caffeine may prepare the body for general alertness and vigorous exertion. However, rather than serve as a reducer of fatigue, caffeine may act in an opposite manner, creating greater weariness and mental exhaustion through its induced arousal effect which in some cases may cause tremors and agitation.[43]

Some research suggests that athletes performing in endurance events may derive benefit from the ingestion of caffeine because of its release of free fatty acids that provide energy in sustained work of longer duration. Theoretically, the fatty acids may spare glycogen, enhance endurance, and reduce the perceived level of exertion.[44] The tolerance levels of caffeine among individuals, young and old, is highly variable, and the drug elicits different rates of stimulation and arousal. Whether the older adult performs in short-term exercise work-outs or long-term endurance programs, low or moderate consumption of such drinks as coffee, tea, or cola probably has a negligible effect on sports and exercise performance (unless the individual manifests cardiovascular symptoms, mental and emotional stress, or renal problems).

It should be quite clear from our earlier discussion that smoking cigarettes or cigars is noxious to the body. The smoker pays a high price for smoking pleasure. Any gains that may result from aerobic exercise regimes are negated by ciliotoxic action that destroys the sweeping action of the cilia in the participant's respiratory passages, causing the lungs to be more susceptible to various infections. Because carbon monoxide enters the blood, ventilatory capacity drops, resulting in hypoxia (oxygen deficiency). Regular exercise or sports participation by the older adult is incompatible with smoking. All forms of tobacco use should be avoided if the senior participant has serious intentions of improving his or her fitness level.

Alcohol is generally viewed by coaches and athletes as a deterrent to elite athletic performance. The same perspective applies to the senior athlete seeking to perform high-level motor skills. As noted earlier, alcohol is a depressant to the nervous system. Although initially it may produce a euphoric state which excites the neural mechanisms and frees the brain of inhibition, this condition is gradually replaced by drowsiness and sedation which decreases mental and sensory alertness required in performing skilled motor tasks. For those senior adults pursuing athletic competition or psychomotor tasks necessitating keen reaction time, alcohol use is inadvisable.

The effect of low or moderate alcohol consumption and exercise upon the cardiovascular system is not conclusive. Again, the variability of individual tolerance appears. Kuland reports that moderate alcohol consumption appears to increase high-density lipoprotein levels and may help to protect against coronary artery disease, as myocardial infarction rates are lower in moderate drinkers than in nondrinkers. However, he hastens to add that this does not justify recommending that nondrinkers start drinking moderately.[45]

The evidence does support the conclusion that alcohol has a retarding effect on fine motor skills and reaction time. These effects can interfere with dynamic and static balance, steadiness, and a variety of intricate everyday tasks. Such fitness parameters are also usually included in structured exercise programs. If the senior adult is experiencing difficulty with coordination and balance ability, alcohol consumption can only exaggerate deficits in these fitness elements.

Summary

The elderly use a greater proportion of drugs and medications than any other single segment of the population. Informed and intelligent use of drugs is essential for the reduction of potential adverse side effects that may accompany the ingestion of common chemical compounds. For example, iatrogenic illness, including organic brain syndrome, can be induced by misuse of psychotropic tranquilizers. Extensive use of diuretics can lead to dehydration. Certain types of antiarthritic drugs can result in gastric dysfunctions.

A good understanding of how drugs work and of their effects on body function helps to reduce the danger of drug toxicity. Ten principles of drug use germane to the elderly population were presented in this chapter. The implementation of the principles requires a coordinated effort involving the senior adult and the physician. Fitness specialists and directors can serve as an important link between the user and medical doctor.

Five types of cardiac pharmacologic agents were discussed, and specific drugs for specific disorders were presented with the benefits and potential side effects indicated.

High blood pressure and the effects of diuretics, vasodilators, and adrenergic blocking agents were described and evaluated. The various types of antiarthritic drugs used to treat rheumatoid arthritis and osteoarthritis also were described, analyzed, and assessed. It was stressed that diabetics need careful regulation of insulin, diet, and exercise to maintain a correct balance of blood sugar concentration in the body. Physically active adults should guard against hypoglycemia since exercise produces an insulin effect of lowering blood sugar levels.

Staying active physically and mentally provides natural buffers against depression, particularly among retired persons. Two principal drug groups used for depression were described—antidepressants and antianxiety agents. Side effects of lightheadedness to more serious consequences, such as organic brain syndrome were discussed.

Despite the physical symptoms of Parkinson's disease, this condition usually does not affect intelligence; however, serious mood swings and depression can occur. Two important drug agents are used to help control its symptoms: Levodopa and anticholinergics. Although these drugs help to restore biomechanical balance in the brain, their effects afford relief, not cure.

Organ brain syndrome (OBS) refers to a group of mental diseases that impair memory and intellectual functioning. A serious cognitive disorder of the brain among adults is Alzheimer's disease. Although various drugs and other treatments have been used for Alzheimer's, only modest improvement in alertness and decrease in confusion have resulted.

The neural stimulating effects of and other physiological responses to caffeine were described and evaluated. Most people can tolerate low and moderate levels of caffeine, but excessive amounts can endanger the cardiovascular system and contribute to hypertension and cardiac arrhythmias.

In addition to the proven causal relationship between smoking and lung malignancies, the chemical compounds in tobacco disrupt cardiovascular functions and lead to coronary heart disease. Older persons are more susceptible to cardiovascular disorders, lung infections, bronchitis, and pneumonia—all of which are exacerbated by smoking.

The temperate use of alcohol probably presents no significant health risk to the older adult. However, excessive use may lead to dependence and addiction, which result in the development of a host of physical and mental dysfunctions.

The relationships between exercise and four specific conditions commonly found among the elderly—cardiovascular disorders, arthritis, diabetes, and depression—were then discussed. Suggestions were offered for selecting and implementing appropriate activities for each condition with respect to how exercise interacts with prescribed drugs. Finally, whether the senior adult consumes one or six different medications for the relief of any ailment, the rule of using a minimum number of drugs with the correct therapeutic dose remains a wise one.

REFERENCES
1. Robert N. Butler and Myrna I. Lewis, *Aging and Mental Health,* 3d ed. (St. Louis: C. V. Mosby, 1982), p. 345.
2. National Indicators Systems, *Report Number 7: Health Economics* (Washington, D.C.: National Center for Health Statistics, October 1981).

3. *Dorland's Medical Dictionary,* 26th ed. (Philadelphia: W. B. Saunders, 1981), p. 405.

4. J. W. Rowe and R. W. Besdine, "Drug Therapy," in Rowe and Besdine, eds., *Health and Disease in Old Age* (Boston: Little, Brown, 1982), p. 39.

5. John G. Gerber, "Drug Usage in the Elderly," in R. W. Schrier, ed., *Clinical Internal Medicine in the Aged* (Philadelphia: W. B. Saunders, 1982), p. 58.

6. H. R. Ochs et al., "Reduced Quinidine Clearance in Elderly Persons," *American Journal of Cardiology* 42 (1978): 481–485.

7. E. Sheridan, R. H. Patterson, and E. A. Gustafson, *Falconer's: The Drug—The Nurse—The Patient,* 7th ed. (Philadelphia: W. B. Saunders, 1982), p. 397.

8. D. A. Chamberlain et al., "Plasma Digoxin Concentrations in Patients with Atrial Fibrillation," *British Medical Journal* 3 (1970): 429–432.

9. Ibid.

10. William D. Poe and Donald A. Holloway, *Drugs and the Aged* (New York: McGraw-Hill, 1980), p. 122.

11. Kenneth A. Conrad and Rubin Bressler, *Drug Therapy for the Elderly* (St. Louis: C. V. Mosby, 1982), p. 249.

12. Rowe and Besdine, "Drug Therapy," p. 47.

13. Roy J. Shephard, *Physical Activity and Aging* (Chicago: Year Book Medical Publishers, 1978), pp. 255–256.

14. Jim Ferstile, "Meeting Notes: Symposium on Future Issues in Exercise Biology, Ann Arbor, Michigan, November, 1981," *The Physician and Sportsmedicine* 10, no. 4 (1982): 133.

15. Conrad and Bressler, *Drug Therapy,* p. 341.

16. H. L. Resnick and J. M. Contor, "Suicide and Aging," *American Journal of Geriatrics* 18 (1970): 152–158.

17. Rowe and Besdine, "Drug Therapy," p. 51.

18. Troy L. Thompson, "Psychosocial and Psychiatric Problems in the Aged," in Robert W. Schrier, ed., *Clinical Internal Medicine in the Aged* (Philadelphia: W. B. Saunders, 1982), p. 37.

19. Michael J. Gaeta and Ronald J. Gaetano, *The Elderly: Their Health and the Drugs in Their Lives* (Dubuque, Ia.: Kendall-Hunt Publishers, 1977), p. 85.

20. Conrad and Bressler, *Drug Therapy,* p. 341.

21. Leon J. Epstein, "Clinical Geropsychiatry," in William Reichel, ed., *Topics in Aging and Long-Term Care*(Baltimore: Williams & Wilkins, 1981), p. 46.

22. Rowe and Besdine, "Drug Therapy," pp. 108–109.

23. Stuart Schneck, "Aging of the Nervous System and Dementia," in Robert W. Schrier, ed., *Clinical Internal Medicine in the Aged* (Philadelphia: W. B. Saunders, 1982), p. 49.

24. E. A. Jacobs et al., "Hyperbaric Oxygen Effect on Cognition and Behavior in the Aged," in J. H. Masserman, ed., *Current Psychiatric Therapies,* vol. 11 (Greene & Stratton, 1971), pp. 100–106; and E. A. Jacobs, H. J. Alvis, and S. M. Small, "Persistence Effects of Intermittent Hyperoxygenation in the Elderly," in W. G. Trapp et al., eds., *Fifth International Hyperbaric Conference,* vol. 1 (Burnaby, Canada: Simon Fraser University, 1974), pp. 439–445.

25. Allan E. Edwards and George M. Hart, "Hyperbaric Oxygenation and the Cognitive Functioning of the Aged," *Journal of the American Geriatric Society* 23, no. 8 (1974): 376–379.
26. A. I. Goldfarb et al., "Hyperbaric Oxygen Treatment of Organic Mental Syndrome in Aged Persons," *Journal of Gerontology* 27 (1974), 212–217; and B. Reisberg, S. H. Ferris, and S. Gershon, "Pharmacotherapy of Senile Dementia," in J. O. Cole and J. E. Barratt, eds., *Psychopathology in the Aged* (Raven Press, 1980).
27. Wilse B. Webb, "Sleep in Older Persons: Sleep Structures of 50–60 Year old Men and Women," *Journal of Gerontology* 37, no. 5 (1982): 581–586.
28. U.S. Department of Health, Education & Welfare, *Smoking and Health: A Report of the Surgeon General* (Washington, D.C.: USGPO, 1979).
29. Ibid., p. 15-5.
30. Ibid., p. 15-7.
31. Ibid., pp. 11–34, 35.
32. U.S. Department of Health, Education & Welfare, *Alcohol and Health: A Special Report to the U.S. Congress* (Washington, D.C.: USGPO, 1974), pp. 27–35.
33. W. Schmidt and J. Lint, "Causes of Death of Alcoholics," *Quarterly Journal of Structural Alcohol* 33 (1972): 171.
34. Erwald Busse and Dan Blazer, *Handbook of Geriatric Psychiatry* (New York: Van Nostrand Reinhold, 1980), pp. 409–412.
35. National Council on Alcoholism, "Criteria for the Diagnosis of Alcoholism," *American Journal of Psychiatry* 129 (1972): 127.
36. Rowe and Besdine, "Drug Therapy," p. 47.
37. Daniel N. Kuland, *The Injured Athlete* (Philadelphia: J. B. Lippincott, 1982), p. 81.
38. D. L. Costill, J. M. Miller, and W. J. Fink, "Energy Metabolism in Diabetic Distance Runners," *The Physician and Sports Medicine* 8, no. 10 (1980): 64–71.
39. Gerald F. Fletcher, *Exercise in the Practice of Medicine* (Mount Kisco, N.Y.: Futura Publishing, 1982), pp. 338–339.
40. Ibid., p. 339.
41. Herbert A. deVries and Gene M. Adams, "Electromyographic Comparison of Single Doses of Exercise and Meprobamate as to Effects on Muscular Relaxation," *American Journal of Physical Medicine* 51, no. 3 (1972): 130–140.
42. Peter J. Van Handel and D. Essig, "Caffeine," in G. Alan Stull, ed., *Encyclopedia of Physical Education, Fitness and Sports: Training Environment Nutrition and Fitness*, vol. 2 (Salt Lake City: Brighton Publishing, 1980), pp. 385–397.
43. Kuland, *Injured Athlete*, p. 60.
44. Ibid., p. 62.
45. Ibid., p. 61.

8

Facilities and Equipment for Activity Programs

INTRODUCTION

Facilities, equipment, and areas of activity programs for older persons range from a room-size all-purpose facility equipped only with a portable record player to a self-contained multipurpose senior center with specialized activity areas. A modern facility is furnished completely to conduct physical exercise, social activities, arts and crafts, recreational activities, cultural and intellectual functions, nutrition programs, physical examination screening, reading and relaxing, and a variety of outdoor sports.

Because activity programs for older persons are found in diverse settings, such as recreational community buildings, churches, housing projects, converted school buildings, and multipurpose senior centers specifically designed for older adults, it is unrealistic to set forth uniform standards for each situation. Program facility planners usually find themselves adapting and modifying existing facilities and areas to meet the physical, social, recreational, intellectual, and cultural needs of their constituent members. Facilities and equipment also vary depending upon the nature of the target population they serve. For example, programs that deal with handicapped and extremely frail elderly require more specialized room designs and wider entrances and exits, in addition to specialty apparatus and equipment to accommodate the functional limitations of this group. Our presentation focuses upon facilities and equipment necessary to conduct successful activity

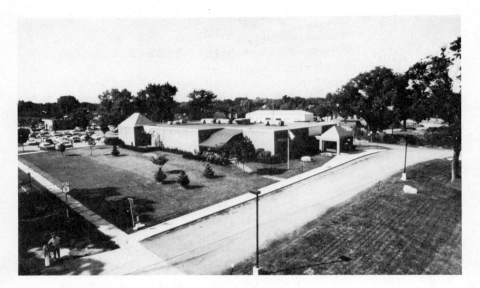

Figure 8.1 Amherst Senior Center—a modern multipurpose senior center. (Courtesy of Town of Amherst Senior Center, Williamsville, N.Y.)

programs for the person living in the community, free from serious disabling conditions, and able to participate at a multipurpose senior center or similar setting.

INDOOR FACILITIES

Main Gymnasium Area

The central core space of a successful fitness program is a gymnasium large enough for general physical and social activities. The size of the area depends upon the number using the facility, types of activities conducted, and anticipated growth. Such a facility can be used for dancing, volleyball, and group games. The room should be large enough to accommodate up to 100 persons for free-moving exercise activities including group calisthenics and social, ballroom, and square dancing. The gymnasium floor size varies from a minimum of 45 × 60 feet to 90 × 110 feet. These dimensions represent comparable sizes of small to large gymnasiums found in high schools.[1]

Budget and funding constraints normally dictate the type and size of an indoor gymnasium facility. Irrespective of size and related trappings, the following principles should be respected when considering the construction of an indoor main gymnasium area:

- Size of the unit is determined by the number of participants using the facility per week and daily average attendance.
- Seating area for spectators should be held at a minimum with seating accommodations close to walls.
- Main floor area, markings, and equipment should be designed for multiple use: volleyball, wall handball, jogging, badminton, group games, and dancing.
- Lavatories and toilet facilities should be located close to the activity area so that they are readily accessible.
- Use of folding doors or partitions should be considered to allow greater flexibility in changing activity area dimensions.
- Ceiling heights should be determined by the activity requirements.
- Adequate storage areas should be conveniently located for security of equipment, such as recorders, balls, wands, mats, etc.
- Activity area should be well-lighted without excessive glare.
- A safe and healthful environment should be a prime concern in facility design and construction.
- Attention should be given to sound control and acoustics—hard surfaces should be balanced with soft absorbing materials to result in reduced reverberation time to enhance good hearing conditions.
- Floor area should be of hard wood or a synthetic surface. New synthetics are desirable when use is extensive or subject to considerable stress (e.g., the setting up of chairs, tables, and miscellaneous items for special events).
- Gymnasium area should be easily accessible to handicapped persons; i.e., with wide doors and entrances, visual clues for the hearing-impaired, sound signal system for sight-impaired, low heights for items such as telephones, mirrors, faucets, lavatories, etc.

Ideally, a main gymnasium should contain the basic features of a modern school or college gym. Such a facility should include appropriate locker and shower service facilities, carefully designed and constructed to provide a safe and pleasant environment for the participants. Attention should also be directed to the need of ensuring privacy in locker room facilities. An adequate number of shower heads, depending upon peak load use, should be provided to prevent crowding and consequently reduce the risk of falling.

Fitness Activity Rooms

It is recognized that budget constraints frequently militate against the inclusion of ancillary facilities in addition to one main gymnasium or activity area. Nevertheless, two other types of activity areas are essential in order to

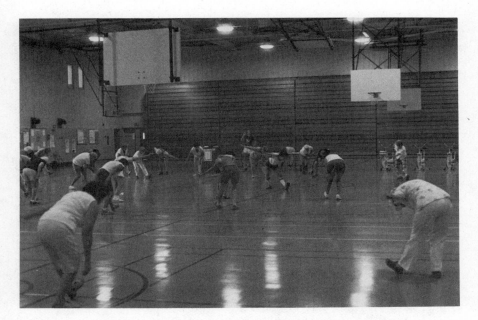

Figure 8.2 An ideal main gymnasium area to accommodate up to 100 senior adults in group activities. (Courtesy of Lifeline Program, University of Southern Maine.)

provide a complete range of fitness activities for the diverse nature, capabilities, and abilities of the senior population: an all-purpose body conditioning room and swimming pool.

All-Purpose Fitness Room. This room should provide space for individual workout modes and individualized prescriptive exercise protocols for the correction of specific musculoskeletal, orthopedic, and other conditions that may prevent senior adults from participating in general group activities. Many people derive greater satisfaction from exercising on an individualized basis using weights, engaging in various calisthenic drills, or simply moving from one type of activity—stretching, situps, etc.—in an unstructured way. Such an activity place offers an opportunity for participants to exercise on their own. This space also allows for personal fitness counseling service between the program director or exercise leader and the participant.

The all-purpose fitness room should be carpeted or covered with a durable resilient material. It should contain such items as mirrors, small floormats, dumbbells, a universal or similar-type weight machine, wall ladders for body mechanics exercises, stationary exercise bikes, barbells, and weight racks.

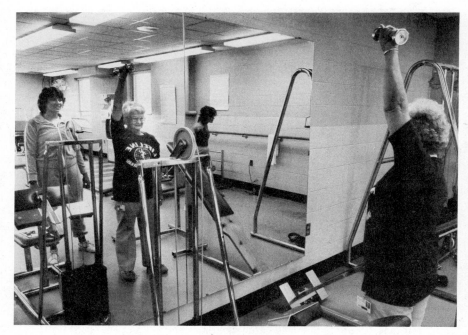

Figure 8.3 Fitness "body shop" equipped with free weight equipment and exercise machines. (Courtesy of Lifeline Program, University of Southern Maine.)

Natatorium. Most programs in multipurpose centers generally use natatorium facilities at the local YMCA, school, or the municipal recreational center. Retirement villages are beginning to provide swimming pools, in addition to other social activity facilities.

Ideally, each senior center should contain its own natatorium. However, most communities and organizations, because of economic considerations, must plan and operate their swimming pools with flexibility that allow many different populations, including school age youth and adults, to use the facility. The following discussion centers upon general guiding principles of pool construction and operation applicable to instructional and recreational needs of the participants, rather than facility requirements for elite competitive swimming programs.

Swimming is a vital part of a fitness program for senior adults. Aquatics allow an exercise outlet for those persons who, for various physical reasons, cannot participate in land activities. Additionally, swimming activities are preferred by many adults without medical limitations.

In most climates, a closed or indoor pool is preferable so that swimming will not be curtailed during the winter months. The sizes of most pools vary from 30 × 60 feet to 60 × 75 feet, although some are Olympic size (50 meters long). Unfortunately, too many pools are 30 feet wide with four lanes, which results in crowding or severely restricts the number of swimmers who can use the facility at one time.

Natatoriums with six to eight lane widths and 75-foot lengths are far more functional from an instructional perspective. Water depths range from 2 feet, 6 inches to 4½ feet at the shallow end, and from 9 to 12 feet at the deep end. Standard water depths of 3 feet, 6 inches (shallow end) and 12 feet (deep end) are recommended to meet the instructional and recreational needs of most swimmers.

Pools equipped with a one-meter diving board should have a minimum of 12 feet in water depth under the end of the board. Minimum diving board water depths of 12 feet should exist from 6 feet back to 20 feet forward of the end of the board, 10 to 15 feet between boards, and 12 feet between the board and side of pool.[2]

Particular attention should be given to lighting, water temperature, ladders into the pool, acoustical quality, and the tile on deck areas. Many natatoriums are notoriously deficient in these features, all of which are important for the safety, comfort, and effectiveness of swimming instruction. One hundred foot candle light is recommended for overhead illumination in an indoor pool, and a greater concentration is advisable over the end walls. Underwater lights add to the esthetic qualities of the pool, but are not necessary from a functional perspective. Many pools contain multiple glass side wall panels that reflect on the water surface and create glare, which can interfere with visual acuity of the swimmer (see Chapter 6). Reflections from the outside should be held to a minimum by an appropriate covering material.

Water temperatures usually range from 78 to 92 degrees, depending upon group needs. For example, skilled swimmers prefer cooler temperatures, of less than 80 degrees. Handicapped swimmers need water temperatures up to 92 degrees for relaxation, floating, and modified forms of water propulsion skills. A range of 80 to 82 degrees is generally acceptable for the safety and comfort of most swimmers. The air temperature should be at least 10 degrees above the water temperature to avoid chilling.

Ladders leading into the pool well should be recessed into the side walls. Rungs and grasping handles should not be placed over the side wall into the water—such installations can cause injury to swimmers in outside lanes.

Too often swimming pools, although beautifully constructed and durable, contain hard surfaces of tile, concrete, and steel—all of which intensify the reverberation of sound. Walls and ceilings should be acoustically treated to allow easy communication between instructor and participants. Sound systems simply amplify voices or music and add to noise pollution when used in untreated acoustical natatoriums.

Pools are constantly wet and slippery. Since the elderly are highly susceptible to falls, and the consequences are far more serious for those over 60 than for younger persons, older adults should not enter swimming pools unless walking areas, approaches to pool ladders, and diving boards are finished with a non-skid material.

The following checklist offers essential guidelines for planning and operational use of indoor natatoriums.

Checklist for Indoor Natatoriums

		Yes	No
1.	Does the facility design and construction meet the special needs and requirements of older adults?	___	___
2.	Has pool construction and operation been approved and checked by the local board of health?	___	___
3.	Are toilet facilities provided for wet swimmers separate from the dry area?	___	___
4.	Is adequate deck space provided around the pool (10–20 feet on each side and ends of pool wall)?	___	___
5.	Does the pool provide adequate illumination and proper acoustics?	___	___
6.	Does pool operation include daily checks of water temperature, water acidity, and chlorine content?	___	___
7.	Does pool use require a qualified lifeguard or instructor at all times?	___	___
8.	Is the bottom of the pool clearly visible at all times during use?	___	___
9.	Does the pool contain adequate lifesaving gear and pool cleaning equipment?	___	___
10.	Does the pool contain adequate overhead clearance for diving (16 feet for one-meter boards)?	___	___
11.	Is reflection of light from the outside and glare held to a minimum?	___	___
12.	Is there proper ventilation?	___	___
13.	Can the humidity of the pool be controlled?	___	___
14.	Does the pool contain a telephone or buzzer for immediate communication in the event of an emergency?	___	___
15.	Does the pool contain depth markings on the side and end walls?	___	___
16.	Are guard rails provided for diving boards?	___	___
17.	Does the pool contain a storage room accessible to the deck for small swimming equipment items?	___	___

Checklist for Indoor Natatoriums

		Yes	No
18.	Does the pool contain adequate drains to avoid puddle formation on the deck?	___	___
19.	Does the pool contain adequate provision for accessibility to ambulance service?	___	___
20.	Are pool decks and edges rounded and smooth, devoid of sharp edges?	___	___
21.	Does the pool entrance provide easy access for wheelchair participants?	___	___
22.	Are general swimming and diving rules for the safe conduct of the participants clearly posted?	___	___

This checklist should be helpful to the program director who is seeking a community swimming facility to enrich the activity offerings for his or her particular senior setting. Local school or YMCA/YWCA facilities are excellent resources that generally offer arrangements of aquatic activities for senior adults.

The aquatics area is a very important part of any fitness program for senior adults. Program planners should strive to include an indoor pool along with other space and activity areas whenever the construction of a new senior center is contemplated.

Indoor Social and Recreational Areas

Satisfying human social and recreational needs is part of implementing the broad concept of health-fitness of senior adults. Thus, adequate space and specific accommodations for the conduct of social and recreational experiences such as arts and crafts, hobbies, music and relaxing, dance, educational activities, reading, drama, television, and special events should be provided.

Although it would be ideal to furnish special rooms for each individual activity, the reality of cost containment dictates application of the modification and adaptation principle, which means that one or two areas can serve a variety of activities. For example, one large room can serve as a social hall, dining hall, and auditorium for group gatherings. Smaller multipurpose rooms may be used for class meetings in various arts and crafts sessions. Each senior setting will reflect its own unique activity interests, talent, and leadership. For example, one local senior center set aside a room for miniature golf, a popular activity among its members. The course itself was built by several talented retired carpenters from the membership. The following discussion covers a sample of facilities to accommodate recre-

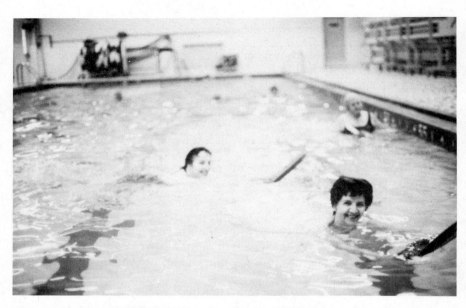

Figure 8.4 A swimming pool with sufficient deck space—ideal for a variety of aquatic activities.

ational activities generally found in multipurpose senior centers and similar settings.

Arts and Crafts Room. Painting, writing, leather work, ceramics, drawing, and graphic and plastic arts are a few examples of the arts and crafts activities found in multipurpose centers and residential settings, including long-term health care facilities. Such activities allow the senior adult to express his or her interests and talent freely; an opportunity to enhance their sensory mechanisms, particularly involving coordinated movements of the eyes and hands; and the potential for social contact.

A separate room for arts and crafts is desirable. Rooms equipped for crafts should have a modern sink and ample storage cabinets, closets, and lockers for the safe deposit of craft materials, unfinished projects, and exhibit items. Base and wall plugs should be furnished for the operation of such items as sewing machines, power tools, and electric irons. Ceramic kilns should be equipped with heavy-duty 220 volt electrical outlets. Bulletin boards and exhibit cases should be available for display of completed projects. A well-lighted area is essential for a successful craft program, and the room should be large enough to allow ample working space.

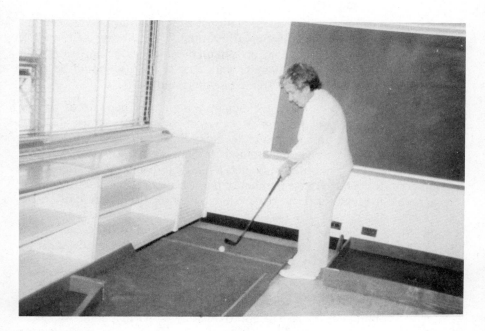

Figure 8.5 Miniature golf course. (Courtesy of Town of Tonawanda Senior Center, N.Y.)

Woodshops. The woodshop is a leisure area for many different kinds of activities, such as antiquing and finishing furniture; repairing tables, chairs, and chests; and building bookcases. Generally, woodcraft is preferred by men, although some women display great interest and talent in this activity. Woodshops require space for large pieces of furniture that will remain in place for several weeks of work. It is recommended that the woodshop be housed in a room separate from other arts and crafts areas because of the prevalence of power tools and assorted machinery necessary for the construction and repair of furniture.

Game and Activities Room. A general game and activities room, approximately 35 × 65 feet, is recommended for a variety of games including pool, table tennis, and other table top games. Such rooms may also be used for special events, such as birthday parties and holiday celebrations. Sufficient storage space should be provided for the various items of game equipment and supplies.

Library and Reading Room. A room should be set aside simply for quiet reading and relaxing. This area should be furnished with comfortable furniture, including tables and chairs for study and writing notes. Such a room may also be used for small group educational cultural affairs. Many seniors enjoy reading in a quiet atmosphere. Essentially, the library and reading room represents a calm place where the senior adult can find satisfying literary and intellectual contentment. This special facility should be well-lighted and contain acoustically treated ceilings and walls.

Dance Studio. Social and square dancing combine the benefits of dance, exercise, music, and socialization. Because of these fitness attributes and popularity, a separate area should be included in the physical plant suitable for a variety of dance modes, including both dancing and folk and rhythmic games using assorted instruments, such as rattles, drums, sticks, cymbals, and tambourines. The average number of participants in a class setting offers a measurement gauge for room size. While budget restraints primarily regulate the size and design of a facility, program planners should aim for the specifications considered ideal for a complete program of dance activities. The Council on Facilities, Equipment and Supplies of the Athletic Institute and the American Alliance for Health, Physical Education, Recreation and Dance recommend the following specifications:

1. Area of 54,000 square feet (54 by 100 feet is suggested) that will accommodate a class of approximately 60 participants.
2. Dance area that is generally rectangular with a length-width ratio of approximately 3 to 2 (e.g., 90 by 60 feet).
3. Ceiling height that is proportional to the size of the room but never lower than 12 feet.
4. Floors of hardwood, such as maple, of random lengths and tongue-and-grooved.
5. Incandescent light rather than fluorescent light.
6. Storage space for sound equipment adjacent to the dance equipment with built-in deposit space for records, tapes, and musical instruments.
7. Heavy-duty wiring for all dance facilities, capable of carrying portable phonographs, additional speakers, tape recorders, and projectors; wall outlets convenient to all areas.
8. Mechanisms for heating and cooling as nearly silent as possible to avoid interfering with the quality of sound and its reception.
9. Wall mirrors along two adjoining walls so that movement can be analyzed from two directions.
10. Chalkboards and bulletin boards for instructional exhibit purposes.[3]

These specifications should accommodate a large group of 60 dancers, so appropriate reductions in room size would be made according to actual number of seniors using the facility. *Therapeutic Dance/Movement* by Caplow-Lindner et al. provides more specific material about dance and its therapeutic effects upon older adults.[4]

Music Room and Lounge. Listening to music offers an opportunity for the senior adult to relax, and serves as a tool for the stimulation of conversation and the development of friendships. A well-functioning senior center contains a music room and lounge equipped with a high-fidelity sound system and a wide assortment of recordings—classical, standard favorites, and contemporary titles. The room should be comfortably furnished projecting a home living room atmosphere, with lounge chairs, lamps, and sofas. A television set should be conveniently placed in a separate area within the room. Individual sound receivers should be available to avoid audio conflicts between stereo listeners and television viewers.

OUTDOOR FACILITIES

Outdoor facilities for senior centers generally follow the design of neighborhood recreational centers. However, facilities and playing areas for highly vigorous play and intense competitive sports are not usually included. The scope, nature of land characteristics, budget allowances, and desired programming determine the specific kinds of outdoor facilities that will surround a senior center. Outdoor facilities for the following activities are discussed here: (1) horseshoes, (2) shuffleboard, (3) bocci, (4) tennis, (5) ice skating, (6) softball, (7) bowling on the green, (8) pitch and put golf, and (9) exercise trails.

Horseshoes

Horseshoe pitching, usually played outdoors, is an activity of moderate energy level appropriate for men and women of all ages. The horseshoe court consists of two boxes, 6 feet square, set flush with the ground. The boxes, as shown in Figure 8.7, can be made using 2-by-4s nailed together. A stake is driven into the center of the box with 14 inches remaining above the surface. The court is laid out over level ground with centers of the boxes 40 feet apart. Clay or dirt should surround the stake to absorb the force of the tossed horseshoe and allow the shoes to stay where they land.

An alternate court with a shortened distance of 30 feet between stakes can be provided to accommodate individuals with lower strength capability. Rubber horseshoes may be substituted for the official 2½-pound metal shoes. Further modifications of the game may substitute plastic rings or bean bags for the use of handicapped or frail elderly persons. Most ambulatory and well-elderly players do not require adjustments in the game or equipment.

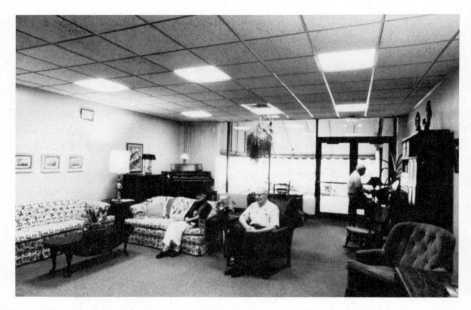

Figure 8.6 Music room and lounge. (Courtesy of Town of Amherst Senior Center, Williamsville, N.Y.)

Shuffleboard

The game of shuffleboard is usually identified with older and retired persons, probably because of the large number of courts found in the sunny climates of Florida. The game itself represents a mild form of exercise that stimulates sensory and body neuromuscular control, equally appropriate for both sexes. Shuffleboard is also an excellent recreational activity for the older adult confined to a wheel chair (see Figure 6.17).

The official game is played on a court 52 feet long and 6 feet wide. Playing surfaces may be concrete or terrazzo. Score surfaces are located at the ends of the court, which are identically marked. Each end contains a triangular scoring area marked according to specifications, as shown in Figure 8.9.

The object of the game is to push one's discs into the scoring areas and to prevent the opposing player from doing likewise. The playing court distance may be shortened or widened; or in further modification, the player can be allowed to use the inside of his or her foot to push or kick the disc. The game may also be played as table shuffleboard. (Seaton's *Physical Education Handbook* provides specific rules, scoring, and strategies employed in the game.[5])

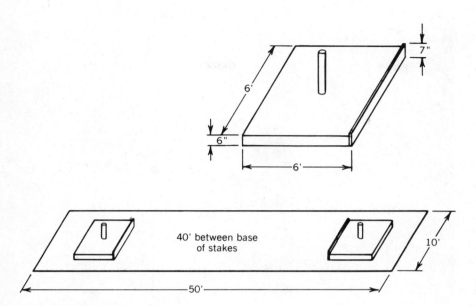

Figure 8.7 Horseshoe court.

Tennis

The game of tennis is no longer confined to the young. Today, there are U.S. Tennis Association (USTA) tournaments for players 80 years of age and older.[6] These tournaments use grass, hard, indoor, or outdoor courts. Tennis requires a high level of fitness and above-average motor skill. Tennis is suitable for seniors who are in good condition and possess some experience in fundamentals of the game.

Kuland et al. studied the long-term effects of playing tennis and found that players had faster simple and total reaction times than less-active counterparts; their total reaction time was similar to that of college sophomores.[7] Other researchers have found bone densities in the dominant arm of senior amateur tennis players to be 8 to 9 percent greater than in the non-dominant arm, suggesting that the greater muscular activity on the dominant side is responsible for bone growth.[8] Such research bodes well for the game and its players as a worthy sport for maintaining physical fitness and retarding or preventing the onset of osteoporosis. Additionally, the elite level of skill and fitness achieved by this group serves as a positive model for other senior adults.

Most multipurpose senior centers do not provide tennis courts for their members. Arrangements are generally made with municipal facilities or private tennis clubs at stipulated fee rates. Ideally, each center should contain

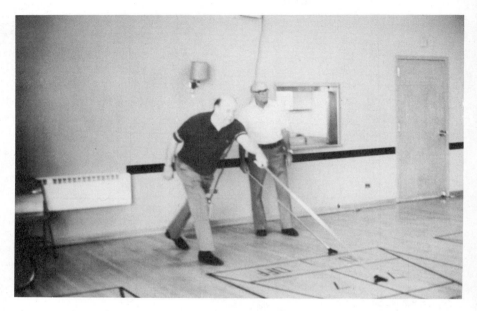

Figure 8.8 Shuffleboard—a mild form of exercise appropriate for older men and women.

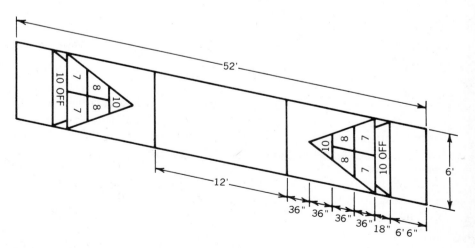

Figure 8.9 Shuffleboard playing area.

its own courts, the number of which may range from two to six depending upon the interest and number of participants. Hard surface, usually asphalt, is probably best from a maintenance viewpoint. Additionally, hard surface courts can be modified for other activities, such as volleyball and ice skating. Figure 8.10 delineates the dimensions of singles and doubles courts. (The *Physical Education Handbook* mentioned above provides details about the rules and regulations of the game.)

Bocci

Bocci is a target sport game, well-known in Italian communities and quite popular in European and American recreational programs. The facilities and equipment are easily and inexpensively acquired, and maintenance is minimal. The rules are simple and quickly understood. The physical requirements are low, and it can be played by men and women of all ages. Court dimensions are approximately 60 × 10 feet.[9] The court is enclosed by 12-inch wooden sides, with slightly higher ends that serve as backstops (see Figure 8.11).

The outdoor surface should be level and contain a mixture of sand and clay (loam). Simple floodlighting is desirable for night play. The equipment consists of eight balls of a diameter of 4½ inches, plus a smaller "Jack ball," 2¾ inches in diameter. A starter player begins the game by tossing the Jack ball from one end of the court any desired distance toward the opposite end. The object of the game is then to toss the larger ball as close to the Jack ball as possible. Balls are delivered with a underhand throw, thrown through the air or bowled, as the player chooses. It is permissible to change the location of the Jack ball by hitting it, and to attempt to knock it away from an

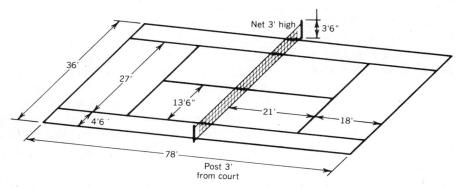

Figure 8.10 Tennis court. Dimensions of a singles court are 78' by 27'. Dimensions of a doubles court are 78' by 36' (4½' alley added to each side).

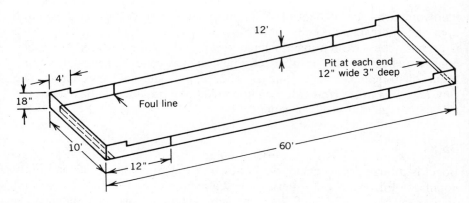

Figure 8.11 Bocci court.

opposing player's ball. One point is awarded for every ball closer to the Jack ball than the closest ball of the opponent. Bocci may also be played indoors using carpet rather than a dirt surface (Figure 8.12). It may be played with or without modification; simply shortening the distance or lowering the winning score rule from 12 to 6 points will allow seniors with limited capacities, or those in wheelchairs, to enjoy the satisfaction of play.

Lawn Bowling

Lawn bowling, also called "Bowling on the Green," originated in England in the twelfth century. The sport is similar to bocci, and the game may have come from a version of bocci played by the ancient Egyptians. Lawn bowling is played on a 120 × 120 foot grass or loam surface. The green is divided into eight 14 × 11-foot rinks with each rink accommodating two to four players. The lawn is surrounded by a ditch or wall 10 to 15 inches wide and 2 to 4 inches deep. A bank approximately 1½ feet high on the outside surrounds the green. The green is slightly sloped in the direction of the ditch. The ditch and bank serve to stop bowls that are thrown too hard.

The equipment consists of wooden balls called bowls, usually made of lignum vitae (extremely hard and heavy wood), and a small ball called a "Jack." The bowl is not round, but unbalanced, which makes it possible for the player to deliver a curve to the bowl. The bowls are 16½ inches in circumference and weigh 3½ pounds. The Jack is 8 inches in circumference and weighs 10 ounces. The bowler starts the game from a mat 22-by-14 inches.

The object of the game is to move the bowl as close as possible to the Jack ball after the Jack is rolled down the green. It is permissible to hit the

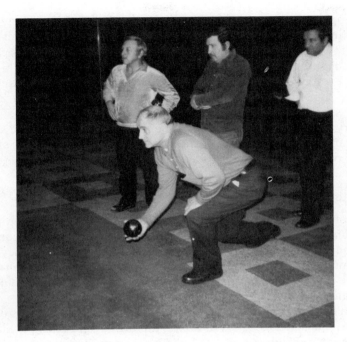

Figure 8.12 Bocci—an excellent motor activity for the maintenance of accuracy and dynamic balance. (Courtesy of Settimo Trivellin and the Italian Heritage Center, Portland, Me.)

opponents' bowls away from the Jack. Points are scored for each bowl closer to the Jack than any bowls of the opponents (one point for each bowl). Twenty-one points usually end the game in singles play, but other arrangements may be made prior to the start of the game.

Exercise Trail

The continued emphasis on health at all ages has inspired a unique mode of fostering physical fitness. Exercise trails, Parcourses, or fitness trails, have been commercially designed to improve cardiovascular efficiency, agility, flexibility, muscular strength and endurance. A trail consists of a number of exercise stations along a walking or jogging course. Trails range from one to two miles in distance and contain 12 to 20 stations.

Most exercise trails are patterned for young adults, and strict conformance to station requirements at each stop would be inappropriate for the senior adult unless the participant is a conditioned and highly skilled athlete.

For example, exercise stations that require wall scaling, jumping shoulder-high barriers, and rope climbing should be omitted. For some older persons, walking through the course may suffice, depending upon the physical capacity and conditioning state of the participant.

The exercise trail for seniors should accent stretching exercises, simple and safe movements that invigorate upper- and lower-body muscular strength, and neuromuscular motor tasks and skills that reinforce upright stationary and dynamic balance. Completion of the course should not stress speed. Participants should be encouraged to finish the trail at their own pace, skipping or adding the exercises as they like.

Ice Skating

Recreational ice skating is suitable for experienced seniors with previous background in the sport. Ice skating is classified as a continuous motor skill—and if the coordinating movements are learned well, they tend to resist "forgetting" (see Chapter 6). Thus, opportunities for leisure skating should be provided when funds allow, because of the strong cardiovascular and dynamic balance benefits to the participant.

Such facilities can be adapted from hard surface tennis courts or volleyball areas. Enclosed ice rinks or arenas are highly specialized facilities that would be impractical as separate buildings in a multipurpose senior center for the express use of senior adults. Many communities contain multipurpose ice arenas to accommodate ice hockey, figure skating, and recreational skating. Program directors should arrange schedules that allow interested and experienced seniors the use of municipal facilities.

Volleyball

Volleyball is a team sport that is universally played throughout the world. It can be played by young or old, men or women, the highly skilled or the unskilled performer. Rules may be modified to fit the needs of the group. For example, allowing one bounce of the ball before a return volley over the net slows the pace of the game. Lighter and softer balls may be used for handicapped players. Volleyball can be altered in a such a way that game play can even be safe for older persons with limited ambulation living in extended health care facilities. For example, using a volleyball net strung across a room, with participants on both sides of the net, and heavy balloons substituted for balls, will enable the frail and unskilled player to participate in a pleasurable exercise activity.

The official court dimensions are 60 feet long and 30 feet wide; the net is 32 feet in length, 3 feet wide, and 8 feet high (see Figure 8.13) for men, 7 feet,

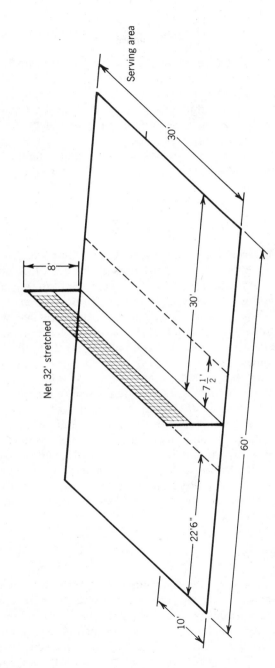

Figure 8.13 Volleyball court.

6 inches high for women. The ball is leather or rubber, 26 to 27 inches in circumference, and 9 to 10 ounces in weight.

Volleyball is both an indoor game and an outdoor sport. Gymnasiums should be floor lined to the dimensions shown in Figure 8.13. Various types of surfaces can be used for outdoor volleyball courts, such as earth, turf, synthetics, and asphalt. Asphalt has several advantages: it is durable; maintenance is easy and inexpensive; when properly installed, the finish is dust-free and drains quickly; and it provides a neat, no-glare, hard surface.[10] Many excellent manuals contain information about volleyball rules, skills, techniques, and team strategy (e.g., *Basic Skills in Sports* by Armbruster et al.).[11]

Miniature Golf

Golf putting offers a mild form of exercise that sharpens hand-eye coordination and accuracy skills. It is particularly suitable for older adults who are unable to participate in vigorous activities because of limiting cardiovascular disorders or musculoskeletal aberrations. The game is an excellent sport for persons with physiological limits because it can be played without undue exertion and with players in control of the pace of the game. Individuals confined to wheelchairs may also participate by stroking the ball from outside the bump boards.

A putting court should include at least a four-hole course, which provides variation in play. Game skills include the use of bump boards for bank shots and proper placement of the ball for tee shots. Table 8.1 and Figure 8.14 show equipment and layout for a four-hole miniature golf course.

This course has a minimum number of holes. Nine-hole miniature courses, designed with various rises, bump boards, and obstacles, provide seniors greater challenges for testing and refining their motor skills. It is not uncommon to find skilled golfers among retired groups. These individuals can serve as excellent resources in the design and construction of different types of courses and their par score values.

Softball

Softball is classified as a moderate to vigorous activity for older adults. This sport is usually pursued into the later years by those individuals who have had some experience in baseball or softball in their earlier life. Much of the popularity of the sport stems from its wide sponsorship by industrial organizations and municipal recreation departments. Most schools and colleges now sponsor softball programs for women, and with the ever-increasing

Table 8.1 Equipment for Four-Hole Putting Course

Item	Quantity
Tee mats	4
Aluminum hole numbers 1-2-3-4 wing blocks	4
Aluminum par markers wing blocks	4
Stainless steel anchor rods	20
4½ ft. × 60 ft. carpet	1 roll
Carpet adhesive	5 gallons
Medium triangle	1
Aluminum bump boards	900 feet
Bumper fasteners	—
Concrete #3000	5½ yards
Reinforcing wire	2 rolls
P-2 putters (35″)	10
P-3 putters (32″)	10
Putting balls (1 doz. each color)	5

Source: R. Adams, "Putt-Putt Golf," *Journal of Health, Physical Education and Recreation* 42, no. 3 (1971): 49. Used with permission.

numbers of females participating in all sports programs, softball participation by older women should steadily expand.

The game itself is a modification of baseball, with the essential differences in the delivery of the pitch, which is an underarm motion, and the requirement that the baserunner advance only after the ball has left the pitcher's hand in his or her delivery. The baserunner is "out" if he or she steps off a base prior to the ball release.

Softball is played on a diamond smaller than a baseball field: the distance between bases is 60 feet and the span from the pitcher's mound to home plate is 46 feet for men and 40 feet for women (see Figure 8.15). A softball game has seven innings, compared to nine in baseball.

Softball fields range from sandlots and pastures to well-kept official diamonds. The best fields have clean diamonds with all grass, weeds, and rocks eliminated.[12] A softball facility that is well maintained can be used in early spring and made playable sooner after a heavy rain storm.

The softball bat is smaller and lighter than the baseball bat: it is not more than 34 inches in length, and less than 2⅛ inches in diameter at its largest part. The ball is approximately 12 inches in circumference and weighs about 6 ounces. The ball cover is leather and it usually contains an inner mixture of rubber and cork or *Kapok*. Softball gloves are made of leather and designed with a larger pocket than found in a baseball glove. The catcher wears a protective mask. Softball is not considered a prime fitness sport, but it does help to enhance agility and stimulate the sensory mecha-

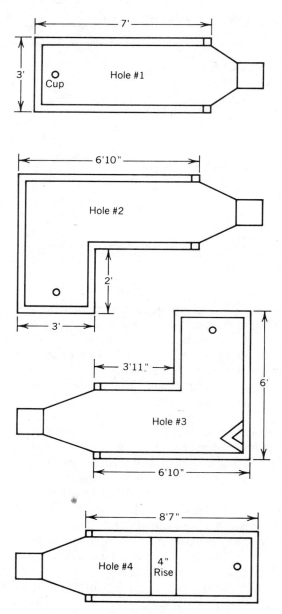

Figure 8.14 Layout for a four-hole putting course. (From F. Adams, "Putt-Putt Golf," p. 49. Used with permission.)

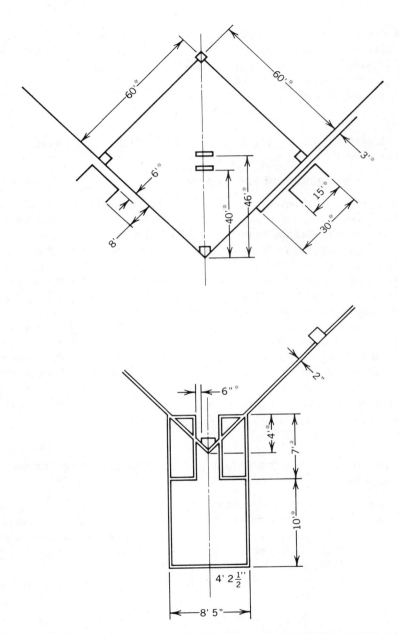

Figure 8.15 Softball playing area. (From K. A. Penman, *Planning Physical Education and Athletic Facilities in Schools* [New York: John Wiley & Sons, 1977], p. 402. Used with permission.)

nisms that control hand-eye coordination. Additionally, the interaction of team play offers an opportunity for good fun and social camaraderie. Modifications such as reducing the length of the running bases or using light and larger balls can be introduced to allow those individuals with lesser physical capacity and ability to play the game (see Table 6.1).

EQUIPMENT AND SUPPLIES FOR FITNESS AND RECREATION PROGRAMMING

Importance of Equipment and Supplies

Most physical and recreational activities need some specific piece of equipment (nonexpendable item used over a period of years) or supply item (expendable item that is replaced periodically). Facilities including gymnasiums and game and activities rooms require teaching and learning materials to encourage maximum participation in a variety of program experiences. Certain pieces of equipment, such as pianos or record players, can serve large numbers of participants, whereas wands, small free weights, and frisbees are necessary for each member of the group to ensure efficient use of activity time. The scope and diversity of activities essentially depend upon the equipment and supplies available.

The following section deals with materials recommended for the implementation of a successful fitness and recreation program. Certain items may be used in long-term care facilities, while others are more appropriate in multipurpose or resident centers for ambulatory seniors without serious acute or chronic diseases.

Determining Factors in the Selection and Purchase of Equipment and Supplies

The overriding factor in the selection and use of any equipment or supply for senior adults is its potential degree of contribution to the health and safety of the participants. For example, heavy metal objects, exercise equipment with sharp or pointed ends, and undersized balls for throwing and catching games should be generally avoided.

The following selection and purchase principles are useful once primary health and safety criteria have been satisfied:

1. *Program of activities.* Selection must include consideration of the type of activities offered. Different types of activities require specific kinds of items.
2. *Facilities and space.* Consideration should be given to materials

appropriate for facilities and space available. For example, items for horseshoes or bocci should not be purchased unless adequate areas are available.

3. *Physical capacity and ability of participants.* Nature and characteristics of functional age and skill level of the group should be considered. For example, larger, softer balls should be selected for beginner and low-level volleyball and softball game play.

4. *Number of participants served.* The number of participants expected to use the equipment or supplies at a given time, and over an extended period, must be considered. This factor is essential for maximum activity participation.

5. *Interests and needs of the participants.* Consideration should be given to particular interests and needs of participants. For example, if program clientele desire and enjoy rhythmic or aerobic exercise activity, greater expenditures for audiotapes, recorders, and other music accompaniment equipment is justified.

6. *Selection of materials should be based upon quality.* Purchase of better grades of material is the best policy—and in the long run, repair and replacement costs are less.

7. *Selection of equipment should be made by competent personnel.* Persons selecting and purchasing equipment should know the advantages and disadvantages of items under consideration. Usually, advice can be sought from the staff member who actually uses the equipment or supply item.

8. *Purchases should be made from reputable and well-established business organizations.* It is wise to deal with firms that have a reputation for fair prices, quality merchandise, and reliable service. Program directors should consult the local Better Business Bureau for specific information about prospective firms under consideration.

EQUIPMENT AND SUPPLIES FOR SPECIFIC FACILITIES

Fitness and recreation programs use a wide variety of equipment and supplies, which can cost thousands of dollars. Thus, it is important to apply the principles suggested above in order to derive returned health-fitness values equivalent to the high cost of the materials purchased. Equipment and supply inventories are developed graudually as the needs and interests of participants emerge. However, certain items are basic, and should be procured as quickly as possible. For example, a record or cassette player is essential for rhythmic exercise programs. Small individual mats are also necessary for the safety and comfort of participants involved in sitting, prone, and supine floor exercises. Each program director will most likely develop a priority listing for material selection and purchase since most organizations are usually under budget limitations. Priorities will vary from one organizational setting to another, depending on the type of activities offered and the available facilities. The checklist items outlined below are suggested (not necessarily in priority order) for the selected facilities described earlier in this chapter:

I. Indoor Facilities
    A. Main Gymnasium Area
        1. Individual Activities and Basic Items
            —Balls—rubber (6 to 8 inches in circumference)
            —Beanbags
            —Exercise wands or short sticks (36″)
            —Individual mats (lightweight—4′ × 6′)
            —Assorted dumbbells (2, 5, and 6 lb. wts.)
            —Regular floor mats (lightweight—6′ × 12′)
            —Low balance beams (variable widths and lengths—2″, 4″, 6″, 8″ and 12″ wide, 10′ long)
            —Frisbees
            —Hoops (plastic)
            —Folding chairs (chair exercises)
            —Soccer balls
            —Ball inflator pump
            —Softballs
            —Plastic bats
            —Tape measure (100′)
            —Basketballs
        2. Sports, Rhythm, and Group Activities
            a. Volleyball
                —Balls
                —Nets
                —Standards rule book
            b. Badminton
                —Nets
                —Rackets
                —Shuttlecocks
                —Standards rule book
            c. Wall Paddle Ball
                —Tennis balls
                —Paddles
                —Rule book

        d. Rhythmic Activity Materials
- Sound System: microphone, record player, cassette player
- Records and tapes
- Cymbals
- Piano
- Rhythm sticks
- Tambourines

        e. Parachute Activity Materials
- 28′ Alternating-color panels (nylon)
- Assorted sponges
- Parachute play records

        f. Bowling
- Plastic balls
- Plastic pins

B. Fitness Activity Areas
  1. All-purpose Fitness Room*
      a. Developmental Exercise Equipment
- Stall bars
- Stall bar bench
- Floor and chest pulley
- Wall weights
- Abdominal sit-up board
- Treadmills with rails
- Rowing machines
- Bicycle exercise machine
- Exercise folding mats
- First aid supplies
- Exercise benches (padded and unpadded)
- Universal-type weight machine

      b. Posture Training Equipment
- Posture training mirror
- Arthrodial protractor
- Posture evaluation grid
- Low balance beam
- Stall bars

      c. Resistance Exercise Equipment
- Dumbbell wagon equipment with dumbbells
- Weight caddy, equipped with disc-type weights

*Selection and number of exercise devices and equipment depend upon the size of the facility, number of participants, and objectives of the program.

—Press bench
—Medicine ball
—Hand chalk
—Multipurpose weight bench
—Leg press machine

d. Testing, Measurement, and Anthropometric Equipment*
—Weight scale
—Wet spirometer
—Skinfold caliper
—Flexometer
—Hand dynamometer
—Chalk board
—Stopwatch
—Exercise timer
—Electric rhythm metronome
—Footstool
—Anthropometric measuring tape
—Shoulder and chest girth measurement calipers
—Mechanical goniometers
—Motor-driven treadmill
—Stadiometer
—Bicycle ergometer
—Step-test bench
—Low balance beam
—Reaction time testing equipment

C. Natatorium
—Kickboards
—Lane markers
—Life buoys and reach poles
—Noseclips
—Goggles and swim caps
—Earplugs
—One-meter diving board
—Clock
—Swim fins
—Rubber balls (for water games)
—First aid supplies
—Telephone or emergency buzzer

*Testing and evaluation center should be in separate area or adjacent room.

D. Social and Recreational Areas

   1. Arts and Crafts Room
- Sketching materials: paper, pencils, tablets
- Ceramic supplies and kiln
- Sewing machine
- Painting and drawing materials, easels
- Work benches
- Storage area for small tools and supplies
- Clay sculpturing material
- Glass etching supplies
- Weaving materials
- Leatherwork supplies; needles, paste
- Knitting and crochet materials
- Mosaic materials for decorating and fittings of murals, plaques, pictures, etc.
- Macramé materials for belts, plant hangers, shades, etc.
- Basketry weaving; frames and reeds

   2. Woodshop
- Workbenches
- Hand power tools
- Storage room for assorted paints and supplies
- Carpentry tools
- Antiquing and finishing supplies
- Saws, screwdrivers, pliers, and assorted screws

   3. Game and Activity Room
- Pool and billiard tables
- Card tables
- Table tennis table
- Storage space

   4. Library and Reading Room
- Sofa and chairs
- Assortment of classic and contemporary books
- Newspapers and magazines
- Encyclopedia
- Unabridged dictionary
- Up-to-date brochures and newsletters about Social Security and community programs affecting senior adults

   5. Dance Studio
- Piano
- Record and cassette players
- Assorted rhythm instruments (rattles, drums, sticks, cymbals, and tambourines)

— Chalkboard
— Bongo drums
— Portable instruments, (e.g., guitar)
  6. Music Room and Lounge
    — High fidelity stereophonic record player
    — Assortment of classical, contemporary and popular recordings
    — Individual ear receivers for listening
    — Television set (adjacent area) equipped with individual sound receivers

II. Outdoor Facilities
  A. Horseshoes
    — Horseshoes (some rubber)
    — Stakes
    — Rule book
  B. Shuffleboard
    — Scoring cards
    — Cues
    — Discs, set
    — Rule book
  C. Tennis
    — Balls
    — Net, posts
    — Rackets
    — Racket presses
    — Rule book
  D. Bocci
    — Balls (lignum vitae or duck pin balls—4½" diameter)
    — Jack (2¾" diameter)
    — Yardstick or flexible ruler
    — Rule book
  E. Lawn bowling
    — Bowls (wooden—16½" circumference)
    — Jack (wooden—8" circumference)
    — Shoes
  F. Exercise Trail
    — Selected exercise stations accenting stretching, balance, and agility activities
    — Walking or jogging trail along exercise stations
    — Instructions with illustrations posted at each station
    — Distance markers at each quarter mile
    — Directional signs at intersections

   —Sneakers
 G. Ice Skating (casual)
   —Skates (nontubular)
 H. Volleyball
   —Balls
   —Net
   —Shoes
   —Rule book
 I. Miniature Golf
   —Putters (32″ and 35″)
   —Golf balls
 J. Softball
   —Balls
   —Bases
   —Bat bag
   —Gloves: catcher's, fielder's, first baseman's

PLANNING FACILITIES FOR THE HANDICAPPED SENIOR ADULT

Considerable attention in recent years has been drawn to the improvement in the quality of life for handicapped individuals of all ages. In the past, buildings were constructed without consideration of persons functioning with vision, hearing, and musculoskeletal limitations. For example, bathrooms with too narrow doorways and entrance steps to buildings created accessibility barriers for wheelchair individuals and discouraged their use of program services. The current philosophy is to allow people to function and live in a least restrictive environment and the most normal or integrated setting feasible.[13] Federal mandates now require that facilities built or renovated with federal funds be accessible to persons with handicapping conditions.

States, cities and towns are supplementing the federal mandate of accessibility through revisions in their building codes and ordinances. Program directors, building committees, and planners should familiarize themselves with the key federal mandates, Public Laws 90–480 and 93–112, which have direct relevance for senior adults, as well as children and youth. The essential points of the legislation are as follows:

- *Public Law 90–480:* "An act to ensure that certain buildings, financed with federal funds, are so designed and constructed as to be accessible to the handicapped, more commonly known as the *Architectural Barrier Act."*
- *Public Law 93–112:* "The Rehabilitation Act of 1973" contains a

nondiscrimination statement on the basis of handicap clause (Section 504) which states, "No otherwise qualified handicapped individual shall, solely by reason of his handicap be excluded from participation in, be denied the benefits of, or be subject to discrimination under any program or activity receiving federal financial assistance. Participants with handicapping conditions must also be provided program opportunities in normal settings appropriate to the maximum degree possible."[14]

The intent of the above laws is to make facilities and programs available and accessible to everyone as a basic right. A composite body of facilities experts assembled by the Athletic Institute and the American Alliance for Health, Physical Education, Recreation and Dance set forth the following concepts that should be considered when planning or adapting facilities for everyone, including handicapped individuals:

- Avoiding making old facilities accessible through addition of new facilities without carefully analyzing how old facilities can be made usable to persons with handicapping conditions.
- Avoiding designs which provide accessibility for part of a facility and create extreme internal barrier problems in other parts of the facility.
- Minimum height factors for mirrors, telephones, lavatories, faucets, elevator buttons, and switch controls should consider their locations as well as populations being served.
- Ramp gradients and turns need to consider all forms of wheelchairs—self-propelled, electric.
- Sufficiently large restrooms with grab bars and accessible sinks and mirrors.
- Low public telephones.
- Low and easily operated water fountains.
- Nonskid floors.
- Elevators, ramps, and/or special lifting devices rather than steps.
- Proper lighting.
- Doors at least 32 inches wide.
- Ramps with a slope not greater than 1 foot rise in 12 feet.
- Hand rails that are smooth, extend 1 foot beyond the top and bottom, and are placed on at least one side of ramps that are 32 inches high.
- Door thresholds flush with the floor.
- Curb-cuts.
- Special and extra large parking spaces for vans and with sufficient space between cars when doors are open.

- Braille markers on elevators and in other key places for information.
- Sound system for emergencies and other program uses.
- Visual warning system for emergencies.
- Pedestrian-operated traffic signals with standardized time-delay to allow deaf or blind persons enough time to cross streets safely.
- Meeting rooms designed so deaf persons can clearly see interpreters, visual display areas, and others in the meeting.
- See through panels in doors, unless privacy is necessary, to allow deaf persons chances to see into rooms before entering.
- Anti-static carpets to avoid interference with hearing aids.
- Flashing light attachments on phones to indicate rings.
- Fire alarm and smoke detection systems attached to strobe lights to ensure that deaf persons are notified of dangers.
- Other emergency messages conveyed graphically—e.g., a sign in an elevator could flash help is on the way should the cab become stuck.[15]

Senior centers and other facilities for social gatherings of yesterday were housed in whatever space was available, such as church halls, converted community centers, and library rooms. Many of these facilities now are obsolete. Specially constructed centers equipped for multiple physical and social functions are now commonplace in the United States.

Many public schools have been converted from classrooms to excellent senior center units. Most centers do not contain standard gymnasiums and natatoriums, unless the facility is a converted school building. Nevertheless, the future bodes well for the inclusion of these necessary facilities in a physical plant designed for older people because of the continuous increase in numbers of this special population. In addition, there is a greater awareness, by society as a whole, about providing preventive programs in maintaining health and fitness through such organizations as multipurpose senior centers and municipal and private recreational organizations. Quality programs require quality support facilities, which include provisions for the handicapped senior adult.

Such mundane elements as parking, building access and entrances, restrooms, telephones, light switches, doorknobs, elevator controls, water fountains, and emergency equipment gear should be easily accessible to persons with limited ambulatory capacity and sensory deficits, all of which tend to increase among the aging. Making common-sense judgments about ways and means of modifying facilities, in collaboration with the involved handicapped person, is a valuable approach to providing usable facilities for the impaired in a normal and integrated setting.

SUMMARY

Facility and equipment design and content vary, depending upon the nature, needs, and interests of the target groups served within the older population. Frail and handicapped elderly require greater specialization in room design, in addition to special apparatus and equipment. A senior center that is fully functional for the well-elderly and for those with limited ambulatory capacity requires a well-planned assortment of indoor and outdoor facilities, equipment, and activity areas. Facility design and content, within a given senior setting, reflects the philosophy of those persons responsible for program development and administration.

This chapter stressed the need for a main gymnasium area as a central facility.

The all-purpose fitness room and natatorium were identified as other important activity stations. The all-purpose fitness room includes equipment for individual workouts, as well as space for the administration and supervision of physical fitness tests. Although most senior centers do not provide natatorium accommodations, these are deemed worthy for inclusion in future senior centers because of the important fitness benefits derived from aquatic activities for older adults.

An arts and crafts room, woodshop, game and activity room, library and reading room, dance studio, and a music room and lounge also were identified as appropriate facilities to satisfy the social and recreation needs of program participants.

Although woodshop activity can be included in the arts and crafts category, it is recommended that wood work, antiquing, and finishing be conducted in a separate area away from the smaller and more fragile equipment necessary for painting, drawing, ceramics, and sculpture. A game and activity room is recommended for billiards, pool, table tennis, and table top games. A library and reading room allows the senior adult to relax and participate in passive activities, alone or with others in a quiet environment. Dance studio dimensions and related equipment were enumerated and discussed. Because of its mental and therapeutic value, a music room and lounge is advocated.

Availability of outdoor facilities represent the other half of a senior center complex designed for a well-functioning program.

Dimensions and playing area specifications were identified for activities from horseshoes to softball.

In order to encourage maximum participation in individual, two-person, and team activities, facilities need nonexpendable items termed *equipment* and expendable items, or *supplies*. Eight determining factors were identified for consideration in the selection and purchase of equipment and supplies.

Building and construction needs of the handicapped senior adult were then discussed. Finally, certain concepts were presented, expressing the current philosophy that it is necessary to enhance the quality of life for handicapped individuals by modifying and adapting structures that are least restrictive, and the most normal in an integrated environmental setting.

REFERENCES

1. John M. Cooper and Clinton Strong, *The Physical Education Curriculum* (Columbia, Mo.: Lucas Brothers Publishers, 1973), p.61.
2. Edward Coates and Richard B. Flynn, eds., *Planning Facilities for Athletics, Physical Education and Recreation* (North Palm Beach, Fla.: Athletic Institute; and Washington, D.C.: American Alliance for Health, Physical Education, Recreation and Dance, 1979), p. 86.
3. Ibid., p. 43.
4. E. Caplow-Lindner, L. Harpaz, and S. Samberg, *Therapeutic Dance/Movement: Expressive Activities for Older Adults* (New York: Human Sciences Press), 1979.
5. C. D. Seaton et al., *Physical Education Handbook,* 7th ed. (Englewood Cliffs, N.J.: Prentice-Hall, 1983).
6. Daniel N. Kuland, David A. Rockwell and Clifford E. Brubaker, "The Long-Term Effects of Playing Tennis," *The Physician and Sportsmedicine* 7, no. 4 (1979): 87–94.
7. Ibid.
8. H. J. Montoye et al., "Bone Mineral in Senior Tennis Players," in *Physician and Sportsmedicine* 9, no. 8 (1981): 43.
9. Elmer D. Mitchell, ed., *Sports for Recreation* (New York: A. S. Barnes, 1952), p. 479.
10. Coates and Flynn, *Planning Facilities,* p. 60.
11. David A. Armbruster, Sr., Frank F. Musker, and Dale Mood, *Basic Skills in Sports for Men and Women,* 6th ed. (St. Louis: C. V. Mosby, 1975).
12. Coates and Flynn, *Planning Facilities,* p. 62.
13. Ibid., p. 192.
14. Ibid., p. 193.
15. Ibid., p. 61.

9

Measurement and Evaluation of Programs for Older Adults: Practical Applications

OVERVIEW

Measurement and evaluation is an integral component of good fitness programs. Base-line data provide initial information and are crucial for establishing individualized exercise prescription. Exit data furnish clues and objective information about program effectiveness. Whatever data we are seeking, the accuracy of assessment depends upon the validity and reliability of the instruments and procedures used.

Another important consideration in measurement and evaluation protocol is related to the purpose of the information sought. If the gerontologist is seeking practical or clinical assessment for broad screening purposes, sophisticated electronic instruments and devices that provide precise figures to thousandths of millimeters are not appropriate. On the other hand, if exact quantitative measurement is desired, valid instruments using stringent research protocol must be employed. For example, indirect testing methods, using the sit-and-reach test (see Figure 9.18), offer adequate base-line data about spinal column flexibility in a field setting. However, if precise data about flexibility variables such as range of motion, amplitude, angular velocity, sequence of movement, or angle of a joint at specific points found in normal and pathological walking patterns are desired, an electrogoniometer (electronic instrument designed to measure angular joint positions while the body is in motion) should be used.

The type of instrument employed and the approach used for measurement differs depending upon: (1) type of information desired, (2) detail required, (3) purpose of the instrument itself, (4) characteristics of the target population, and (5) skill and competence of the evaluator.

Measurement and evaluation should not be considered an end product; that is, facts and figures should not be collected merely for the sake of establishing a record of performance to be filed in the evaluator's office. Fitness testing, evaluation, and assessment are means to an end—to maintain and improve specific physical parameters of older adults discussed in this text for sustaining mobility, independence, and life enrichment. There are several specific reasons for using tests as part of the evaluative process:

- to determine base-line data for initial exercise prescriptive programming.
- to determine the physical fitness status at various points in the program.
- to motivate the participant—help create interest in program activities.
- to analyze needs, strength, and weaknesses of specific fitness parameters.
- to assess the attainability of desired program objectives.
- to determine the value of exercise types and procedures for specific avowed purposes.
- to assist the participant to assess his or her level of performance.
- to provide clues for the program director to evaluate program content and effectiveness.

When evaluating older persons, relevance and meaningfulness of the test should be considered. For example, measurement of explosive strength in a standing broad jump may be a valuable strength parameter for young people in determining power, but it is of little interest to a 65-year-old gentleman who needs enough strength for a leisurely walk to a friend's home or flexibility necessary to work in his vegetable garden.

BASIC MEASUREMENT CONCEPTS

In order for the program evaluator to derive meaningful and accurate information from physical fitness tests, four basic concepts must be involved in evaluation: *validity, reliability, objectivity,* and *norms.* Whether the evaluator is assessing muscular strength or joint range of motion, these statistical concepts must be considered before intelligent judgments can be made about a particular test or the effectiveness of its results.

Validity

A test has validity if it measures what it is supposed to measure. For example, when measuring the range of the shoulder or the knee joint motion, it is invalid to generalize that the individual is flexible or inflexible based upon the scores derived from one or two measurements. Flexibility is specific to a particular joint; that is, a person can be limber in one joint and quite inflexible in another body articulation region. Another example of validity would involve comparing data of the same test on two different population groups. For instance, comparing flexibility scores between arthritic and nonarthritic senior adults to determine typical flexibility ranges among older persons is a vain procedure that will elicit spurious information. Older persons are a diverse and heterogeneous group and must be classified according to their individual capacity before tests of any sort are administered.

Simple scale weighing is another procedure that can give invalid information about a person's leanness or fatness. For example, older persons past 60 tend to be lighter due to decreases in muscle and bone densities, yet, they may also be fatter—which can result in overall reduced weight since adipose tissue is less heavy than muscle and bone. Thus, when assessing body fat, weight measurement alone will not yield valid data about body composition. Thus validity of measurement is affected by the characteristics of the instrument, the purpose of the test, and the method used to collect the data.

Reliability

Test reliability refers to the ability to obtain consistent results with repeated measurements. Some measures demand similar results, other calculations need exact duplication of scores depending upon nature and purpose of the administered test. For example, precision and accuracy of a weight scale are essential factors for correct interpretation of body weight. If the scale reads 150¼ lbs. on the first reading, and 150½ on a second reading immediately following the first trial, the scale is unacceptable as a reliable weighing instrument. On the other hand, blood pressure readings can be reliable without showing exact duplication of scores since actual variations occur from one reading to another, and such figures may be acceptable to the evaluator depending upon established pressure ranges.

Reliability may also be affected by methods of performing a test. For example, if the individual is doing sit-ups with legs straight in the first trial and then executes the same exercise with legs bent, the reliability coefficients between the two tests would be low because it is more difficult to perform the exercise with legs bent than straight (assuming that other variables remain constant).

Another source of error that affects reliability of measurement lies with the tester. For example, when body fat content is determined using a skinfold caliper, it is not uncommon for inconsistency of scores to occur.[1] Although the instrument may be precise and accurate, the tester's failure to master the technique of measurement can result in a low reliability coefficient, consequently lessening the validity of the test. Practicing on the same subjects using the correct technique decreases the probability of low reliability of the tester. A detailed discussion of body composition measurement using skinfold calipers is presented in a later section of this chapter.

Objectivity

Test objectivity and reliability are similar concepts, but not identical. Reliability refers to a situation in which only one examiner is repeating the same test on the same group of subjects and then comparing the results, while objectivity refers to two or more examiners comparing their results.[2] For example, in skinfold measurement, if the two sets of skinfold scores gathered by two testers agree, it can be concluded that the skinfold test is objective. Any test that is not high on objectivity and reliability should be dropped, particularly when using data for research purposes.[3] It is obvious that the application of unreliable or nonobjective tests caused by using inaccurate instruments or improper techniques destroys the value of evaluation and complicates the process of making intelligent judgments in assessing the benefits or ineffectiveness of a particular test at hand.

Norms

Norms represent a standard to which obtained data can be compared. The purpose of norms is to provide information that helps interpret the significance of the data in relation to the attainment of scores made by individuals of a sample population. A problem may arise when dealing with older persons, for, as noted previously, the elderly constitute a diverse and heterogeneous group, and the practitioner or researcher must be cautious in generalizing when comparing test results involving the elderly of the same chronological age. Certain individuals may be under drug therapy, others may have chronic disabilities, such as arthritis or cardiovascular conditions, which affect physical performance. Norms must be specific to the group that is being studied and should contain a sufficient number of subjects to assure the reliability of the established scores. Their application is dependent upon the representativeness of the tested sample. For example, the data gathered about strength, flexibility, and motor performance from a sampling of institutionalized residents in a long-term care facility are not applicable to the well-elderly living independently at home.

Although national norms provide clues to performance levels about certain fitness parameters within given samples, such standards only offer indirect evidence at best because of the plethora of variables that can influence the validity and reliability of set standards. Evaluators would probably gain more meaningful models of performance (norms) if such measurement data were taken from their local situation within a specific group over an extended period of time. It should be remembered that norms are temporary, representing scores at a particular time and under a given set of circumstances. As such, standards determined 30 years ago for older adults need updating and revision to accommodate societal changes that affect the characteristics and abilities of the tested subjects.*

FIELD-BASED ASSESSMENT VERSUS RESEARCH ASSESSMENT

Selection criteria for field-based and research evaluative instruments can be similar in certain characteristics and quite different in other ways. Whether the investigator chooses a field-based or research instrument, tools, devices, procedures, and techniques should satisfy the basic requirements of validity, reliability, and objectivity.

Essentially, research modes demand absolute precision, accuracy, and freedom from bias using the scientific method of inquiry when solving a problem. For example, using a sophisticated electrogoniometer for recording the range of motion and other flexibility patterns on a goniogram provides valid and reliable information about body joints at rest and in motion. However, such instruments are expensive and require some knowledge of electronic phenomena and biomechanics—in addition to the possibility of posing an obtrusive and uncomfortable testing situation for the older adult participating in field-based testing in such environments as multipurpose senior centers. Such devices are not considered practical for everyday fitness programs in community-based settings. On the other hand, mechanical goniometers or Leighton Flexometers, shown in Figure 9.14 and 9.16, are less costly, bulky, and simple to use when the correct protocol is followed. The ensuing discussion focuses upon practical instruments and techniques that can be applied in a field-based or clinical setting, as contrasted

*See Barry L. Johnson and Jack K.Nelson, *Practical Measurements for Evaluation in Physical Education* (Minneapolis: Burgess Publishing, 1979) for an expanded discussion of validity, reliability, objectivity, and norms.

with instrumentation systems found in university or hospital research laboratories.

Criteria for the Selection of Practical Assessment Instruments

Assessment systems may be classified into two broad categories: qualitative and quantitative. Qualitative analysis of a movement or motor skills entails the identification and assessment of action components as a whole. The quality of performance is *subjectively* rated by the evaluator. Such procedures are appropriate when analyzing and correcting errors in walking, bending, or climbing stairs, or when the senior adult is participating in swimming, volleyball, horseshoes, bowling, etc.

Quantitative analysis implies determining the exact numerical components of a motor skill or action. Data is collected *objectively* using valid and reliable instruments focusing upon a particular component of a total motor performance. Quantitative measurement depends on the precision, accuracy of instrumentation, and expertise of the tester, not upon the subjective judgment of the tester. For example, using the Leighton Flexometer for flexibility measurement or a hand dynamometer for grip strength will yield quantitative numerical data, rather than a judgmental assessment. Each of these approaches can be used effectively by the practitioner depending upon his or her objectives.

The choice of selecting a qualitative or quantitative instrument and approach for practical use involves the following considerations:

- Instrument should be *reliable* and *valid*.
- Technique should be *simple*.
- Instrument should be relatively *inexpensive* and require *minimum maintenance*.
- Instrument and technique should be *nonthreatening* and acceptable to the participant.
- Instrument should be *portable*, not bulky.
- Instrument should be *safe* to use.
- Instrument should be appropriate to the *nature* and *capabilities* of the targeted population.
- Purpose of the instrument should be *understood* by the *evaluator* and the *client*.
- Formulas and statistical procedures used should be easily *computed* and *understood*.
- Test should be *relevant* to the daily lives of the older adult.

The evaluator should remember that we are dealing with an at-risk population. Instruments and testing protocols must consider the safety and well-being of the senior adult as a *first* responsibility. For example, maximum stress tests of cardiovascular endurance for the typical unconditioned senior adult present an undue risk in field-based programming and are inappropriate for typical retirement centers. Such fitness testing protocols should be reserved for the exceptional adult, and conducted in research or hospital environments under the careful supervision of medical and technically qualified personnel.

The intelligent use of tests requires a pattern of *consistency* using valid and reliable instruments. This process implies an orderly manner of selecting, analyzing, and comparing data germane to a targeted population.

MEASUREMENT OF SPECIFIC FITNESS COMPONENTS

Measuring and evaluating specific physical components embraces the concept of *functional fitness*. Certain fitness authorities would classify balance and neuromusuclar coordination as performance skills and not true fitness parameters. Others subscribe to the notion that the only genuine measure of physical fitness is heart-lung efficiency. Still other experts would argue that flexibility is primarily an inherited trait.[4] Rather than categorize these fitness components as performance-based or physical fitness attributes, this discussion centers on those parameters relevant to the effective functioning of the human machine in work, play, and everyday living tasks irrespective of their motor performance or physical fitness labels.

Measurement of Cardiorespiratory Efficiency

From our discussion of cardiovascular and pulmonary functions in Chapters 4 and 5, it is evident that cardiorespiratory evaluations entail objective measurements of heart rate and blood pressure. The field-based methods of using the basic formula of 220 minus age and procedures of determining heart rate by monitoring the pulse beat have been described in considerable detail. The presentation now focuses upon instrumentation systems and types of equipment used to measure heart rate and blood pressure.

Bicycle Ergometer. A common way of determining heart rate is by measuring the amount of "work" performed on a stationary bicycle or ergometer. This activity can load the heart and respiratory muscles from low to high degrees depending upon the prescribed resistance load and rate of pedaling. The stationary bike is used for exercise stress testing at submaximal or maximum levels in field-based settings, and is also widely found in physiological laboratories.

Figure 9.1 exhibits a model designed for testing purposes that features a

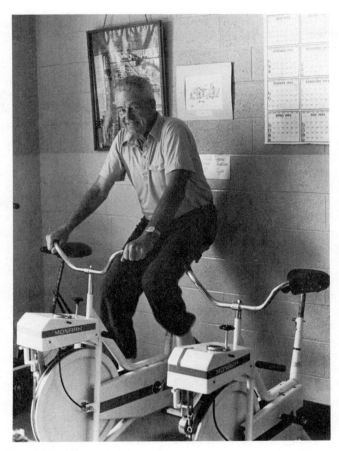

Figure 9.1 Exercise bicycle ergometer.

Newton scale showing kilopounds and Newton units, built-in speedometer and odometer, and a handwheel to adjust braking resistance. Other related equipment necessary to determine exercise work loads includes: (1) metronome, (2) stop watch, and (3) clock to determine work-time. If blood pressure measures are used in the protocol, a sphygmomanometer is also necessary (see Chapter 4).

In bicycle ergometer tests, the subject attempts to pedal at a constant rate—in time with a metronome. The energy output is accelerated by increasing the braking resistance. The load is adjusted by varying the tension (braking resistance) of a belt running around the rim of the wheel while the subject pedals. Most bike testing procedures have two- to three-minute stages, and resistance is increased by 100 or 150 to 300 kpm/min. per stage. Older and less fit persons begin at a 100 or 150 to 300 kpm/min. power output and increase by 100 or 150 kpm/min. per stage.[5]

The YMCA has developed a submaximal stress test that consists of three three-minute stages. The first stage starts at 300 kpm/min. for men and 150 kpm/min. for women. Depending upon intensity (heart rate response and sex), the second stage increases to a higher rate beyond 150 kpm/min. The third stage is increased even further depending upon heart response. The intensity increases every three minutes unless the heart rate does not level off. The heart rate and blood pressure are taken at the end of every second and third minute. Subjects pedal at 50 revolutions per minute (rpm). The basic formula of 220 minus age is used to establish maximum heart rate response. Maximum heart rate, workloads, and exercise heart rate for first and second stages are plotted on a chart which yields the subject's maximum O_2 uptake and fitness level. Details of the test procedure and explanatory charts for estimating VO_2 max are found in the *The Y's Way to Physical Fitness*.[6]

Unlike the treadmill, where the speed is controlled by the technician, bike pedaling depends upon the subject, so it is important to motivate the participant to maintain a constant rate of pedaling. Bicycle ergometers are portable and their cost is considerably less than that of treadmill devices. In certain cases subjects may be unaccustomed to bicycle pedaling and may have to stop prematurely due to thigh fatigue. Other forms of submaximal stress tests such as the treadmill or step tests are presented in the following sections. Overall, if the correct protocol is followed with careful monitoring, submaximal bicycle ergometer tests can provide accurate and useful information for programming individualized exercise prescriptions.

Treadmill Testing. Treadmill devices are the most widely used mode of evaluating cardiorespiratory efficiency in testing facilities within the United States.[7] The treadmill has an advantage over the cycle ergometer since the subject keeps up with a moving belt, pre-regulated by the tester, instead of working to the cadence of the metronome—and is therefore less likely to be influenced by motivation and interest. Most treadmills have adjustable belt speed and the capacity to provide variable inclinations of grade to allow progressive increments of work loads.

The treadmill device probably also has an advantage over the cycle ergometer from a motor coordination standpoint since bicycle movements require greater leg coordination than walking. On the other hand, the bicycle ergometer has the following advantages over the treadmill:

- Less expensive.
- Requires little space.

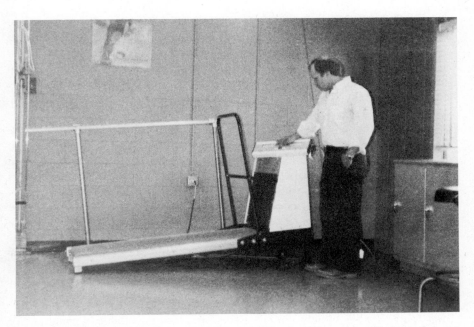

Figure 9.2 Treadmill testing apparatus. (From the Physical Therapy and Exercise Science Laboratory, State University of New York at Buffalo.)

- Easily transported.
- Easier to take heart rate.
- Requires little or no training in learning sessions.
- External work is known.[8]

Several protocols are frequently used employing the treadmill, such as the Bruce, Balke, Ellestad, Naughton, and the National Exercise Project Treadmill tests. Each of these tests meets the basic exercise requirements set forth by the American College of Sports Medicine and the American Heart Association, which recommend that the initial work load for deconditioned individuals be graded and should not exceed three MET Units. Work loads should increase gradually and should not progress more than one to two METS per increment. Each stage of the test should last for a minimum of one minute.[9]

The Bruce protocol is a commonly used test featuring a multi-stage treadmill progression from a slow walk upgrade to jogging on stepping grades until the subject's activity is limited by fatigue or other factors. The protocol begins at a slope of 10 percent and a speed of 1.7 miles per hour. It contains seven stages, and few nonathletes progress beyond the fourth stage.[10] The Naughton Test is recommended for older less-fit and cardiac patients.[11] This test starts the subject at 1 mph and progresses to 2 mph with a grade increase of zero to 22 percent. The total test requires one-half hour. Although there are a number of variations to treadmill testing, it is advisable to use the constant speed tests (increasing grade with belt speed held constant) when testing nonathletic, and persons unfamiliar with the equipment.

Treadmill testing, when used for medical screening and evaluation, requires competent and professional personnel, well-versed in anatomy, physiology, equipment calibration, and electrocardiographic protocol. These procedures are used for medical evaluations and must be monitored by a physician. Thus, for practical field-based settings such elaborate systems may not be feasible. Treadmill testing with ECG capabilities should be reserved for settings with trained technical personnel (e.g., prescribed by the American College of Sports Medicine) and clinical environments usually found in hospitals or research laboratories under the control and surveillance of an attending physician. The work of Wilmore et al. and the other reseachers cited throughout this section provide further details about the advantages and disadvantages of various treadmill stress testing equipment and protocols.[12]

Step Tests. If a bicycle ergometer or treadmill is not available, a rough index of conditioning may be attained by using a step test. Such a test requires a bench ranging in height from 16 inches to 20 inches, adjusted according to the subject's height (see Figure 9.3 and Table 9.1).

The individual steps up and down on the bench at a rate of 30 times per minute for a total of four minutes. At fatigue or the completion of the test,

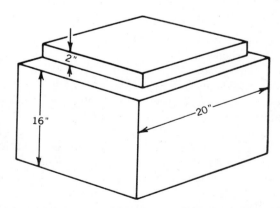

Figure 9.3 Bench used for modified Harvard step test. (From G. F. Fletcher and J. D. Cantwell, *Exercise in the Management of Coronary Heart Disease* Springfield, Ill.: Charles C. Thomas, 1971, p. 46. Used with permission.)

Table 9.1   Bench Test Determination of Post-Exercise Pulse Recovery

	Subject Height	Bench Height	
	5 ft, 3 in to 5 ft, 9 in	15 in	
	5 ft, 9 in to 6 ft	18 in	
	over 6 ft	20 in	

Total Pulse Counts[a]	Recovery Index	Fitness Grade
> 198	< 61	Poor
171 to 198	61 to 70	Fair
150 to 170	71 to 80	Good
133 to 149	81 to 90	Very Good
< 133	> 90	Excellent

[a]Total Pulse Count = total number of pulse beats during first 30 seconds of each of the first three minutes following exercise.
Source: G. F. Fletcher and J. D. Cantwell, *Management of Coronary Heart Disease*, p. 47. Used with permission.

the subject rests in a sitting position for one minute and his or her pulse is then taken during the first 30 seconds of each of the following three minutes. The three numbers are added together and a pulse recovery index and fitness grade are scored according to Table 9.1.

The master two-step test represents an inexpensive cardiovascular diagnostic and rehabilitation test that has been used for more than 40 years.[13] This test is a variation of the bench step test and requires a two-step apparatus with each step 9 inches high and about 10 inches deep. The width of the steps is 20 to 24 inches. In performing the test, the subject ascends to the top of the two-step apparatus and walks down the other side, which is counted as one trip. The steps are retraced to perform a second, third, and fourth trip until the end-point of the exercise is reached. The task is to complete the trips if possible in three minutes. The test is terminated before its completion upon signs of fatigue or distress. The number of trips required have been standardized for age, sex, and weight (15 to 79 yrs) with tabular data in Fletcher and Cantwell's *Exercise and Coronary Heart Disease*. Such tests should be monitored by a physician with an exercise technical assistant using electrocardiographic equipment; this electronic requirement constricts its use by exercise leaders in a field-based environment.

Measurement of Body Composition

Adipose is one of the most variable tissues found in the body. Because fat tissue peaks in early childhood and again in late maturity, with a decline past 70 years of age, comparisons and norms of fat data must be made using persons from similar populations. For example, generalizing about fat content of persons past 60 based on scores generated measuring young adults or middle-aged people will yield misleading information. Not only do fat characteristics differ among age groups, but distinct differences between males and females, as well as in site patterns, exist within the older population. For example, among older adults, loss tends to be centripetal; that is, fat is lost earlier and to a greater degree from the extremities, and is maintained more consistently and longer on the trunk.[14] Females generally show a greater skinfold thickness pattern throughout the life cycle.[15] These variable adipose patterns are also influenced by individualistic somatotype, nutrition, and activity level. Thus, tables and norms reflecting fat amounts at several body points should be interpreted as general clues to obesity or leanness rather than absolute standards.

Hydrostatic Weighing. This method of determining leanness/fatness ratio represents an indirect procedure of estimating body composition. The technique requires total immersion of the subject in water and consequently necessitates specialized equipment. The system applies the Archimedes principle: i.e., an object will displace a volume of water equal to its own volume. The volume of water displaced can be measured and its weight determined. Dense objects will displace less water per unit of weight. For example, one pound of bone or lean meat will displace less water than one pound of fat. By weighing an object on land and then while totally submerged, its density can be ascertained. This is accomplished by computing the object's specific gravity.

$$\text{Specific gravity} = \frac{\text{weight of an object}}{\text{weight of an equal volume of water}}$$

Because an object's loss of weight in water equals the weight of the volume of water it displaces, specific gravity can also be defined as the ratio of the weight of an object in air over its loss of weight in water.

$$\text{Specific gravity} = \frac{\text{weight of an object in air}}{(\text{weight in air} - \text{weight in water})}$$

Experiments have established that fat has a specific gravity of 0.90; in other words, its weight for a specific volume is less than the weight of a like volume of water. Experiments have also established that fat-free tissue has a specific gravity of 1.10. Because the animal bodies, including the human body, consist of fat and fat-free tissue, their specific gravity must range between 0.90 and 1.10.

Specific gravity is a measure of the weight of an object in relation to its volume or its density.

$$\text{density} = \frac{\text{weight}}{\text{volume}}$$

Thus, it becomes obvious that a person's specific gravity is basically a measure of the proportion of fat to lean tissue in his or her body. The weight of the total body fat is determined by multiplying the total body weight by the percent of body fat using an established equation. Other factors such as water, temperature, and residual volume (the air in the lungs) must also be measured to correct the buoyancy effect upon the underwater weight.

Although this method of determining body fat is an accurate technique, the use of such procedures is restricted to hospital and research laboratory settings because of the prohibitive equipment costs and technical skills necessary for measuring and collecting the data. Additionally, such assessment methods may intimidate senior adults, particularly those individuals who are less skillful at holding their breath underwater. When accuracy is essential, this procedure offers a valid means of measuring body fat.*

Practical Adipose Measurement. Body shape and adipose dimensions for young and older persons can be determined by simple girth measurements and skinfold caliper procedures. Calipers are particularly well-suited for older people since this instrument is innocuous and easy to use and interpret.

Chest, abdominal, arm, and leg circumference provide objective data about size and shape. Caliper techniques furnish evidence about adipose tissue. Although girth measurements yield configurative data, this procedure does not distinguish differences between muscular and fatty tissue. Girth size may be due to adipose deposits or concentrated stores of muscle mass. Since fat is inactive tissue, and muscular fibers provide the energy source for human mobility, maintenance of a sensible state of muscular tone and hypertrophy is vital as one advances in chronological years.

The skinfold caliper shown in Figure 9.4 is a valid instrument to determine subcutaneous (skinfold) thickness. However, careful attention is needed with the technique. Variability of skinfold scores greatly depends upon the objectivity of the tester's procedure. Careful and consistent bite depths of the subcutaneous folds must be observed using a calibrated caliper with jaw face pressure of 10 gm/mm^2.

*For further details about hydrostatic weighing, see John Piscopo and James A. Baley, *Kinesiology; The Science of Movement* (New York: John Wiley & Sons, 1981), Chapter 3.

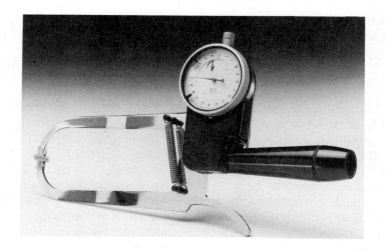

Figure 9.4 The Harpenden skinfold caliper. (Courtesy of British Indicators, Ltd. St. Albans, Herts, England

The skinfold caliper measurement technique provides a quick and accurate estimate of body fat and should be part of the body composition evaluative process of older persons. The resultant data, in conjunction with other anthropometrical measurements such as height, weight, and girth measurements, can provide an effective way to appraise the leanness/fatness status of an individual.

The ease and rapidity with which a fold of skin is located and lifted are important factors in site selection of skinfolds. Based on the author's experience and that of other skinfold caliper researchers, the following body areas are recommended, fulfilling the criteria of ease, accuracy, and rapidity of measurement:[16]

> *Posterior arm.* With subject standing, measurement is made at the fold parallel to the long axis of the preferred arm, over the triceps, halfway between the olecranon and acromial processes (Figure 9.5a).
>
> *Abdomen.* With subject standing, measurement is made with skinfold oriented laterally approximately 5 cm. to the right of the navel (Figure 9.5b).
>
> *Scapula.* With subject standing, measurement is made at the fold diagonally from the vertebral column toward the inferior angle and slightly toward the midline of the body (Figure 9.5c).

The upper posterior arm is a popular measurement location and can give reliable estimates when only one site is to be measured. Additionally, this surface area can be measured without the subject having to disrobe.

A fourth site, located in the chest area, may also be used in males:

Chest. With the subject standing, measurement is made at the fold parallel to a line from the right nipple and uppermost point of the axillary fold (5 cm. from the nipple) (Figure 9.5d).

Measure of the chest skinfold is rather awkward in females, and may be omitted.

Skinfold Measurement Technique. The skinfold is lifted with the thumb and index finger and held while the caliper is applied approximately one cm. away. A firm hold on the skinfold is preferred, with the caliper jaws applied in such a way that the critical pressure on the skinfold is exercised by the constant surfaces of the instrument, not by the observer's fingers. Measurements are highly dependent upon caliper pressure until at least 10 gm/mm^2 between the jaw faces is reached. The positioning of the contact plates on the fold is an important consideration. Keys and Brozek state that when the plates are placed at the very bottom of the skinfold, the values will be larger than when the fold proper is measured.[17] These researchers recommend that the vertical depth of the skinfold at which the thickness is to be measured be about one-half of the preliminary estimate of the skinfold thickness. All skinfolds should be measured carefully at least three times before the final value is recorded.

Interpretation of Skinfold Size. The manner in which subcutaneous fat is distributed over the body from early childhood to old age undergoes considerable change. For example, fat tissue tends to accumulate in the abdominal area and diminish in the extremities in advanced age. Differences occur between older males and females—older women retain larger thickness of skinfolds in the abdominal region over a longer period of time than males, as indicated in Figure 9.6.

When comparing fat fold measurements with norms, the data should be matched with similar population age groups and sex because of the variability throughout the life span. Most tables of norms focus upon young and middle-aged people, and absolute judgment regarding fatness or leanness should be approached with caution. For example, a 20-mm. fat fold size in the abdominal area of a 65-year-old male may be perfectly normal, but this figure could indicate a propensity toward obesity for an 18-year-old person.

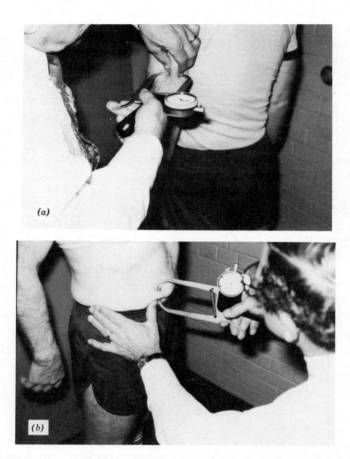

Figure 9.5 Measuring skinfolds: (a) measuring posterior arm skinfold; (b) measuring abdominal skinfold; (c) measuring scapula skinfold; (d) measuring chest skinfold.

Studies involving men and women from 16 to 72 years of age have served as a basis for generating prediction equations in estimating total body fat.[18] Jackson adapted regression equations based upon the above research and developed percent body fat estimate tables for men and women (see Tables 9.2 and 9.3).[19] These tables are currently used as standards in National YMCA programs. Examples of skinfold measurements using the sum of four selected sites for men, and three locations for women, are shown below:

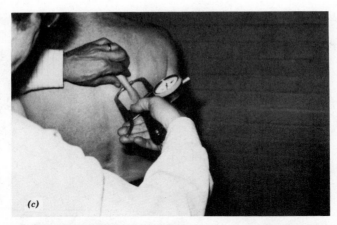

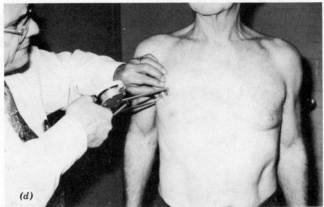

Example 1. Subject A:—Male 58 years old

Chest	21 mm
Ilium	28 mm
Abdomen	33 mm
Axilla	20 mm
Total	102 mm

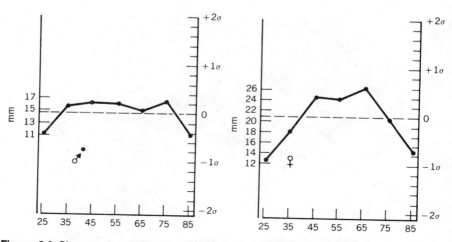

Figure 9.6 Changes in paraumbilical skinfold thickness with age and sex. The fold is thicker in the female, and the maximum reached later in life. (From E. C. Finch and L. Hayflick, eds., *Handbook of the Biology of Aging,* (c) 1977 by Van Nostrand Reinhold Co, New York, p. 198. Reprinted by permission of the publisher.)

Example 2. Subject B:—Female 58 years old

Ilium	25 mm
Abdomen	30 mm
Triceps	18 mm
Total	73 mm

Using Table 9.2, which is the sum of four skinfolds, a total of 102 mm and age 58 at last birthday gives a percent fat of 26.7 percent. Using Table 9.3, which is the sum of three skinfolds, a total of 73 mm at age 58 gives a percent fat of 31.1 percent.

It should be noted that the ilium (hip) skinfold (see Figure 9.7), which is the diagonal fold just above the crest of the ilium, is used in totaling the skinfolds, and the triceps site is deleted in the Y model for men. The axilla site is (see Figure 9.8) is also incorporated into the summation instead of the scapula location.

What is the ideal body fat content for the senior adult? It has been suggested that for men it should be under 20 percent and for women under 30 percent from a health risk standpoint. These figures probably are too large, if the goals sought are for posture, aesthetic, or physical training purposes. Tables 9.2 and 9.3 offer estimates only and should not be considered to be final. We have yet to show scientifically that moderate leanness or fatness

Table 9.2 Percent Fat Estimates for Men (Sum of Four Skinfolds: Chest, Ilium, Abdomen, Axilla)

Sum of 4 Skinfolds	18 to 22	23 to 27	28 to 32	33 to 37	38 to 42	43 to 47	48 to 52	53 to 57	58 and older
					Age To Last Year				
8–12	1.9	2.5	3.2	3.8	4.4	5.0	5.7	6.3	6.9
13–17	3.3	3.9	4.5	5.1	5.7	6.4	7.0	7.6	8.2
18–22	4.5	5.2	5.8	6.4	7.0	7.7	8.3	8.9	9.5
23–27	5.8	6.4	7.1	7.7	8.3	8.9	9.5	10.2	10.8
28–32	7.1	7.7	8.3	8.9	9.5	10.2	10.8	11.4	12.0
33–37	8.3	8.9	9.5	10.1	10.8	11.4	12.0	12.6	13.2
38–42	9.5	10.1	10.7	11.3	11.9	12.6	13.2	13.8	14.4
43–47	10.6	11.3	11.9	12.5	13.1	13.7	14.4	15.0	15.6
48–52	11.8	12.4	13.0	13.6	14.2	14.9	15.5	16.1	16.7
53–57	12.9	13.5	14.1	14.7	15.4	16.0	16.6	17.2	17.9
58–62	14.0	14.6	15.2	15.8	16.4	17.1	17.7	18.3	18.9
63–67	15.0	15.6	16.3	16.9	17.5	18.1	18.8	19.4	20.0
68–72	16.1	16.7	17.3	17.9	18.5	19.2	19.8	20.4	21.0
73–77	17.1	17.7	18.3	18.9	19.5	20.2	20.8	21.4	22.0
78–82	18.0	18.7	19.3	19.9	20.5	21.0	21.8	22.4	23.0
83–87	19.0	19.6	20.2	20.8	21.5	22.1	22.7	23.3	24.0
88–92	19.9	20.5	21.2	21.8	22.4	23.0	23.6	24.3	24.9
93–97	20.8	21.4	22.1	22.7	23.3	23.9	24.5	25.2	25.8
98–102	21.7	22.3	22.9	23.5	24.2	24.8	25.4	26.0	26.7
103–107	22.5	23.2	23.8	24.4	25.0	25.6	26.3	26.9	27.5
108–112	23.4	24.0	24.6	25.2	25.8	26.5	27.1	27.7	28.3
113–117	24.1	24.8	25.4	26.0	26.6	27.3	27.9	28.5	29.1
118–122	24.9	25.5	26.2	26.8	27.4	28.0	28.6	29.3	29.9
123–127	25.7	26.3	26.9	27.5	28.1	28.8	29.4	30.0	30.6
128–132	26.4	27.0	27.6	28.2	28.8	29.5	30.1	30.7	31.3
133–137	27.1	27.7	28.3	28.9	29.5	30.2	30.8	31.4	32.0
138–142	27.7	28.3	29.0	29.6	30.2	30.8	31.4	32.1	32.7
143–147	28.3	29.0	29.6	30.2	30.8	31.5	32.1	32.7	33.3
148–152	29.0	29.6	30.2	30.8	31.4	32.1	32.7	33.3	33.9
153–157	29.5	30.2	30.8	31.4	32.0	32.7	33.3	33.9	34.5
158–162	30.1	30.7	31.3	31.9	32.6	33.2	33.8	34.4	35.1
163–167	30.6	31.2	31.9	32.5	33.1	33.7	34.3	35.0	35.6
168–172	31.1	31.7	32.4	33.0	33.6	34.2	34.8	35.5	36.1
173–177	31.6	32.2	32.8	33.5	34.1	34.7	35.3	35.9	36.6
178–182	32.0	32.7	33.3	33.9	34.5	35.2	35.8	36.4	37.0
183–187	32.5	33.1	33.7	34.3	34.9	35.6	36.2	26.8	37.4
188–192	32.9	33.5	34.1	34.7	35.3	36.0	36.6	37.2	37.8
193–197	33.2	33.8	34.5	35.1	35.7	36.3	37.0	36.8	38.2
198–202	33.6	34.2	34.8	35.4	36.1	36.7	37.3	37.9	38.5
203–207	33.9	34.5	35.1	35.7	36.4	37.0	37.6	38.2	38.9

Source: L. D. Golding, C. R. Myers, and W. E. Sinning, eds., *The Y's Way to Physical Fitness,* rev. ed. (National Board of YMCA, 1982), p. 102. Used with permission.

Table 9.3   Percent Fat Estimate for Women (Sum of Three Skinfolds: Triceps, Abdomen, and Ilium)

Sum of 3 Skinfolds	18 to 22	23 to 27	28 to 32	33 to 37	38 to 42	43 to 47	48 to 52	53 to 57	58 and older
8–12	8.8	9.0	9.2	9.4	9.5	9.7	9.9	10.1	10.3
13–17	10.8	10.9	11.1	11.3	11.5	11.7	11.8	12.0	12.2
18–22	12.6	12.8	13.0	13.2	13.4	13.5	13.7	13.9	14.1
23–27	14.5	14.6	14.8	15.0	15.2	15.4	15.6	15.7	15.9
28–32	16.2	16.4	16.6	16.8	17.0	17.1	17.3	17.5	17.7
33–37	17.9	18.1	18.3	18.5	18.7	18.9	19.0	19.2	19.4
38–42	19.6	19.8	20.0	20.2	20.3	20.5	20.7	20.9	21.1
43–47	21.2	21.4	21.6	21.8	21.9	22.1	22.3	22.5	22.7
48–52	22.8	22.9	23.1	23.3	23.5	23.7	23.8	24.0	24.2
53–57	24.2	24.4	24.6	24.8	25.0	25.2	25.3	25.5	25.7
									27.1
58–62	25.7	25.9	26.0	26.2	26.4	26.6	26.8	27.0	37.1
63–67	27.1	27.2	27.4	27.6	27.8	28.0	28.2	28.3	28.5
68–72	28.4	28.6	28.7	28.9	29.1	29.3	29.5	29.7	29.8
73–77	29.6	29.8	30.0	30.2	30.4	30.6	30.7	30.9	31.1
78–82	30.9	31.0	31.2	31.4	31.6	31.8	31.9	32.1	32.3
83–87	32.0	32.2	32.4	32.6	32.7	32.9	33.1	33.3	33.5
88–92	33.1	33.3	33.5	33.7	33.8	34.0	34.2	34.4	34.6
93–97	34.1	34.3	34.5	34.7	34.9	35.1	35.2	35.4	35.6
98–102	35.1	35.3	35.5	35.7	35.9	36.0	36.2	36.4	36.6
103–107	36.1	36.2	36.4	36.6	36.8	37.0	37.2	37.3	37.5
108–112	36.9	37.1	37.3	37.5	37.7	37.9	38.0	38.2	38.4
113–117	37.8	37.9	38.1	38.3	39.2	39.4	39.6	39.8	40.0
118–122	38.5	38.7	38.9	39.1	39.4	39.6	39.8	40.0	
123–127	39.2	39.4	39.6	39.8	40.0	40.1	40.3	40.5	40.7
128–132	39.9	40.1	40.2	40.4	40.6	40.8	41.0	41.2	41.3
133–137	40.5	40.7	40.8	41.0	41.2	41.4	41.6	41.7	41.9
138–142	41.0	41.2	41.4	41.6	41.7	41.9	42.1	42.3	42.5
143–147	41.5	41.7	41.9	42.0	42.2	42.4	42.6	42.8	43.0
148–152	41.9	42.1	42.3	42.8	42.6	42.8	43.0	43.2	43.4
153–157	42.3	42.5	42.6	52.8	43.0	43.2	43.4	43.6	43.7
158–162	42.6	42.8	42.0	43.1	43.3	43.5	43.7	43.9	44.1
163–167	42.9	43.0	43.2	43.4	43.6	43.8	44.0	44.1	44.3
168–172	43.1	43.2	43.4	43.6	43.8	44.0	44.2	44.3	44.5
173–177	43.2	43.4	43.6	43.8	43.9	44.1	44.3	44.5	44.7
178–182	43.3	43.5	43.7	43.8	44.0	44.2	44.4	44.6	44.8

Source: Golding, Myers, and Sinning, *Y's Way to Physical Fitness,* p. 83. Used with permission.

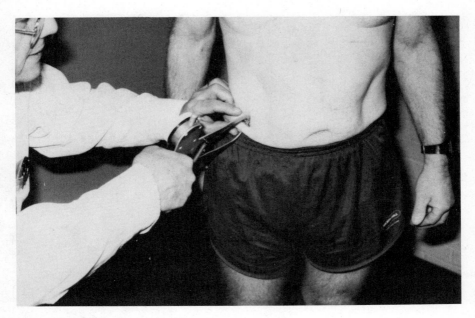

Figure 9.7 Measurement of the hip skinfold.

significantly affects longevity, but we do know that gross obesity increases mortality and morbidity in both sexes. Until definitive mortality evidence about obesity is produced, it appears advisable to keep skinfolds within a pinch of an inch (about 26 mm) at all measurement sites.

Measurement of Muscular Strength and Endurance

When evaluating strength, two general types should be considered: isometric and dynamic. Isometric strength measurement involves testing various muscle groups in a single all-out effort, essentially without significant motion. For example, grip strength testing is the quantifying of an isometric muscular contraction of the forearm flexors.

Dynamic strength grading is based on muscular task with a continuous flow of motion, usually in a repetitive pattern. Assessing sit-ups is one dynamic muscular test, usually to evaluate flexors of the trunk and abdominal muscles. Another way of looking at strength testing is from maximum force that can be exerted in a *single effort,* or a force that is *sustained* over a period of time. Each of these types of muscle strength tests can be performed statically or dynamically. For example, the grip strength test, using a hand dynamometer, is classified as a static test of muscular strength, apply-

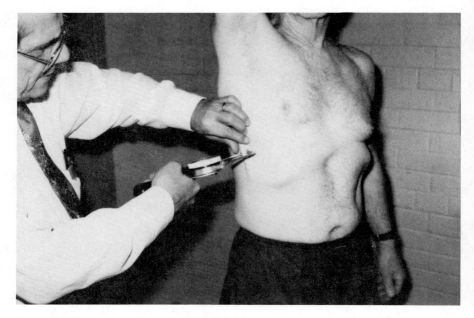

Figure 9.8 Measurement of the axilla skinfold.

ing maximum effort for about 5 to 10 seconds. Conversely, completing a dynamic series of sit-ups within a prescribed period of time is a test of muscular endurance. Thus, it can be seen that muscle contraction can be exerted statically (muscle strength) in one burst of energy or produced in a sustained or continuous manner (muscle endurance). Each of these types should be measured when evaluating older adults.

Measurement of Muscular Static Strength. Static strength measures may involve many muscle groups and various body regions, such as arm and leg extension, back extension, trunk flexion, and other joint movements whereby tension is applied in a single effort of maximum contraction. The measurement of total body strength is not practical in a field-based situation because of the time factor, assemblage of various testing devices, and— perhaps its most significant disadvantage—obtrusive nature of multiple test procedures to the senior adult.

A simple test that can be done quickly and represents a fairly good measure of body static strength is the hand grip strength test. A grip dynamometer is used to measure the muscular torque (grip) of the hand and forearm as shown in Figure 9.9. The instrument is constructed with an aluminum frame; the dial is calibrated in kilograms with two indicating point-

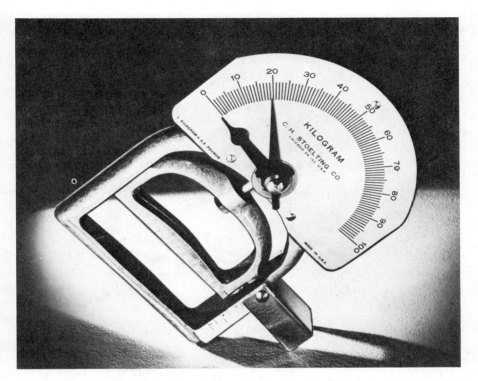

Figure 9.9 Hand dynamometer for measuring hand and forearm grip strength. (Courtesy of Stoelting Co., 1350 South Kostner Avenue, Chicago, Ill.)

ers employed: one pointer, having a range from 0–100 kg. indicates the momentary pressure, the second remains at the maximum pressure location and can be returned to zero manually. Reliability coefficients have been reported in the 0.90s, indicating that there is a satisfactory degree of reliability and that the scale does measure from zero to 100 kilograms.[20]

Chalking the hand to allow a firm grasp on the instrument should precede the actual test. The subject is allowed to move while squeezing the dynamometer (Figure 9.10). Two trials should be made with each hand, with a short rest period between trials permitted. The better score of the two trials should be counted.

Norms for grip strength have not been well documented for persons beyond the seventh decade; however, a comprehensive strength study of more than 6000 healthy males and females from age 10 to 69 was completed by Montoye and Lamphiear.[21] These researchers established percentile scores for the sum of grip strengths, and provide noteworthy guidelines for

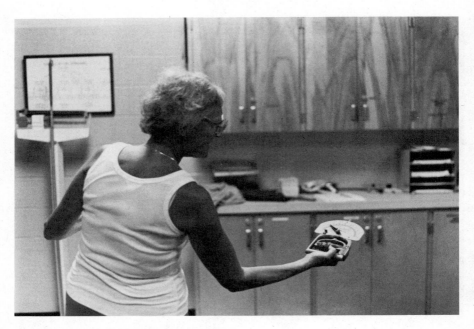

Figure 9.10 Testing hand/forearm strength.

interpreting test scores. Table 9.4 presents the percentile scores from age 10 to 59 years. It should be noted that Table 9.4 indicates scores up to 59 years. Caution is advised when using these scores for comparison with actual results of age groups beyond 60. Adjustments should be made for advanced years, reducing each decade by about 5 percent for men and 10 percent for women.

Measurement of Muscular Endurance. This form of sustained muscular work can be done isometrically (maintaining pressure on a grip dynamometer) or isotonically (continuing to raise and lower a load). Two practical measures of muscular endurance that are appropriate for persons over 50 are the modified push-up and bent-knee sit-up tests.

The modified push-up determines muscular endurance of the arms and shoulder girdle, while the bent-knee sit-up tests the stamina of the trunk flexors and abdominal muscles. Caution should be applied when interpreting the results of these two measures, as such movements place the small individual with shorter arms and legs at a lever advantage (see Chapter 5). At best, such tests provide approximate information about arm, shoulder, trunk, and abdominal muscle endurance. Norms have yet to be developed to

Table 9.4 Percentile Scores for Sum of Grip Strengths (Kg)

Percentile											Age						
	10	11	12	13	14	15	16	17	18	19	20–24	25–29	30–34	35–39	40–44	45–49	50–59
Males																	
90	34	42	52	69	89	96	106	111	117	118	122	123	124	123	123	116	110
80	30	37	47	60	80	90	99	105	106	113	115	115	115	115	115	108	102
70	26	34	41	53	72	84	95	99	101	109	110	110	110	109	108	104	96
60	24	32	38	48	66	80	91	93	98	104	105	107	106	106	103	99	93
50	22	29	34	44	61	76	87	89	96	101	102	103	102	102	100	95	89
40	20	26	31	42	58	73	84	85	93	98	99	100	98	98	97	91	85
30	18	23	30	39	54	69	78	81	90	94	94	95	95	93	93	82	81
20	15	21	27	34	49	64	74	76	86	90	89	90	90	88	87	81	75
10	11	16	23	28	39	55	68	70	81	84	80	81	82	79	81	75	66
Mean	23.6	30.2	37.4	47.5	64.3	76.6	87.6	91.5	97.1	102.0	102.9	103.6	103.4	101.9	101.4	95.6	89.4
SD	8.8	9.9	11.9	14.4	18.1	15.1	15.5	18.2	15.5	13.7	16.8	15.6	16.8	17.3	16.1	16.1	16.1
N	104	116	120	97	97	92	106	85	55	54	212	198	221	248	203	126	144
Females																	
90	30	37	44	49	65	60	58	61	59	63	61	67	65	66	64	64	57
80	25	33	40	44	50	54	53	54	55	59	57	62	60	69	58	57	52
70	22	30	36	41	48	49	49	50	52	54	53	57	57	55	54	53	48
60	20	27	33	38	44	45	48	47	49	50	50	53	53	53	51	52	45
50	18	25	31	36	41	43	43	44	46	48	48	49	49	51	49	49	43
40	17	23	28	34	39	41	41	42	43	46	45	48	47	49	47	47	40
30	15	20	26	32	36	38	39	39	39	42	42	46	44	46	43	44	38
20	14	17	22	30	32	36	36	36	36	39	38	43	41	43	40	40	34
10	10	12	18	26	27	31	33	31	31	36	34	37	36	36	36	34	30
Mean	19.9	26.2	32.5	37.8	43.6	45.7	45.8	46.8	47.1	49.9	48.7	52.2	51.5	51.9	50.0	50.0	44.0
SD	7.5	9.7	10.9	9.5	13.4	10.8	10.1	12.1	9.7	10.3	9.8	10.7	11.4	11.6	11.1	10.7	9.8
N	73	102	114	83	85	89	89	64	48	47	195	192	179	208	148	98	88

Source: H. J. Montoye and D. K. Lamphiear, "Grip and Arm Strength in Males and Females, Age 10 to 59," *Research Quarterly* 48, No. 1 (1977), 109–120. Used with permission.

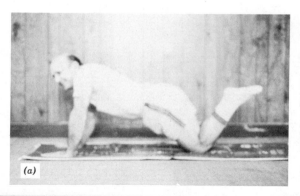

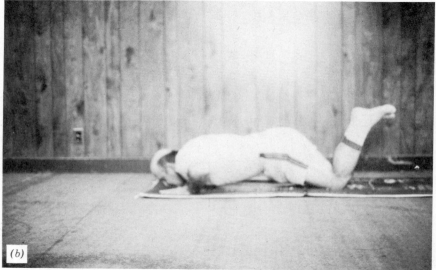

Figure 9.11 Modified push-up.

account for variations in trunk and arm lengths among individuals. Caution is also advised for persons with symptoms of back pain. Such individuals should not engage in any full sit-up exercise tests because of possible injury to the lumbar spine and surrounding tissues (see Chapter 3).

Modified Push-up Test. This upper body test requires flexion and extension of the elbows. Since elbow extension is too rigorous for older persons performing in a standard position with legs extended, the modified posture shown in Figure 9.11 is recommended. This position removes most of the weight from the upper body.

A mat should be placed on the floor to lessen knee discomfort. The subject starts from a straight arm position and lowers the body until the chest touches the mat; this is followed (without stopping) by a return to the straight arm support (see Figure 9.11). The back should not sag throughout the exercise. The test is terminated if the participant stops to rest or if the arms are not completely extended upon returning to the starting position. The score is the number of correct push-ups completed. Table 9.5 presents approximations of push-up values for males and females from ages 20 to 69 years.

It should be noted that the values presented in Table 9.5 represent the standard position for men (full front support without resting on knees), and a lesser knee angulation for the modified position shown in Figure 9.11 for women. These differences should be considered when interpreting push-up scores. Norms using the push-up style with the knee support as shown as not available at the present time.

Bent Knee Sit-up Test. This muscular endurance test provides an appropriate measure of trunk flexor strength, and, to some degree, the rectus abdominus external and internal oblique muscles. Although timed exercise bouts may be difficult for senior adults, this test requires counting the number of sit-ups that can be completed within one minute. The participant should assume a supine position on a mat (important for prevention of lower spine bruise) with knees flexed approximately 60 degrees, heels 15 to 18 inches apart, and hands clasped behind the head as shown in Figure 9.12a. At the signal, the participant should attempt to complete as many sit-ups as possible, with elbows touching the opposite knee, within one minute. A partner should hold the feet on the floor and count for the performer. The participant should be instructed to breathe naturally to avoid the Valsalva effect (see Chapter 4). The total number of repetitions are counted and compared with Table 9.6.

Measurement of Flexibility

Several techniques and methods have been developed to measure joint range of motion. Devices such as the mechanical goniometer and Leighton flexometer are used to determine direct flexion and extension. Indirect methods of determining flexibility are usually integrated into a battery of physical fitness tests. Two simple indirect measures of trunk flexibility are shown in Figure 9.13.

The method utilized depends upon the purpose of gathering mobility data. Employing indirect methods is generally acceptable in determining gross measurement when precision is not necessary. The mechanical

Table 9.5 Push-up Muscular Endurance Test Standards[a]

Age	Males					Females[b]				
	Excellent	Good	Average	Fair	Poor	Excellent	Good	Average	Fair	Poor
20–29	55-above	45–54	35–44	20–34	0–19	49-above	34–48	17–33	6–16	0–5
30–39	45-above	35–44	25–34	15–24	0–14	40-above	25–39	12–24	4–11	0–3
40–49	40-above	30–39	20–29	12–19	0–11	35-above	20–34	8–19	3–7	0–2
50–59	35-above	25–34	15–24	8–14	0–7	30-above	15–29	6–14	2–5	0–1
60–69	30-above	20–29	10–19	5–9	0–4	20-above	5–19	3–4	1–2	0

[a]These values represent approximations, since actual norms are not available.
[b]Modified push-up.

Source: M. L. Pollock, J. H. Wilmore, and S. M. Fox III, Health and Fitness through Physical Activity (New York: John Wiley & Sons), 1978, p. 109. Used with permission.

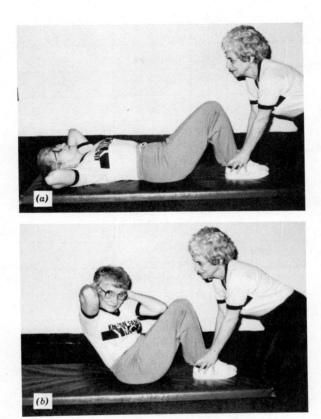

Figure 9.12 Sit-up test.

goniometer and Leighton flexometer are generally used for therapeutic and training purposes when greater precision in degrees of joint angulation is necessary.

Mechanical Goniometer. A popular device for measuring joint flexibility in educational and clinical settings is the universal goniometer. Fundamentally, this tool is a protractor that has a fulcrum or axis with two lever arms attached. One of the arms is movable and is placed in line with the changing part of the body to be measured. Several variations of goniometers are available. Figure 9.14 illustrates three common types currently used by physical educators and allied health professionals.

The mechanical goniometer selected should: (1) be durable with solid construction (stainless steel preferred); (2) be easy to read with clear mark-

Table 9.6. Sit-up Muscular Endurance Test Standards[a]

Age	Males					Females				
	Excellent	Good	Average	Fair	Poor	Excellent	Good	Average	Fair	Poor
20–29	48-above	43–47	37–42	33–36	0–32	44-above	39–43	33–38	29–32	0–28
30–39	40-above	35–39	29–34	25–28	0–24	36-above	31–35	25–30	21–24	0–20
40–49	35-above	30–34	24–29	20–23	0–19	31-above	26–30	19–25	16–18	0–15
50–59	30-above	25–29	19–24	15–18	0–14	26-above	21–25	15–20	11–14	0–10
60–69	25-above	20–24	14–19	10–13	0–9	21-above	16–20	10–15	6–9	0–5

[a]These values represent approximations, since actual norms are not available. Test is timed for 60 seconds.

Source: Pollock, Wilmore, and Fox III, *Health and Fitness,* p. 110. Used with permission.

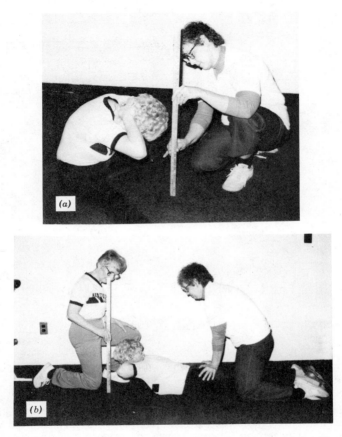

Figure 9.13 (a) indirect method of measuring trunk flexion (lower back); (b) indirect method of measuring trunk extensors (upper back).

ing in degrees ranging from zero to 180 or 360, depending on type; (3) have a movable arm with an adjustable pivot to allow for tightening at a fixed position after flexion or extension point is measured; and (4) have degree readings numbered in two directions from zero to 180 and/or 360 degrees and from 180 and/or 360 to zero degrees. The lever arms should be approximately 15 inches long for upper and lower limbs. Finger joint goniometers should be three to four inches in length.

Although many variations in goniometer types exist, two basic kinds are preferable for general use: a 360-degree stainless steel goniometer with 15-inch lever arms, and 180-degree-type with 4-inch lever arms. These instru-

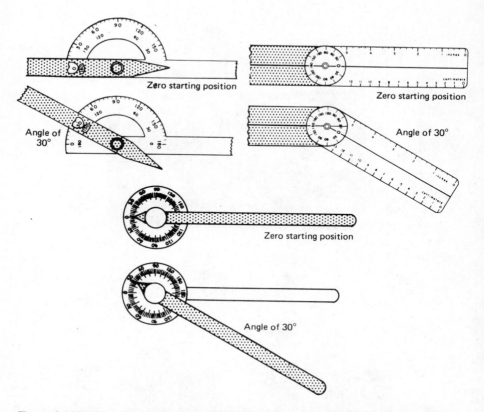

Figure 9.14 Various types of goniometers: (a) metal finger type; (b) 180-degree type; (c) 360-degree type. (From C. V. Heck, E. E. Hendryson, and C. R. Rowe, *Joint Motion: Method of Measuring and Recording* [Chicago: American Academy of Orthopaedic Surgeons, 1965], p. 9. Used with permission.)

ments can measure arm, leg, trunk, and finger articulations with reasonable accuracy.

The mechanical goniometer can yield valid information provided the tester uses the instrument correctly and in a consistent fashion. It is particularly important when measuring obese individuals that joint landmarks be carefully identified as reference points. In certain cases, excessive soft tissues may prevent the correct positioning of the instrument; therefore, other devices such as the Leighton flexometer should be employed to insure accurate measurement.

Several methods exist to interpret the actual degree range of motion. Scores may be determined by subtracting complete flexion from full extension or expressing flexibility in terms of maximum flexion and extension.

One method that can be recommended is the neutral zero method offered by the Committee for the Study of Joint Motion of the American Academy of Orthopedic Surgeons and the American Orthopaedic Association. The principles involved are as follows:

1. All motions of a joint are measured from zero starting positions. Thus, the degrees of motion of a joint are added in the direction the joint moves from the zero starting position. (See Figure 9.15).
2. The extended "anatomical position" of an extremity is therefore accepted as zero degrees, rather than 180 degrees.
3. The motion of the extremity being examined should be compared to that of the opposite extremity. The differences may be expressed in degrees of motion as compared to the opposite extremity, or in percentages of loss of motion in comparison with the opposite extremity.
4. A distinction is made between the terms *extension* and *hyperextension*. *Extension* is used when the position opposite to flexion, at the zero starting position, is a natural motion. This is present in the wrists and shoulder joints. If, however, the motion opposite flexion at the zero starting position is an unnatural one, such as that of the elbow or knees, it is referred to as *hyperextension*.[22]

Figure 9.15 illustrates typical joints using the zero neutral method. Studies indicate that a well-informed tester using a reliable and well-constructed tool can measure flexibility with high reliability.[23]

Joint ranges of motion continue to defy definitions of "average." Variations in physique, age, and sex, and even temperament appear to affect flexibility among individuals. Therefore, flexibility norms should be interpreted as, at best, rough guides in assessing flexibility. Table 9.7 presents estimates in average ranges of joint mention.

Leighton Flexometer. The accuracy and reliability of flexibility measurement was improved with the development of the Leighton flexometer by Jack R. Leighton of Eastern Washington College.[24] Leighton pointed out the limitation of linear measurement devices such as the goniometer. He argued that tall persons have longer segments than shorter persons. Therefore, longer segments moving through the same arc (range of motion) would give greater linear measurements (caliper measurements); and the arcs formed (angular measurement) by longer body segments from their starting positions might actually be equal to, greater than, or less than those of shorter segments.

The instrument shown in Figure 9.16 consists of a weighted 360-degree dial and a weighted pointer mounted in a case.[25] The figure illustrates posi-

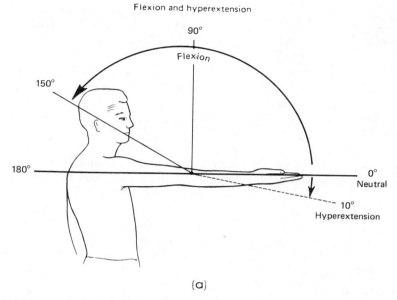

(a)

Figure 9.15 (a) elbow; (b) fingers; (c) ankle. (From Heck, Hendryson, and Rowe, pp. 9, 27, 69. Used with permission.)

tion one and position two following the prescribed procedure established by Leighton.

Sit-and-Reach Test. Because flexibility is specific to the joint, selection of joint ranges for measurement will depend upon the objectives sought. Trunk flexion has been used for many years as a test of flexibility because of its association with low back pain and accompanying reduction of hip flexibility and elasticity of the hamstrings. A simple sit-and-reach test, which was developed by Dr. Barry L. Johnson of Corpus Christi State University (Texas) and is used by the YMCA, is recommended for adults without serious orthopedic handicaps.[26]

The trunk flexion or sit-and-reach test is a quick and practical procedure that provides significant information about the stretchability qualities of the low back and posterior muscles of the upper legs (hamstrings)—two regions that tend to become more rigid with advancing age, especially among men. The administration of the test requires a yardstick to measure the distance reached (a line drawn at right angles to the 15-inch mark), and a piece of tape to keep the measuring instrument in place on the floor. (See Figure 9.17).

The participant assumes a sitting position as shown in Figure 9.18, with the yardstick between the legs and legs extended at right angles to the taped

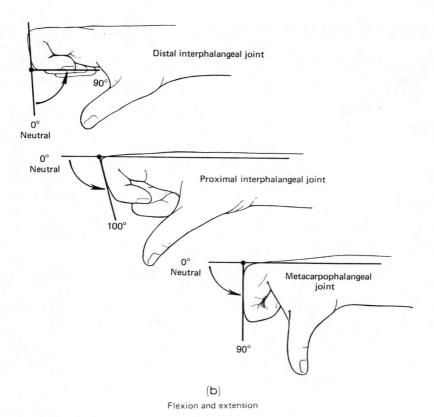

(b)

Flexion and extension

Table 9.7　Average Ranges of Joint Motion

Joint	Average in Degrees	Joint	Average in Degrees
Elbow		*Shoulder*	
Flexion	150	Forward Flexion	180
Hyperextension	0	Horizontal Flexion	135
		Backward Extension	60
Forearm		Abduction	180
Pronation	80	Adduction	75
Supination	80		
		Hip	
Wrist		Flexion	120
Extension	70	Extension	30
Flexion	80	Abduction	45
Ulnar Deviation	30	Adduction	30
Radial Deviation	20		
		Knee	
Thumb[a]		Flexion	135
Abduction	70	Hyperextension	10
Flexion			
I-P Joint	80	*Ankle*	
M-P	50	Flexion	
M-C	15	(Plantar Flex.)	50
Extension		Extension	
Distal Jt.	20	(Dorsiflexion)	20
M-P	0		
M-C	20	*Spine*	
		Cervical	
Fingers		Flexion	45
Flexion		Extension	45
Distal Jt.	90	Lateral Bending	45
Middle Jt.	100	Thoracic & Lumbar	
Proximal Jt.	90	Flexion	80
Extension		Extension	20–30
Distal Jt.	0	Lateral Bending	35
Middle Jt.	0		
Proximal Jt.	45		

[a]I-P Joint = interphalangeal joint; M-P = metacarpophalangeal joint; M-C = carpometacarpal joint.

Source: Heck, Hendryson, and Rowe, *Joint Motion,* pp. 81–86. Used with permission.

line on the floor. Heels of the feet should touch near the edge of the taped line, about 10 to 12 inches apart.

The participant slowly reaches forward with both hands as far as possible on the yardstick, holding this position momentarily; finger tips should be in contact with the yardstick (Figure 9.18 b). The score is the most distant point reached on the yardstick with the best of three trials recorded. The participant should warm up before attempting the test, which should result in a better score and lessen the danger of a pulled muscle. The YMCA has established general norms for adult males and females applicable to ages 46 and older. Caution is advised when comparing a subject's performance with the norms shown in Table 9.8, because of the wide range of joint motion among individuals of varying physiques and age groups.

Measurement of Balance and Equilibrium

The nature of balance characteristics was discussed in considerable detail earlier. At present, standardized balance tests for the well-elderly are not available, except for those medical tests usually administered to diagnose various types of pathological conditions associated with vertigo and assorted states of disequilibrium. Most standard tests are designed for children and young adults. Therefore, this discussion is focused on the modification and adaptation of tests used for younger groups.

Balance and equilibrium is not a general characteristic, but a quality that is composed of specific abilities including stationary and dynamic balance, and their subordinate categories of upright and inverted components. Stationary and dynamic balance are particularly relevant to the everyday functional living skills of senior adults.

Stationary Balance Test. Stationary balance requires the individual to hold the body in a controlled static position with a minimum of extraneous movements.

Various tests of balance such as the Bass stick test, which requires the subject to stand on a stick 1 inch wide, 1 inch high, and 12 inches long on one foot with eyes closed, have been devised.[27] Fleishman developed a similar device and protocol for testing upright stationary balance, which he labeled *gross body equilibrium*.[28] Each of these stationary tests, which require the participant to stand on the balls of the feet with eyes closed on a slightly raised platform, present an undue safety risk for persons past 60, particularly heavy individuals. The one-foot balance stand with eyes open and arms raised sideward is suggested as an appropriate test of upright stationary balance for senior adults.

One-Foot Balance Stand. The objective of this test is to evaluate upright stationary balance of the participant while supported by the preferred leg (Figure 9.19). The participant stands on one foot within a prescribed area 15 inches by 15 inches, eyes open with arms raised sideward (used as a balance pole to assist in maintaining balance). Eyes should be focused at a particular point (on an opposite wall) to provide a point of visual reference. At a given signal, the performer attempts to balance on one foot for 15 seconds without

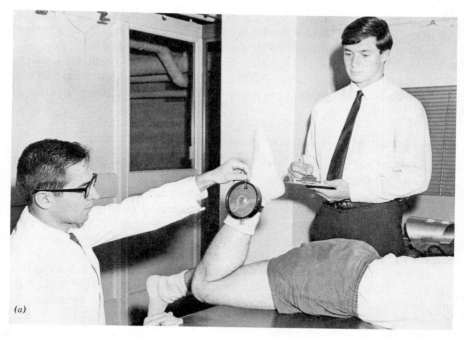

(a)

Figure 9.16 Leighton flexometer—complete knee extension: (a) position one—flexion; (b) position two—extension. (From J. Piscopo and J. A. Baley, *Kinesiology: The Science of Movement* [New York: John Wiley & Sons, 1981], pp. 506–507. Used with permission.)

moving or falling. In the absence of norms, the following checklist can be used to evaluate the proficiency of the participant:

One-Foot Balance Checklist	Yes	No	Comments
1. Can the participant balance 15 seconds on one foot?	___	___	_____
2. Does the participant show control and steadiness?	___	___	_____
3. Does the participant use his or her arms effectively to control balance?	___	___	_____
4. Does the participant use vision effectively to control balance?	___	___	_____
5. Does the participant show signs of dizziness while balancing?	___	___	_____
6. Does the participant show reasonably good form while balancing?	___	___	_____

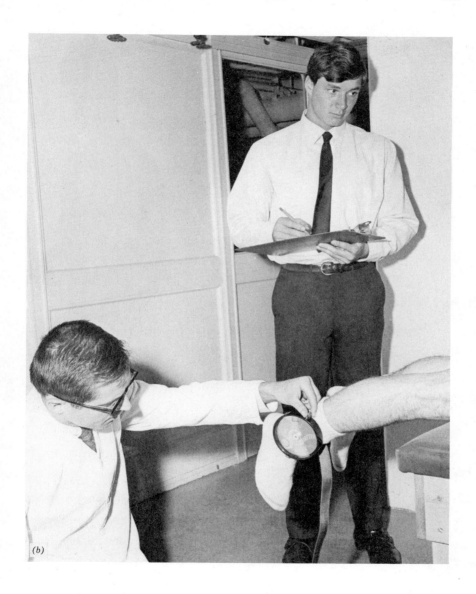

(b)

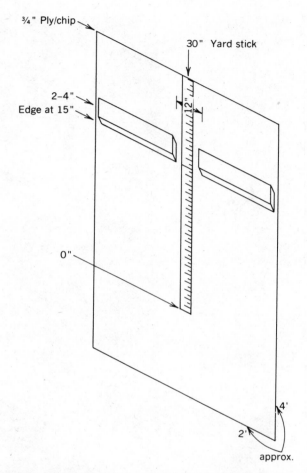

Figure 9.17 Flexibility board specifications. (From Golding, Myers, and Sinning, *Y's Way to Physical Fitness*, p. 102. Used with permission.)

This test requires a stopwatch to check the time limit, and a spotter, standing slightly behind the participant, ready to assist if necessary. Each of the items is scored with a "yes" or "no" and supplemented with a subjective interpretive statement (such as "excellent," "good," "fair," "weak," or "failure"). The checklist offers an opportunity to appraise the quality of upright stationary balance with a degree of specificity in analyzing and correcting errors in upright balancing efficiency.

Dynamic Balance Test. The distinguishing variable between stationary and dynamic balance involves a moving pattern of the body. Dynamic balance

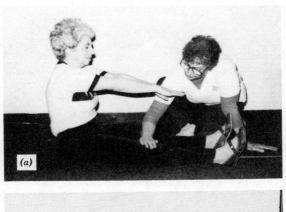

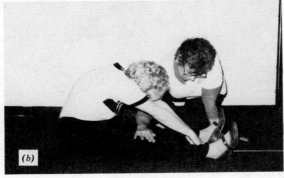

Figure 9.18 Sit-and-reach test: (a) starting point; (b) ending point. (From Golding, Myers, and Sinning, *Y's Way to Physical Fitness*, p. 102. Used with permission.)

Table 9.8 Flexibility Norms 46 Years and Older

Percentage Ranking	Trunk Flexion (inches)	
	Male	*Female*
95 Excellent	20	22
85 Good	17	19
75 Above average	15	18
50 Average	13	15
30 Below average	11	14
15 Fair	8	11
5 Poor	5	9

Source: Adapted from Golding, Myers, and Sinning, *Y's Way to Physical Fitness*, p. 108. Used with permission.

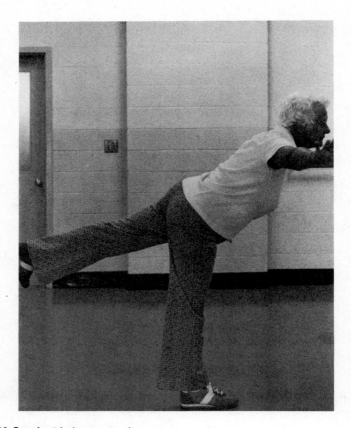

Figure 9.19 One foot balance stand.

requires constant gross changes in posture. These changes are in stance or moving actions depending on the nature of the motor skill. For example, such actions as walking, jumping, or leaping from one point to another entail dynamic balance functions.

Various types of dynamic tests have been devised, such as the Springfield Balance Beam Walking Test and the Bass Stepping Stone Test.[29] The Springfield Test, developed by Harold Seashore, consists of walking nine beams of equal length and height, but varying widths from four to one-fourth inches. The objective is to walk ten steps on each of the progressively narrower beams in a heel-to-toe fashion with hands on hips. The Stepping Stone Test was developed by Ruth Bass in 1939 and is still used with various modifications by physical educators. Essentially, this test measures the ability to jump from one designated position to another in a zig-zag fashion—

using one leg, then leaping on the opposite leg, landing on designated circled targets.* The problem with these tests is that such measures are designed to assess balance of young adults; consequently standard directions and achievement levels are inappropriate for older persons, save the unusual super senior athlete. A modification of the beam walking test is suggested as a practical measure for evaluating upright dynamic balance of older adults.

Modified Beam Walk Test. The objective of this test is to evaluate the participant's ability to walk on a narrow low beam 10 feet long, 4 inches wide, and 4 inches high. The beam walk test does not require any elaborate equipment and can be set up inexpensively (see Figure 5.23). The participant should be instructed to walk along the beam with eyes focused at the end of the beam and arms raised sideward, walking in a heel-to-toe fashion to the end of the beam.

The following checklist can be used to evaluate the performance efficiency of upright dynamic balance.

Modified Beam Walk Test Checklist	Yes	No	Comments
1. Can the participant walk the entire length without falling off the beam?	____	____	_____
2. Does the participant walk in a natural heel-to-toe manner without shuffling?	____	____	_____
3. Does the participant need help during the walk?	____	____	_____
4. Does the participant use his or her vision capabilities effectively as a point of reference?	____	____	_____
5. Does the participant use his or her arms effectively as a balance mechanism?	____	____	_____
6. Does the participant mount and dismount the beam in a controlled manner?	____	____	_____

Measurement of Reaction-Movement Time

Loss of brain cells coupled with the hardening of the vessels within the brain itself affect the quality of neuromuscular response in voluntary skeletal and motor skill movements. Reaction time, which is inherently involved with nerve-muscle control, generally slows down—but at different rates among adults, depending upon the genetic endowment and developmental and en-

*See Piscopo and Baley, *Kinesiology,* for a detailed description of the test.

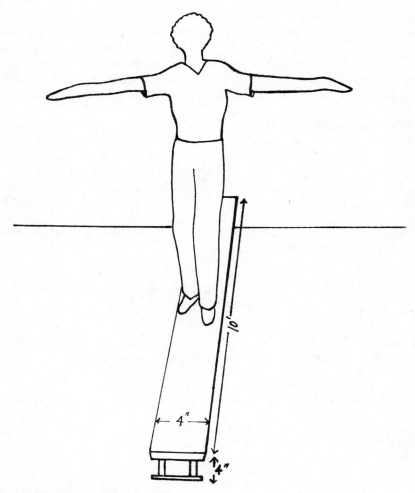

Figure 9.20 Modified beam walk test.

vironmental milieu of the individual. Older persons who actively participate in racket sports and handball have faster reaction time than older inactive people (see Chapter 3).

Speed in response to movement entails two integral components: reaction time and movement time. *Reaction time* is defined as the period from the presentation of a stimulus (which can be auditory, visual, or tactile, taste, smell, or pain) to the beginning of the muscular response. *Movement time* is the actual time from the beginning of the muscular response to a stimulus through the accomplishment of the motor task.[30]

It would seem that persons who possess fast reaction time also exhibit fast movement time; however, studies show that a low correlation exists between these two variables.[31] Simply stated, although an individual may immediately react to a stimulus, quick perception does not ensure fast muscle movement to a motor task. The reaction time component particularly relates to the efficiency of the central and *autonomic nervous system,* whereas movement time entails the *muscular component* of the neural mechanisms that actually result in the production of a physical movement or a composite of reaction-movement time called *response time.* For example, the total time from the moment a driver sees a traffic light turn red until the car actually stops constitutes the response time.

Differentiation in measurement of reaction time and movement time can be made using devices such as internal timers, photoelectric cells, stimulus lights, and other electronic circuitry apparatus. Although such instrumentation systems can yield valid and reliable data about reaction time and movement time, this equipment, because of its expense, is not practical in the majority of field-based settings. Nevertheless, a simple test that can give meaningful information about reaction and movement time is available. Nelson developed a measuring device that is both simple and inexpensive.[32] His Nelson Reaction timer* is based on the law of constant acceleration of freefalling bodies and consists of a stick that is scaled to read in time as computed from the following formula:

$$\text{Time} = \sqrt{\frac{2 \times \text{distance the stick falls}}{\text{acceleration due to gravity}}}$$

The Nelson Hand Reaction Test.† The objective of this test is to measure the speed of reaction with the hand in response to a visual stimulus. The age level that can be tested extends from kindergarten upward. The only limiting factor is related to the subject's ability (or inability) to catch a falling stick with the fingers (see Figure 9.21). The equipment required is a Nelson Reaction Timer, a table, and a chair or desk chair.

The subject sits with the forearm and hand resting comfortably on the table or desk chair. The tops of the thumb and index finger are held in a ready pinch position about three or four inches beyond the edge of the table

---

*The Nelson Reaction Timer, Model RT-2 © Copyright, 1965 by Fred Nelson, P.O. Box 51987, La.

†Complete details about the test may be found in Johnson and Nelson, *Practical Measurements,* pp. 246–248.

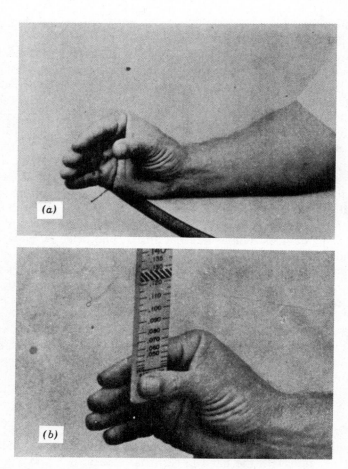

Figure 9.21 Nelson reaction time test: (a) position of the hand and fingers; (b) ready position with thumb as base line; (c) scoring the Nelson hand reaction test (0.170 seconds in this example). (From B. L. Johnson and J. K. Nelson, *Practical Measurement for Evaluation in Physical Education* [Minneapolis, Minn.: Burgess Publishers, 1979], p. 247. Used with permission.)

(Figure 9.21 a). The upper edge of both the thumb and index finger should be in a horizontal position. The tester holds the stick-timer near the top, letting it hang between the subject's thumb and index finger.

    The base-line should be even with the upper surface of the participant's thumb (Figure 9.21 b). The participant is directed to look at the *concentration zone* (black-shaded area between 0.120 and 0.130 lines) and is instructed to react by catching the stick, pinching the thumb and index finger together,

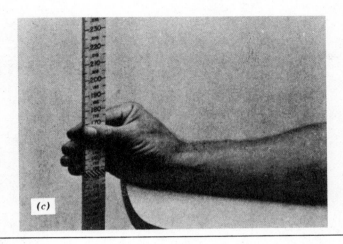

when it is released. The subject should not look at the tester's hand, nor be allowed to move the hand up or down while attempting to catch the stick. Twenty trials are given. Each drop is preceded by a preparatory command of "ready." When the subject catches the timer, the score is read just above the upper edge of the thumb (Finger 9.21 c). The five slowest and the five fastest trials are discarded, and the average of the middle ten is recorded as the score. Numbers on the timer represent thousandths of a second. Scores may be recorded to the nearest 5/1000 of a second.[33]

Norms for senior adults are not available at this time; however, Johnson and Nelson report average reaction time of college men at 0.16 with a range of 0.13 to 0.22, and the average of small children (first graders) at about 0.26.[34] Based upon the generalization that reaction time and movement time does slow beyond the young adult years, we can assume that scores above 0.22 can be expected on the Nelson reaction timer, barring handicapping conditions of poor vision and hearing or severe joint problems. Table 9.9 shows the results of a variety of research reaction time tests with scores recorded from those in their 20s up to 80s. In every case, reaction time is gradually reduced from the teens to late maturity.

It would be imprudent, at this time, to indicate specific typical scores for the older persons in the absence of valid norms. However, extreme scores or inability to catch the stick do signal impaired hand reaction and movement time.

A foot reaction test using the same reaction timer stick can be used with a similar testing procedure. The subject sits on a table or bench with the timer on the wall, using the ball of the foot to stop the stick as it is dropped.*

*For specific details, see Johnson and Nelson, *Practical Measurements*, p. 246.

Table 9.9 Simple Reaction Times (In Seconds)

Author	Type of Reaction[a]	Teens	20s	30s	40s	50s	60s	70s	80s	Percentage Changes 20s–50s	20s–60s	20s–70s	Notes
Miles (1931a)	Press key in response to sound	—	.23	.24	.22	.20	.28	.30	.28	−13	22	30	100 subjects; fewer in the 20s and 80s than other ranges. The 20s ranged from 25 to 29 only.
	Release key in response to sound	—	.21	.22	.22	.22	.23	.26	.28				
	Lift foot in response to sound	—	.22	.22	.24	.24	.26	.27	.30				
DeSilva (1936)	"Brake reaction time" in a test designed to simulate car driving (subject raised foot pedal and transferred it to brake on seeing red flash of a traffic light)	.418	.418	.428	.442	.455	.465	—	—	9	11	—	2000 subjects. The range of the items is 16–19 and of the 60s, 60–65. The figures are approximate only, having been taken from a graph included in DeSilva's paper.
Fleandt et al. (1956)	Press button in response to light	.228	.201	.201	.217	.212	.217	.245	.353	5	8	22	The age ranges were 11–14, 21–24, 29–36, 39–47, 49–56, 59–67, 69–79, and 80–88. Each of the 120 subjects gave five readings. The two extremes of these were excluded and the scores were the means of the remaining three.

Study	Experiment[a]											Notes
Pierson and Montoye (1958)	Lift hand to light	.28	.26	.27	.28	.32	.34	.33	—	23	31	—	400 male subjects aged 8–85. Figures read off graph. Those for subjects under 11 years not shown.
Hugin, Norris, and Shock (1960)	Flex left foot to touch on right foot	.210	.178	.177	.184	.192	.214	.222	.229	8	20	25	Responses measured from muscle action potentials.
	Reflex to scratch on foot	.088	.090	.101	.099	.101	.099	.097	.095				
	abdomen	.060	—	.071	—	.065	.059	.074	.082				
Jalavisto et al. (1962)	Press contact in response to light	—	.235	—	—	.287	—	.320	—	22	—	36	Age groups 20–26, 44–64, 65–83.
	Catch ruler when dropped (visual clue)	—	.210	—	—	.242	—	.250	—				
	Catch ruler—further experiment												
	Visual cue only	—	.195	—	—	.236	—	—	—	—	25	43	Subjects all women. Age groups 12–17, 18–21, 22–38, 39–54, 55–69, 70–84.
	Visual and tactile	—	.137	—	—	.287	—	—	—				
	Tactile only	—	.121	—	—	.160	—	—	—				
Hodgkins (1962)	Release key to light	.224	.203	.214	.240	—	.253	.307	—	—	25	—	

[a] All reactions are made with the hand unless otherwise stated.

Source: Adapted from A. T. Welford, "Motor Performance," in J. E. Birren and K. W. Schaie (Ed.), *Handbook of the Psychology of Aging.* Van Nostrand Reinhold Co., New York, pp. 464–65, with permission.

References for Table 9.9 (Simple Reaction Times)

DeSilva, H. R. "On an Investigation of Driving Skill." *Human Factor* 10 (1936): 1–13.

Fieandt, K. von; Huhtala, A.; Kulberg, P.; and Searl, K. "Personal Tempo and Phenomenal Time at Different Age Levels." *Reports from the Psychological Institute,* no. 2. University of Helsinki, 1956.

Hodgkins, J. "Influence of Age on the Speed of Reaction and Movement in Females." *Journal of Gerontology* 17 (1962): 385–389.

Hugin, F.; Norris, A. A.; and Shock, N. W. "Skin Reflex and Voluntary Reaction Times in Young and Old Males." *Journal of Gerontology* 15 (1960): 338–391.

Jalavisto, E.; Forsen, A.; Lindqvist, C.; Makkoven, T.; and Tallqvist, M. "Age and the Simple Reaction Time in Response to Visual, Tactile, and Proprioceptive Stimuli." *Annals of Academy Science Fenniae Series A, V, Medica,* no. 96 (1962).

Miles, W. R. "Correlation of Reaction Time and Coordination Speed with Age in Adults." *American Journal of Psychology* 43 (1931): 377–391.

Pierson, W. R., and Montoye, H. J. "Movement Time, Reaction Time and Age." *Journal of Gerontology* 13 (1958): 418–421.

PROGRAM EVALUATION

We have presented various methods, instruments, and procedures for measuring basic fitness parameters essential for the maintenance of mobility and ambulation of the senior adult. A parallel component, which is equal to the specific tests of functional ability, must also be included. This evaluation segment entails the assessment of *program content*.

Each organization has its unique objectives that are derived from a basic philosophy and geared to the capacity and abilities of the participating senior adults. Irrespective of the senior environment, several common principles and concepts apply when evaluating the effectiveness of a health-fitness program. Although the listing below is not exhaustive, it does provide a basic philosophy from which program goals can be generated:

- To adopt the concept of health that is expressed by the World Health Organization: "Health is a state of complete physical, mental, and social well-being, and not merely the absence of disease or infirmity."
- To view each senior adult as a whole person recognizing the many varied differences and changing needs of the population.
- To plan, implement, and evaluate programs using an interdisciplinary and multidisciplinary team approach.
- To provide a variety of services in order to maximize the physical, social, psychological, intellectual, and spiritual well-being of the participants.
- To promote and respect the integrity and dignity of the senior adult by maximizing his or her power of choice and self-direction.
- To recognize that aging is a normal process of maturation, not a pathological disease sequence.

After the basic philosophy and objectives of a senior setting have been formulated, successful programs should establish mechanisms whereby continuous and systematic evolutions can be implemented. Such assessments generally include three program elements: (1) the participant, (2) the activity program, and (3) relations with the community.

The Participant

The central focus of any successful program remains on the senior adult participating in the services offered by the organization. Certain programs require evaluations daily, others only weekly, monthly, or at longer time periods, depending upon the type of services. For example, the frail elderly living in an extended health care facility require daily assessment of their general health status, whereas the well-elderly participating in multipurpose senior centers need only initial assessment with periodic review ranging from every six weeks to twice per year, depending upon the specific fitness objectives desired. Evaluative reports about the participant usually include the following information:

- Number and frequency of senior adults using the facility.
- Nature of program participation; e.g., involvement in physical exercise activities, social activities, crafts, arts, etc.
- Functional ability of the participant in an individual and group setting.
- General rate of improvement in participating activities.
- General attitude about program activities.

A card file system for each member should be established and periodically updated. This procedure offers an excellent method of assessing the level of the participant's involvement in the organization's activities. Figure 9.22 illustrates a progress record of activities. Such forms should be modified to reflect the activities of a particular setting, and may include more information about the participant depending upon objectives and services offered.

The Activity Program

This segment of program evaluation deals with the scope and magnitude of activities offered. Revealing statements and questions should be included about the nature and type of activities which serve the needs and interests of the participants. The following self-checklist (Figure 9.23) can assist the evaluator to identify strengths and weaknesses of the program.

This checklist contains the major elements for the assessment of program content and quality. Other items, which may be unique to a particular senior community setting, should be added when appropriate.

Relations with the Community

A quality program strives to establish a positive relationship with the community it serves. One effective way of doing this is to keep senior adults well informed about the program activities of the organization. Monthly program schedules and newsletters are excellent devices to keep participants and other community agencies informed.

Cooperative efforts and projects between the senior center or facility and civic organizations, such as the Rotary and Kiwanis Clubs, should also be encouraged. Community volunteers and personnel of surrounding institu-

Figure 9.22 Resident's progress record in activities. (From T. Merrill, *Activities for the Aged and Infirm* [Springfield, Ill.: Charles C Thomas, 1967], p. 41. Used with permission.

Name of Resident: _____

Age: _____   Birthday: _____

Physical Condition:

   Ambulatory _____   Hearing _____   Coordination _____—Good

                                                                           —Poor

   Semi-

     Ambulatory _____   Visual handicaps _____   Muscular Control ____—Good

   Bedfast ____ Use of Arms and Hands _____   Mental Condition ____—Good

Activities:—

Occupation:—

Hobbies:—

Interests:—

Social:—

Church:—

Club or Lodge affiliation:—

Dates introduced to activities:—

Dates:—

Comments on Reaction:—   Activities:—

                                   Attitude: Nonreceptive _____

                                             Receptive _____

                                     Interest: Good _____

General Benefits and Improvements: Indifferent _____

_____

Signed by professional worker

Figure 9.23 Checklist used to evaluate strengths and weaknesses of the Activity program.

Criteria	Poor (1)	Fair (2)	Good (3)	Very Good (4)	Excellent (5)
1. Does the program contain a diversity of activities to meet the needs and interests of all its participants?	——	——	——	——	——
2. Does the program contain an adequate balance of physical, psychosocial, intellectual, and spiritual activities?	——	——	——	——	——
3. Are the activities compatible with the philosophy and objectives of the organization?	——	——	——	——	——
4. Do the activities offered meet the needs of both sexes and of varied socioeconomic groups?	——	——	——	——	——
5. Does the program contain an appropriate balance of individual and group activities?	——	——	——	——	——
6. Does the program reflect considerable interest, enthusiasm, and satisfaction by the participants?	——	——	——	——	——
7. Does the program include volunteers and other senior adult leaders with unique talents in the conduct of activities?	——	——	——	——	——

Figure 9.23 Continued

Criteria	Poor (1)	Fair (2)	Good (3)	Very Good (4)	Excellent (5)
8. Is the program directed by professionally qualified leadership compatible with the job requirements?	——	——	——	——	——
9. Are the activities scheduled at appropriate times during the day and evening hours?	——	——	——	——	——
10. Does the program offer activities whereby participants have an opportunity to learn new intellectual and motor skills?	——	——	——	——	——
11. Is the activity area large enough and properly equipped for the safe conduct of various social and recreational activities?	——	——	——	——	——
12. Does the facility contain a gymnasium or fitness activity area, as well as ready access to a natatorium?	——	——	——	——	——
13. Are all potential safety hazards, including lighting, furniture arrangements, floor composition, stairs, and passageways, reduced to a minimum to allow easy access to and from one point to another in the facility?	——	——	——	——	——

Figure 9.23 *Continued*

Criteria	Poor (1)	Fair (2)	Good (3)	Very Good (4)	Excellent (5)
14. Are procedures for emergency situations that may arise clearly defined and known by the staff and participants?	___	___	___	___	___
15. Does the facility contain adequate toilet accommodations that can be quickly reached and easily used?	___	___	___	___	___
16. Is the equipment used in good working order?	___	___	___	___	___
17. Does the program of activities reflect evidence of careful planning?	___	___	___	___	___
18. Does the program of activities reflect good communications among staff members?	___	___	___	___	___
19. Is the facility and program adequately funded?	___	___	___	___	___
20. Is the facility attractive and amenable to a relaxing ambience?	___	___	___	___	___

tions of higher learning can enrich program offerings, and simultaneously create a greater awareness and interest in the well-being of the older adult. The following queries can serve as important reminders when assessing the effectiveness of a program community relations:

- Do volunteers from the community assist in implementing programs of organization?
- Is favorable support provided by the local news and television media?

- Are joint projects between the senior setting organization and other civic organizations regularly promoted?
- Are community or agency facilities accessible and utilized when not available at the senior center or residence (e.g., is the Y or high school natatorium used for aquatic activities)?
- Have advisory councils and committees been formed with members of senior setting and citizens from community serving in joint membership?
- Are newsletters and announcements of special program activities regularly sent to local governmental officials?

Effective and productive services for the elderly are maximized when an institution's activities are continually evaluated from the participant, program, and community relations perspectives. Each segment can reinforce the others when sound programming principles are followed.

Summary

Meaningful measurement and evaluation systems provide valuable information about the effectiveness of an organized fitness program. They should be directly related to the objectives sought. Careful attention to validity, reliability, and objectivity of instruments and procedures used must be observed by the tester before definitive conclusions can be made about fitness conditions of the mature adult. Norms represent standards from which data can be compared. Norms must be specific to group that is under study and should involve a sufficient number of subjects to assure the reliability of the recorded data.

Field-based assessment tools and research instrumentation systems were described and compared in the first part of this chapter. Whether the tester is using a sophisticated electrogoniometer or a simple mechanical goniometer for flexibility testing, the basic requirements of validity, reliability and objectivity must be satisfied.

Essentially, research modes demand absolute precision, accuracy, and freedom from bias using the scientific method of inquiry in solving a particular problem. Conversely, field-based testing instruments and procedures applied in a practical setting may not require such exactness. Two broad categories of practical assessment systems were considered: qualitative and quantitative. Each system can be used effectively in field-based testing situations, but the overriding elements must be the safety and well-being of the senior adults.

Measurement and evaluation of six fitness elements were presented: (1) cardiovascular efficiency, (2) body composition, (3) muscular strength and endurance, (4) flexibility, (5) balance and equilibrium, and (6) reaction time.

The bicycle ergometer, treadmill test, and step test protocols were described and compared.

Two methods of measuring body composition were described: hydrostatic weighing and skinfold measurement technique. Although hydrostatic weighing offers greater accuracy in assessing body adipose content, the skinfold method is preferred in a field-based environment because of the prohibitive cost of and technical expertise required by the densiometric procedures. Tables with illustrative norms were provided, but it was pointed out that such tables are estimates of body fat composition and should not be considered finite.

The measurement of muscular strength and endurance was examined from two broad categories: isometric and dynamic. The hand grip strength dynamometer was recommended as an instrument for measuring muscular strength of older adults because of its portability and unobtrusive test characteristics. The modified push-up and bent-knee sit-up tests are appropriate measures of muscular endurance for senior adults.

Three methods and techniques used to measure flexibility were described: mechanical goniometer, the Leighton Flexometer, and the sit-and-reach test. The goniometer and flexometer provide greater accuracy and precision and should be used when measures of multi-joint ranges are desired.

Upright stationary and upright dynamic balance were identified as two important fitness elements for evaluation. The modified one-foot balance stand and the modified beam walk tests were suggested for senior adults.

Reaction-movement time is considered an important fitness parameter among the elderly. Response time is a combination of reaction time and movement time, each component resulting from an integration of neural and muscular mechanisms. The Nelson Hand Reaction Test was selected as a simple and quick measure of hand reaction in response to a visual stimulus.

The final section of this chapter dealt with overall program evaluation applicable to a variety of senior settings. Three elements are central to program assessment: (1) the participant, (2) the activity program, and (3) relations with the community. Several rating charts and a checklist were presented to evaluate each program element.

REFERENCES

1. Wayne E. Sinning, "Use and Misuse of Anthropometric Estimates of Body Composition," *Journal of Physical Education and Recreation* 51, no. 2 (1980): 43–45.
2. Donald K. Mathews, *Measurement in Physical Education,* 4th ed. (Philadelphia: W. B. Saunders, 1973), p. 26.
3. Gladys M. Scott, "Instrument: Software," in A. W. Hubbard, ed., *Research*

Methods in Health, Physical Education and Recreation, 3d ed. (Washington, D.C.: American Association for Health, Physical Education and Recreation, 1973), p. 106.

4. John L. Marshall et al., "Joint Looseness: A Function of the Person and the Joint," *Medicine and Science in Sports and Exercise* 12, no. 3 (1980): 189–194.
5. Terry Jopke, "Choosing An Exercise Testing Protocol," *The Physician and Sportsmedicine* 9, no. 3 (1981): 141–144.
6. L. A. Golding, C. R. Myers, and W. E. Sinning, eds., *The Y's Way to Physical Fitness,* rev. ed. (Chicago: National Board of YMCA, 1982).
7. Jopke, "Exercise Testing Protocol," p. 141.
8. Gerald F. Fletcher and John D. Cantwell, *Exercise and Coronary Heart Disease,* 2d ed. (Springfield: Charles C Thomas Publishers, 1979), pp. 72–121.
9. *Guidelines for Graded Exercise Testing and Exercise Prescription,* 2d ed. (Philadelphia: American College of Sports Medicine, 1980); and *Exercise Testing and Training of Apparently Healthy Individuals: A Handbook for Physicians* (New York: American Heart Association, 1972).
10. Fletcher and Cantwell, *Exercise and Coronary Heart Disease,* p. 77.
11. J. P. Naughton, "Methods of Exercise Testing," in Naughton and H. K. Hellerstein, eds., *Exercise Testing and Exercise Training in Coronary Heart Disease* (New York: Academic Press, 1973), pp. 79–91.
12. J. Wilmore et al., "What Do Stress Tests Show?" *The Physician and Sportsmedicine* 8, no. 9 (1980): 45–56; Jopke, "Exercise Testing Protocol," Fletcher and Cantwell, *Exercise and Coronary Heart Disease;* and *Exercise Testing and Training.*
13. *Exercise Testing and Training,* p. 28.
14. Isadore Rossman, "Anatomic and Body Composition Changes with Aging," in C. E. Finch and L. Hayflick, eds., *The Biology of Aging* (New York: Van Nostrand Reinhold, 1977), p. 197.
15. John Piscopo and James A. Baley, *Kinesiology: The Science of Movement* (New York: John Wiley & Sons, 1981), p. 513.
16. John Piscopo, "Obesity: A Noteworthy Method of Assessment," *New York Journal of Health, Physical Education and Recreation* 20 (1967): 24–27.
17. Ancel Keys and Josef Brozek, "Body Fat in Adult Men." *Physiological Reviews* 33 (1953): 245–325.
18. A. S. Jackson and M. L. Pollock, "Generalized Equations for Predicting Body Density of Men," *British Journal of Nutrition* 40 (1978): 497–504; and J. V. G. A. Durnin and J. Womersley, "Body Fat Assessed from Total Body Density and Its Estimation from Skinfold Thickness: Measurements on 481 Men and Women Aged from 16 to 72 Years," *British Journal of Nutrition* 32 (1974): 77–96.
19. Golding, Myers, and Sinning, *Y's Way to Physical Fitness,* pp. 82–83.
20. Barry L. Johnson and Jack K. Nelson, *Practical Measurements for Evaluation in Physical Education* (Minneapolis: Burgess Publishing, 1979), p. 113.
21. Henry J. Montoye and Donald F. Lamphiear, "Grip and Arm Strength in Males and Females, Age 10 to 69," *Research Quarterly* 48, no. 1 (1977): 109–120.
22. *Joint Motion: Method of Measuring and Recording* (Chicago: American Academy of Orthopaedic Surgeons, 1965).

23. Margaret L. Moore, "Clinical Assessment of Joint Motion," in Sidney Licht, *Therapeutic Exercise,* 2d ed. (Baltimore: Waverly Press, 1965), pp. 128–162.
24. Jack R. Leighton, "A Simple Objective and Reliable Measure of Flexibility," *Research Quarterly* 13 (May 1942): 205–216; and Jack R. Leighton, "An Instrument and Technic for the Measurement of Range of Joint Motion," *Archives of Physical Medicine and Rehabilitation* 36 (September 1955): 571–586.
25. Jack R. Leighton, "The Leighton Flexometer and Flexibility Test," *Journal of the Association for Physical and Mental Rehabilitation* 20 (May-June 1966): 86–93.
26. Golding, Myers, and Sinning, *Y's Way to Physical Fitness,* pp. 101–102.
27. Piscopo and Baley, *Kinesiology,* p. 302.
28. Ibid.
29. Harold C. Seashore, "The Development of a Beam Walking Test and Its Use in Measuring Development of Balance in Children," *Research Quarterly* 18 (December 1947): 246–259; and Ruth I. Bass, "An Analysis of Components of Tests of Semicircular Canal Functions and Static and Dynamic Balance," *Research Quarterly* 10 (May 1939): 33–51.
30. Piscopo and Baley, *Kinesiology,* p. 163.
31. Leon E. Smith, "Reaction Time and Movement Time in Four Large Muscle Movements," *Research Quarterly* 32 (March 1961): 88–92; and Joseph B. Oxendine, *Psychology of Motor Learning* (New York: Appleton-Century-Crofts, 1968), p. 318.
32. Johnson and Nelson, *Practical Measurements,* p. 246.
33. Ibid.
34. Ibid.

A

Selected Exercises for Older Adults

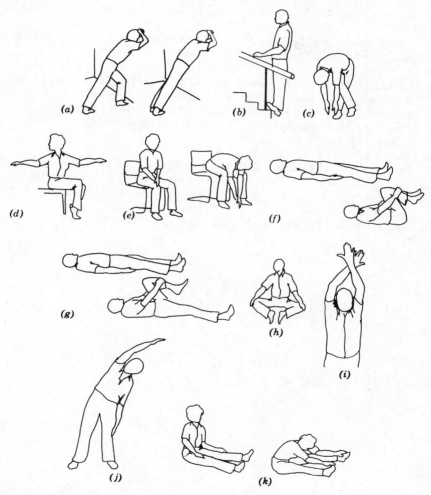

Figure A-1 Flexibility exercises: (a, b) calf and heel cord stretch; (c) hamstring stretch; (d) trunk twister; (e) low back stretch; (f) supine curl-up (g) alternate leg low back stretch; (h) abductor (groin) stretch; (i) shoulder stretch; (j) lateral (side) trunk stretch; (k) low back and hamstring stretch.

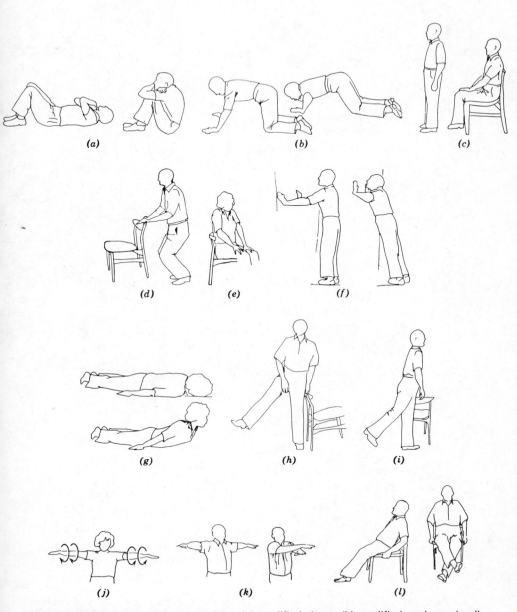

Figure A-2 Strength-building exercises: (a) modified sit-up; (b) modified push-up; (c, d) strengthening upper anterior (front) leg muscles; (e) shoulder shrugs; (f) modified push-up in standing position; (g) strengthening upper posterior (back) extensor muscles; (h) hip abduction; (i) hip extension; (j) arm circles; (k) arm flings; (l) leg cross-over.

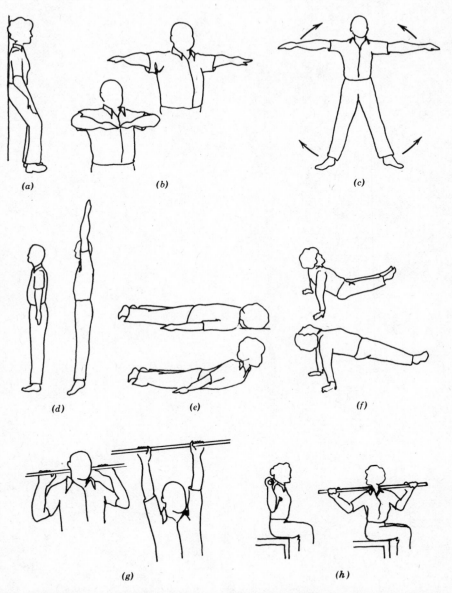

Figure A-3 Posture and physique exercises: (a) wall press—back and buttocks against wall; (b) wing stretcher—arms flung sideward; (c) angel stretch—supine on floor; (d) full body stretch—rising up on toes; (e) upper back stretcher; (f) arch support—stretching and strengthening hips, abdominals, chest; (g) lowering broomstick behind neck—strengthening deltoid (shoulder) muscles; (h) trunk twister with broomstick—sitting position.

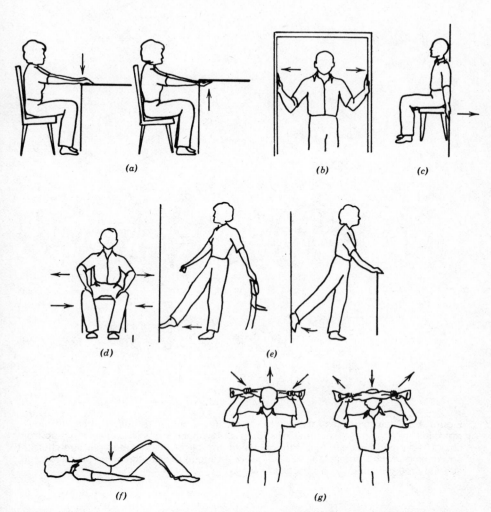

Figure A-4 Isometric exercises, with participant counting aloud, breathing rhythmically, pressing or holding static position for 5–6 seconds without excessive strain: (a, b, c) upper extremities; (d, e) lower extremities; (f) abdominal; (g) neck "iso" with towel.

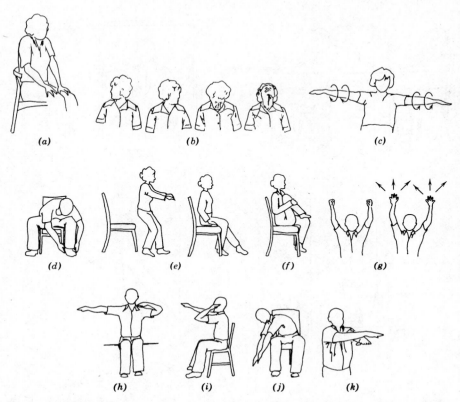

Figure A-5 Chair exercises for the frail elderly: (a) shoulder shrugs; (b) head turning—right, left, down, up; (c) shoulder rotations; (d) low back stretcher; (e) walk-get-up from chair; (f) hip and knee stretcher; (g) overhead arm raiser, hand and finger stretcher; (h) arm flexing in the frontal plane (side); (i) arm flexing in the sagittal plane (front/back); (j) alternate toe touching; (k) arm scissor swings.

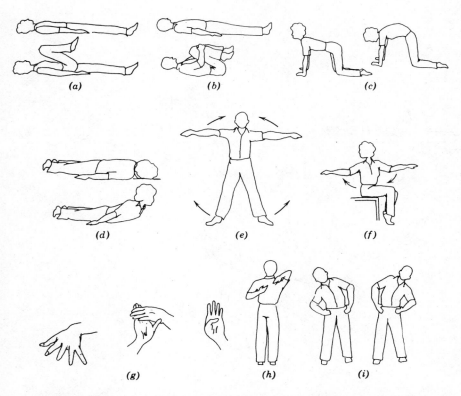

Figure A-6 Exercises for arthritic conditions: (a) supine position—alternate leg flexion on the trunk; (b) supine position—drawing knees up and gently rocking forward and backward; (c) cat stretch; (d) upper back stretcher; (e) supine position—abducting and adducting arms and legs (angel stretch); (f) trunk twister and toe raise; (g) wrist, hand, finger stretcher; (h) over and under shoulder stretcher; (i) lateral (side) trunk twister.

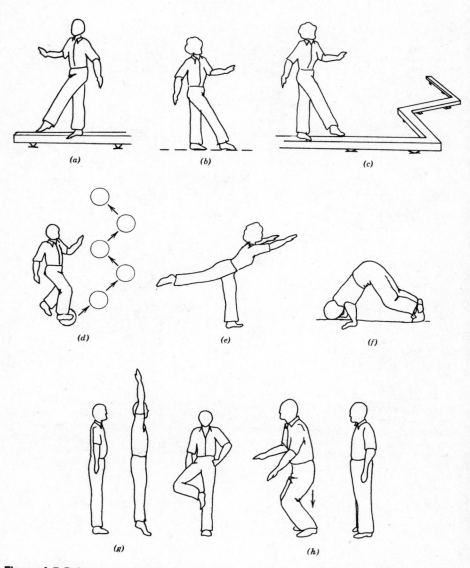

Figure A-7 Balance and equilibrium exercises: (a) beam walking; (b) line walking (on floor); (c) zig-zag beam walking; (d) zig-zag alternate step hopping; (e) one-foot balance stand; (f) modified head stand; (g) diver's balance stand; (h) stork stand; (i) half squat, return to stand.

APPENDIX B

Organizations Sponsoring Tournaments and Athletic Competition for Senior Athletes*

UNITED CYCLING FEDERATION
USCF Building 4
1750 East Boulder St.
Colorado Springs, CO 80909
Conducts national open road championships from 55–80 kilometers, and time trial championships of long distances, for veteran men and women.

UNITED STATES VOLLEYBALL ASSOCIATION (USVBA)
1750 East Boulder St.
Colorado Springs, CO 80909
Sponsors senior division for men and women with age divisions starting at 35 (men) and 30 (women).

UNITED STATES MASTER'S SWIMMING (USMS)
155 Pantry Road
Sudbury, MA 01776
Sponsors annually Master's swimming championships.

---

*For a comprehensive listing of sport opportunities for senior athletes, the reader is referred to the following source: David A. Field, "Opportunities for Senior Athletes," *Journal of Physical Education, Recreation, and Dance* 53, no. 6 (1982): 81–83.

UNITED STATES TENNIS ASSOCIATION (USTA)
51 East 42nd St.
New York, N.Y. 10017
Sponsors national championships on grass, clay, hard, and indoor surfaces for men
and women ranging from ages 35 to 80 +.

SUNFISH SAILING
Steven H. Baker
P.O. Box 1345
Waterbury, CN 06720
Sponsors annual senior competition from ages 40 to 75 +.

NATIONAL FIELD ARCHERY ASSOCIATION (NFAA)
Route 2, Box 514
Redlands, CA 92373
Sponsors programs for over-55 age group. Golden Bowmen and Golden Bowwomen
have annual sectional and national championships.

AMERICAN BOWLING CONGRESS (ABC)
5301 South 76th St.
Greendale, WI 53129
Senior league program for A: 70 +, B: 65–69, C: 60–64, and D: 55–59 categories.

FIELD HOCKEY ASSOCIATION OF AMERICA (FHAA)
1750 East Boulder St.
Colorado Springs, CO 80909
Occasional competition for seniors—no age divisions.

UNITED STATES GOLF ASSOCIATION (USGA)
Golf House
Far Hills, New Jersey 07931
Sponsors three annual senior national championships for men and women: (1) senior
amateur; (2) senior women's amateur, and (3) senior open. Age range from 50 to
65 +.

UNITED STATES HANDBALL ASSOCIATION
4101 Dempster Street
Skokie, IL 60076
Conducts state, regional, and national tournaments. Classifies its competitors as
follows: Master, 40–49; Golden Masters, 50–59; and Super Masters, 60 +.

UNITED STATES RACQUETBALL ASSOCIATION (USRA)
4101 Dempster Street
Skokie, IL 60076
Sponsors regional and national championships for singles and doubles competition
for men and women. Age groups range from 30 to 65+.

NATIONAL ASSOCIATION OF AMATEUR OARSMEN
4 Boathouse Row
Philadelphia, PA 19130
Sponsors Master's national championships in single sculls, double sculls, and four
with coxswain. Age groups range from 27 to 65+.

UNITED STATES AMATEUR CONFEDERATION OF ROLLER SKATING
(USACRS)
7700A Street
P.O. Box 83067
Lincoln, NE 68501
Invites competitors of all ages and both sexes. Competition is conducted on state,
regional, and national levels.

AMATEUR SOFTBALL ASSOCIATION (ASA)
2801 N.E. 50th St.
R.R. Box 4, Box 385
Oklahoma 73111
National headquarters does not sponsor a senior division, but many cities encourage
leagues for older men.

UNITED STATES SQUASH RACQUETS ASSOCIATION (USSRA)
211 Ford Road
Bala Cynwyd, PA 19004
Sponsors national and regional tournaments for men 50–54, 55–59, and 60+.

THE INTER-LAKE YACHTING ASSOCIATION
P.O. Box 435
Vermilion, OH 44089
Sponsors yachting programs for all ages and both sexes.

SENIOR SPORTS INTERNATIONAL, INC.
5670 Wilshire Blvd., Suite 360
Los Angeles, CA 90036
Sponsors organized tournaments in archery, badminton, basketball, bowling, canoeing, cycling, darts, skating, decathlon, handball, tennis, swimming, and other individual, two-person, and team sports.

NATIONAL SENIOR SPORTS ASSOCIATION (NSSA)
1900 M Street, N.W.
Suite 350
Washington, D.C. 20036
Publishes a senior sports newsletter and magazine. Offers instructional clinics and materials.

PRESIDENT'S COUNCIL ON PHYSICAL FITNESS AND SPORTS (PCPFS)
Washington, DC 20201
Conducts conferences on health and fitness for older adults to stimulate interest in athletic competition for seniors.

APPENDIX C

Medical History Form
Entrance to Senior
Lifeline

NAME: _____ DATE: _____

1. Have you any medical complaints at present? i.e., lower back pain, arthritis, neck pain, etc. _____

2. What major illnesses required hospitalization? (give dates) _____
   _____
   _____

3. Smoking status (circle one)
   a. never smoked
   b. smoke now
   c. smoked in past, not now

4. History of cardiovascular disease:

   NO   YES   Personal, if so, what _____
                _____

   NO   YES   Family history, if so, what _____
                _____

   NO   YES   Other _____
                _____

5. (Muscular history) Present or previous injury:
   a. NO
   b. YES
   c. If yes, specify _____

6. (Bone–joint history) Bone or Joint Disease:
   a. NO
   b. YES
   c. If yes, specify _____

7. Place a checkmark by each of the following ailments which apply to you:

   _____ Frequent dizziness
   _____ Hernia
   _____ Diabetes
   _____ Physical impairments, if any please specify _____
   _____

8. On the average how many times do you visit your physician each month? ____

9. How many times do you take medication each week? _____

10. Do you have any limitations not mentioned previously that will place limitations on complete participation in the Senior Lifeline fitness program? _____

Source: Courtesy of Senior Lifeline Program, University of Southern Maine.

D

Suggested Format for Consent Form
Informed Consent

I understand that the purpose of this (project or program) is to enhance my health-fitness status.

I verify that my participation as a participant is fully voluntary, and no coercion of any sort has been used to obtain my participation.

I understand that I may withdraw from the (project or program) without prejudice or malice at any time during the involved period or session.

I have been informed of the procedures and methods that will be used in the (project or program), and understand what will be necessary for me as a participant.

I understand that my participation will remain anonymous unless expressed name permission is given by me.

Signed: _____

Date: _____

APPENDIX E

Senior Lifeline Physical Activity Profile

NAME: _____ DATE: _____

    We would like to know more about you in order to improve our fitness program, and to meet your individual needs. Please fill in the following:

1. What was/is the nature of your employment (i.e., manufacturing, sales, teacher)?
   _____

   Year of retirement if applicable _____

2. How would you rate the physical activity you perform/performed at work (check one)?

   _____ little (sitting, typing, driving, talking)
   _____ moderate (standing, walking, bending, reaching)
   _____ active (light physical work, climbing stairs)
   _____ very active (moderate and physical work, lifting, etc.)

3. My physical activity during the "working hours" of the day has:

   _____ stayed the same
   _____ decreased
   _____ increased

4. What physical and recreational activities are you presently involved in (i.e., dancing, swimming, walking, bowling, etc.)? How often? _____

432

5. My goal(s) for joining a "Lifeline" fitness program is:

_____ to lose body fat
_____ to keep staying active
_____ because my doctor advised me to
_____ because I am concerned about my health (blood pressure, arthritis, bad back, etc.)

6. Check the activity you participate in and place the appropriate category next to the activity:

A   if total time spent is less than 15 minutes (3 times/day)
A+   if total time spent is at least 20 minutes (3 times/week)
A++   if the activity is sustained for more than 20 minutes (3 times/week)

_____ walking   _____ swimming   _____ golf
_____ jogging   _____ dancing   _____ other _____

7. How would you best describe your present level of fitness? (Components of fitness being flexibility, strength, cardiorespiratory condition and body fat composition.)

_____ excellent   _____ average
_____ good   _____ poor
_____ fair   _____ no health problems present

8. (Social, classroom) Would you be interested in attending an informal coffee hour to be scheduled once a month which would cover a short interesting topic.
YES   NO

If so, check categories of interest and also make suggestions:

_____ weight control and diet
_____ back care
_____ nutrition
_____ aerobic exercises
_____ proper equipment (shoes, running attire for winter or summer)
_____ warm up exercises for racquetball, tennis, walking, golf, etc.
_____ stress management
_____ blood pressure
_____ cholesterol
_____ smoking
_____ flexibility
_____ other categories of interest, please list _____
_____
_____

9. (Social) The social aspect of Senior Lifeline may be explored further by giving a check to those type(s) of extracurricular activities you would be interested in.

I would be interested in finding out more about:

_____	social brunch	_____	evening social
_____	hobby hour	_____	leading a physical fitness
_____	Senior Lifeline Club Presi-		class myself or with an as-
	dent, Vice President, Sec-		sistant
	retary and Treasurer		
_____	other _____		

10. Please respond as to how beneficial this interview was in your eyes, and what improvements you would like to see in the future:

_____ quite interesting and helpful

_____ well organized

_____ a waste of time

_____ very confusing

_____ other comments _____

A SELF FITNESS—*REPORT*

_____ 1. What is your sex? (please enter "M" for male, "F" for female)

_____ 2. Your age?

_____ 3. Are you presently exercising regularly? (enter "YES" or "NO")

_____ 4. Do you tire easily from climbing stairs? ("YES" or "NO")

_____ 5. Are you able to lift a bag of groceries comfortably?

_____ 6. How many city blocks do you walk on an average day?

_____ 7. Do you walk unassisted? ("YES" or "NO")

_____ 8. How many hours of sleep do you average per night?

Source: Courtesy of Senior Lifeline Program, University of Southern Maine.

F

Adult Fitness Program Nutrition Profile

NAME: _____ DATE: _____

   The staff of Lifeline considers nutrition to be an important aspect of this exercise program. In order that attention can be given to your total health, we ask that you complete this nutrition profile. The information will be used to assist you in achieving and/or maintaining adequate food, nutrient, and calorie intake.

   If you have questions regarding your eating habits, feel free to ask the staff, or have one of them make an appointment with Lifeline's Consultant Dietitian.

   Please describe in the space provided below a typical 24-hour food intake, listing kinds of food eaten, method of preparation (fried, broiled, etc.), amount eaten (½ cup, 3 oz., etc.), and where the meals are usually eaten. Include beverages and water consumed.

(continued next page)

MORNING MEAL	TIME: _____	PLACE EATEN: _____	MID-MORNING SNACKS
MIDDAY MEAL	TIME: _____	PLACE EATEN: _____	MID-AFTERNOON SNACKS
EVENING MEAL	TIME: _____	PLACE EATEN: _____	EVENING SNACKS

Circle the following items if used and indicate amount taken in a 24-hour period:

Sugar _____   Tea _____
Candy _____   Soda _____
Chips, etc. _____   Alcohol _____
Milk _____   Vitamins _____
Coffee _____

Please list any medications you are taking at the present time: _____

Source: Courtesy of Senior Lifeline Program, University of Southern Maine.

APPENDIX G

Height and Weight Tables

1983 Metropolitan Height and Weight Tables

Men					Women				
Height		Small	Medium	Large	Height		Small	Medium	Large
Feet	Inches	Frame	Frame	Frame	Feet	Inches	Frame	Frame	Frame
5	2	128–134	131–141	138–150	4	10	102–111	109–121	118–131
5	3	130–136	133–143	140–153	4	11	103–113	111–123	120–134
5	4	132–138	135–145	142–156	5	0	104–115	113–126	122–137
5	5	134–140	137–148	144–160	5	1	106–118	115–129	125–140
5	6	136–142	139–151	146–164	5	2	108–121	118–132	128–143
5	7	138–145	142–154	149–168	5	3	111–124	121–135	131–147
5	8	140–148	145–157	152–172	5	4	114–127	124–138	134–151
5	9	142–151	148–160	155–176	5	5	117–130	127–141	137–155
5	10	144–154	151–163	158–180	5	6	120–133	130–144	140–159
5	11	146–157	154–166	161–184	5	7	123–136	133–147	143–163
6	0	149–160	157–170	164–188	5	8	126–139	136–150	146–167
6	1	152–164	160–174	168–192	5	9	129–142	139–153	149–170
6	2	155–168	164–178	172–197	5	10	132–145	142–156	152–173
6	3	158–172	167–182	176–202	5	11	135–148	145–159	155–176
6	4	162–176	171–187	181–207	6	0	138–151	148–162	158–179

Source of basic data: 1979 Build Study, Society of Actuaries and Association of Life Insurance Medical Directors of America, 1980.

To Make an Approximation of Your Frame Size

	Height in 1" heels	Elbow
	Men	Breadth

Extend your arm and bend the forearm upward at a 90 degree angle. Keep fingers straight and turn the inside of your wrist toward your body. If you have a caliper, use it to measure the space between the two prominent bones on *either side* of your elbow. Without a caliper, place thumb and index finger of your other hand on these two bones. Measure the space between your fingers against a ruler or tape measure. Compare it with these tables that list elbow measurements for *medium-framed* men and women. Measurements lower than those listed indicate you have a small frame. Higher measurements indicate a large frame. Weights at ages 25–59 based on lowest mortality. Weight in pounds according to frame (in indoor clothing weighing 5 lbs. for men and 3 lbs. for women; shoes with 1" heels).

Height in 1" heels	Elbow Breadth
Men	
5'2"–5'3"	2½"–2⅞"
5'4"–5'7"	2⅝"–2⅞"
5'8"–5'11"	2¾"–3"
6'0"–6'3"	2¾"–3⅛"
6'4"	2⅞"–3¼"
Women	
4'10"–4'11"	2¼"–2½"
5'0"–5'3"	2¼"–2½"
5'4"–5'7" 2⅜"–2⅝"	
5'8"–5'11"	2⅜"–2⅝"
6'0"	2½"–2¾"

Source: In Brief 6, no. 1 (Spring 1983). Courtesy of Metropolitan Life Insurance Co. Used with permission.

Procedure for Trio-Badminton, A Modified Game for Senior Citizens

Boundaries: Use doubles lines.

Number of players: Three; two play side-by-side in the forecourt and follow all the doubles rules and regulations; one backup player covers the back court. Remain in these positions throughout the game.

Number of points to the game: 15. Set score when tied at 13 or 14 according to doubles play.

Serving order: The game is started as in doubles: first side to serve has only one "down" before opponent's serve.

Play always starts first in the right hand court as a team begins term of service. The forecourt players take their turn followed by the backcourt player who serves only to the backcourt player on the other team. This player serves according to singles play: from the right court if the score is even; from the left court if the score is odd. (This is the only departure from the doubles rules.)

Play: Immediately after the service and return of the serve any member on the side the shuttlecock is on may contact the bird.

As playing skills increase, positions on the court can be shifted effectively. Doubles play can take place by eliminating the third player (the one in backup position). Singles play can result by eliminating the forecourt players and playing to 11 points. Lines for singles will be the farthest boundary in the backcourt and the inner sideline.

Source: Courtesy of Dorothy Chrisman, *Body Recall, Inc.,* College Post Office Box 363, Berea, KY 40404.

Glossary

Acetylcholine A hormone released by the parasympathetic and skeletal nerve endings, which lowers blood pressure, increases peristalsis, and activates muscles.

Addiction Habituation to some practice, especially the alcohol or drug habit.

Aerobic Muscular work that requires the presence of oxygen, such as jogging a two-mile event.

Aerobic power Refers to the amount of oxygen used (liters or milliliters per kilogram of body weight) per unit of time (usually a minute).

Ageism Refers to a disparaging image of someone simply because of his or her advanced age.

Aging The maturational changes that occur with advancing age.

Agonist muscle A muscle responsible for a specific movement.

Alcoholic One addicted to chronic drinking of excessive amounts of alcohol to the extent that it interferes with his or her health.

Amino acids Any one of a large group of organic compounds with the basic formula NH_2—R—COOH. They form the chief structure of proteins, and several are essential in human nutrition.

Anaerobic Muscular work of short duration that does not depend upon the presence of oxygen, such as running a 50-yard dash.

Analgesic An agent that alleviates pain without causing loss of consciousness.

Angina Spasmodic choking, or suffocative pain; angina pectoris.

Ankylosing spondylitis An inflammatory disease of the spine that leads to obliteration of the vertebral joints.

Anorgasmia Failure to experience orgasm in coitus.

Antagonistic muscle A muscle that directly opposes the action of another muscle.

440

Antianginal agent   Drug used for acute attacks of angina pectoris and prophylactic therapy, such as nitrites/nitrates or coronary vasodilators.

Antiarrhythmic agent   Drug used in the treatment of individuals with arrhythmia, such as quinidine, lidocaine, and propranolol.

Anticoagulant agent   A drug or substance that serves to prevent the coagulation of blood, such as coumarin and heparin.

Antihypertensive   Drug used to lower blood pressure, usually falling into one of three categories: (1) diuretics, (2) vasodilators, and (3) adrenergic blocking agents.

Antimalarial drug   Agent used to treat malaria and certain forms of arthritis, such as rheumatoid arthritis.

Anxiety   A state of apprehension and fear, accompanied by restlessness and uncertainty.

Aortic stenosis   Narrowing of the aortic orifice of the heart or the aorta itself.

Arrhythmia   Any variation in the normal rhythm of the heart beat.

Arteriosclerosis   A group of diseases characterized by thickening or hardening and loss of elasticity in arterial walls.

Arteriosclerotic brain disease   An excessive thickening and rigidity of the arteries leading to, and in, the brain.

Arthritis   A broad term used to cover rheumatism, as well as approximately one hundred different conditions that cause aching and pain in the joints and connective tissues, with or without inflammation.

Asymptomatic   Showing no evidence of symptoms of disease.

Ataxia   Incoordination of muscular action.

Atherosclerosis   A common form of arteriosclerosis in which deposits of yellow plaque containing cholesterol and fatty substances form within the inner portion of the arteries.

Autoantibody   Antibodies produced by the body formed in response to stimulation by an antigen, which reacts to overcome the toxic effects of a specific substance.

Autonomic nervous system   Part of the nervous system that regulates the functions of certain internal organs independent of will power. It consists of two main divisions: sympathetic, and parasympathetic.

Ballistic stretching   Quick, jerky type of stretching exercise, such as fast alternate toe touching movements.

Basal metabolic rate   The energy expenditure of the body under conditions of complete rest.

Beta-adrenergic blocking agent   Drugs used in the treatment of hypertension to block receptor responses to nerve impulses.

Biofeedback   Technique of providing visual or auditory information about how autonomic processes of the body are functioning.

Blood platelets   Spheroidal or ovoid light-gray bodies found in the blood which are important in blood coagulation.

Blood pressure   The force with which the blood distends the walls of the arteries; dependent upon the heart action, elasticity of arteries, volume and viscosity of the blood.

Bone accretion   Development of bone hypertrophy—increase in bone mass and density.

Bone resorption   A type of bone loss characterized by decreased mineral mass and increased bone porosity.

Bursitis   Inflammation of a sac-like cavity filled with viscid fluid around joints (bursa), occasionally accompanied by calcium deposits.

Calorie   A unit of heat; the amount required to raise the temperature of one kilogram of water one degree Centigrade.

Carbohydrate loading   A nutritional regimen followed before competition to enhance endurance by adjusting carbohydrate intake from low levels to high dosages of foods such as bread, spaghetti, potatoes, and sugar.

Carcinogenic   Capable of producing a malignant growth resulting in metastases or cancer.

Cardiac output   Volume of blood expelled by either ventricle of the heart per unit of time.

Cardiomyopathy   A general term designating a disease of the heart, often of unknown cause.

Catecholamines   Hormones secreted by the nerve endings of the sympathetic nervous system; also called adrenalin and noradrenalin.

Cholinergic   A term applied to those nerve fibers that liberate acetylcholine at the neural-muscular junction, when a nerve impulse passes.

Chromatin   The protoplasmic substance of the cell's nucleus, which is stainable and forms the network of nuclear fibrils.

Closed skill   A motor skill in which the environment of the activity does not change, such as bowling.

Concentric exercise   A force generated by muscles resulting in shortening contraction; e.g., biceps shorten concentrically in elbow flexion.

Conductive hearing loss   Impairment usually caused by faulty mechanical transmission of sound from external and middle ear mechanisms into the internal ear.

Cortical bone   The compact part of the bone shaft that surrounds the marrow (medullary cavity).

Cortisol   A steroid hormone, which plays a role in fat and water metabolism, affects muscle tone and the excitation of nerve tissue, increases gastric secretion response to injury, and impedes cartilage production.

Crystallized intelligence   A type of intelligence which is a result of cultural assimilation and influenced by formal and informal educational factors throughout the life span; presumed to increase with age unless some disease is present.

Decibel   A unit used to express the intensity of a sound wave.

Decubitus   A common type of pressure sore suffered by individuals who spend long periods of time in bed.

Delirium tremens   A form of alcoholic psychosis characterized by acute mental and emotional distress, and gastrointestinal symptoms; trembling, anxiety, and disorientation may be present.

Diastolic pressure   The lowest level to which arterial blood pressure falls—relaxation phase of cardiac activity.

Digitalis The dried leaf of digitalis purpurea which acts as a powerful cardiac stimulant, and is used to increase the force of heart contraction.

Disc degeneration The loss of structural and functional soundness of the vertebral disc.

Diuretic An agent that increases the secretion of urine.

DNA Deoxyribonucleic acid, found in all living cells, which carries the genetic information of organisms.

Dopamine A catecholamine found in the basal nuclei of the brain.

Drug tolerance Adaptation by the body that lessens responsiveness to a drug on continuous administration.

Drug toxicity Capacity of a drug to dangerously impair body functions or to damage body tissues.

Dyspnea Difficult or labored breathing.

Eccentric exercise A type of muscular tension that occurs in controlled lengthening, such as elbow extension of the biceps in lowering a cup or glass to the table.

Edema Excessive accumulation of fluid in the tissue spaces.

Edentulous Without teeth; having lost the natural teeth.

Embolism The occlusion of a blood vessel caused by a clot or plug, obstructing circulation.

Emphysema A pathological accumulation of air in tissues or organs; applied especially to the lungs—characterized by loss of lung elasticity, shortness of breath, distended lung air sacs, and chest expansion.

Encoding information A psychological term that refers to the process of learning and storing information in the mind.

Endorphin Hormonal secretion of the pituitary gland associated with mood changes such as "runner's high."

Enzyme A catalytic substance formed by living cells, having a specific action in promoting a chemical change.

Ergot A dried sclerotium of claviceps purpurea; ergot alkaloids are used in the treatment of migraine.

Essential hypertension Persistently high arterial blood pressure occurring without a discoverable organic cause.

Estrogen A female hormone produced by the ovaries and adrenal glands.

Flatulence The presence of excessive amounts of air or gases in the stomach or intestines.

Fluid intelligence A type of intelligence that involves the ability to reorganize one's perception; considered to reflect functioning or neurological structures; increases until the cessation of neural maturation.

Frigidity A general term applied to female sexual inadequacy—lack of libido; unsatisfactory response or coldness in a woman.

Functional age Refers to the proficiency of the individual to perform mental and physical tasks as contrasted to chronologic age, which measures time units since birth.

Generic drug A drug not protected by a trademark, usually descriptive of its chemical structure; also known as general or public drug.

Geriatrics   A branch of medical science dealing with diseases, dysfunctions, and disabilities of older people—a part of gerontology.

Gerontology   A field of scientific study dealing with the study of biological, psychological, and sociological components of aging.

Gerontophobia   Persistent dread or morbid fear of growing old.

Glucose   A simple sugar having the formula C_6—H_{12}—O_6; a form of carbohydrate that is transported by the blood and metabolized in the tissues.

Glycogen   Form of carbohydrate stored within the body—a complex animal starch built up of large numbers of glucose molecules found in the liver and muscles.

Glycoside agent   Plant alkaloids such as digitalis, used for treating congestive heart failure; improves blood supply to the organs and helps to relieve edema (swelling).

Gold compounds   A class of drugs, sodium thiomalate (gold salts), used in the treatment of rheumatoid arthritis.

Gout   A metabolic arthritic disorder of body chemistry associated with elevated amounts of uric acid in the blood.

Heberden's nodes   A form of arthritis in the smaller joints, accompanied by nodules around the distal finger joints.

Hemiplegia   Paralysis affecting one side of the body.

High-density lipoproteins   A combination of a lipid and protein containing more protein and less cholesterol and triacylglycerides.

Homeostasis   A tendency of the body to maintain internal cellular environmental stability and constancy.

Hyperbaric oxygenation   A procedure intended to improve mental functioning by enhancing oxygen supply to the brain cells in certain cases of psychosis and cerebral vascular insufficiency.

Hyperglycemia   Excess sugar in the blood.

Hyperlipidemia   Excess fat in the blood.

Hypertension   Generally, a symptomless disease characterized by abnormal and persistent states of high blood pressure.

Hypoglycemia   A condition produced by an abnormally low glucose content in the blood, which may lead to headache, confusion, hallucination, bizarre behavior, and, ultimately, convulsions and coma.

Hypokalemia   Abnormally low level of potassium concentration in the blood.

Hypothalamus   An endocrine gland that regulates water balance, body temperature, sleep, food intake, and the development of secondary sex characteristics.

Iatrogenic illness   An adverse disorder or illness occurring as a consequence of treatment by a physician.

Impotence   Lack of penile erectile capacity in the male, which prevents copulation.

Incontinence   Inability to control excretory function of the bladder or bowels.

Intermediate care facility (ICF)   A health care facility staffed and equipped to provide technical nursing care by or under the supervision of a licensed practical nurse. Residents usually are ambulatory, and require few nursing procedures.

Inverse stretch reflex   A neural phenomenon that allows a muscle to relax after a slow, steady stretch movement.

Ischemic heart disease Deficiency of blood supply to the heart muscle due to an obstruction or constriction of the coronary arteries.

Isometric exercise The development of a muscle contraction without skeletal movement—exercise in which force is exerted against an immovable object.

Isometric strength Refers to the ability to apply maximum strength without movement.

Isotonic exercise A dynamic exercise accompanied by changes in muscle length; e.g., flexing or extending the biceps in elbow movements.

Isotonic strength Refers to the ability to apply maximal strength through a range of motion.

Kegel exercises A set of exercises designed to relieve urinary stress incontinence; often results in increased female orgasmic responsiveness.

Kg-m A unit of work equal to the energy required to move one kilogram through a distance of one meter.

Kinesiology The science of movement, based on applied anatomy, neuromuscular physiology, and mechanics.

Kinesthesia A position sense; an awareness of position and movements of body segments or the whole body as a unit.

Kyphosis A postural condition characterized by an increased convex curve in the upper back; also called thoracic or dorsal kyphosis.

Lactic acid A fatiguing metabolite of the lactic acid system resulting from the incomplete breakdown of glucose (sugar); the byproduct of anaerobic metabolism.

Lactic acidosis A condition in which excessive acids accumulate in the body resulting in a diminution of alkali reserve in the blood.

Lean body mass Body weight minus the weight of body fat.

Lethargy Quality or state of being drowsy, dull, sluggish; lack of energy.

Libido Sexual desire.

Light adaptation Ability of the eye to adjust itself to variations in the intensity of light; e.g., adapting vision in the dark (night vision), adjusting vision in sunlight or bright illumination.

Long-term care facility Extended health care facility; a nursing home.

Lipofuscin Any one of a class of fatty pigments formed by the solution of a pigment in fat.

Low-density lipoproteins A combination of a lipid and protein containing more cholesterol and triacylglycerides, and less protein.

Ludotherapy A medical term used to express treatment by games and physical activities for individuals manifesting psychological problems.

Macroscopic Visible with the naked eye without the use of a microscope.

Maximum heart rate The heart rate measured at the highest exercise intensity attained.

Melanin Dark pigment found in the skin and hair; produced by metabolic activity of certain specialized cells.

Ménière's syndrome A disease of the internal ear (labyrinth) characterized by tinnitus, deafness, and acute attacks of vertigo.

Meprobamate   An antidepressant drug used in the treatment of neuroses and as a muscle relaxant; an effective tranquilizer for emotional disturbances.

MET unit   A unit of measurement of heat production by the body—one MET is the equivalent of the resting oxygen consumption (VO_2) which is approximately 3.5 ml/kg. min (1 MET = 3.5 ml/kg. min).

Metabolism   The sum of all the physical and chemical processes by which a living organism is produced, utilized for maintaining life.

Microscopic   Extremely small size; visible only by use of a microscope.

Mitochondria   Small granules or rod-shaped structures found in the cells, which form the principal sites of the generation of energy resulting from the oxidation of foodstuffs.

Monoaminal oxidase inhibitors   A class of drugs used to treat depression and various phases of manic depressive psychoses—rarely used as first agents for therapy of depressive illness.

Monosaccharide   Any carbohydrate whose molecule cannot be split into simpler carbohydrates (a simple sugar).

Morbidity   Proportion of sickness or of a specific disease in a geographical locality; incidence of sickness.

Mortality   Relative frequency of death, or death rate in a district or community; incidence of deaths.

Motor ability   Proficiency of an individual to perform a wide range of motor skills extending from everyday living tasks to elite athletic sports.

Motor capacity   Refers to the maximum capacity potential of an individual to succeed in a motor skill.

Multipurpose senior center   A community-sponsored organization where older adults participate in a variety of social, physical, and cultural activities and programs.

Muscle atrophy   Shrinking, diminution in muscle size and strength; antithesis of hypertrophy.

Muscle hypertrophy   An increase in muscle fiber size and strength.

Muscular endurance   Refers to the ability of the individual to perform repeated muscular contractions, such as a number of sit-ups within a set time limit.

Muscular strength   Refers to the ability of a muscle or muscle group to apply maximal force with a single contraction.

Myocardial infarction   Necrosis of heart muscle tissue due to interference of blood flow to the area as in coronary thrombosis.

Myogenic tone   Residual firmness when a muscle is at rest, resulting from the effects of exercise.

Myotatic reflex   A muscle spindle reflex, which, by its stretch effect, excites a muscle to contract automatically.

Myth   Traditional or legendary story about a person or event without a basis of fact; an invented idea, or concept lacking evidence.

Negative work   Work done by a muscle that is eccentrically contracting while lengthening—e.g., biceps while lowering a glass to a table, or action of hamstrings while walking downstairs.

Neurofibrillary tangles A thickening and twisting of the neurofibril network within the nerve cell of the cerebral cortex of the brain.

Neurogenic tone Aspect of muscle tonus which provides a continuous barrage of low-level neural impulses that enhance muscular firmness.

Nosocomial infection Disease or condition pertaining to, or originating in, a hospital.

Open skill A motor skill in which the environment of the activity is constantly changing, such as basketball.

Organic brain syndrome A group of mental disorders caused by, or associated with, impairment of brain tissue function.

Orthostatic hypotension Weakness on rising to an erect position (*see* postural hypotension).

Osteoarthritis A common form of arthritis called "wear-and-tear" disuse of the joints; usually mild, and not usually inflammatory.

Osteoblast Cells of mesodermal origin related to the formation of bony tissue.

Osteoblastic growth Increase in bone cellular activity associated with the production and repair bone.

Osteomalacia Softening and reduction of bone strength due to decreased mineralization.

Osteopenia A state in which bone mass is reduced below normal.

Osteophyte An excessive bony growth or projection.

Osteoporosis Loss of skeletal mass and density due to demineralization of bone substance.

Overweight A state of heaviness that may be caused by increased muscle mass and bone size and density—not necessarily excess body fat.

Oxygen uptake The ability of the body to use oxygen, technically called *maximum aerobic power*.

Paraplegia Paralysis affecting the legs and lower part of the body.

Peripheral vascular circulation Refers to blood flow and circulation to body extremities.

Phlebitis Inflammation of a vein.

Piezoelectric The development of electrical charges by certain bone crystals when subjected to strain.

Pitch The quality of sound dependent on the rapidity (frequency) of vibrations that make the sound.

Popranolol Beta-adrenergic blocking agent used in the treatment of cardiac arrhythmias.

Positive work Work accomplished by muscles used concentrically against gravity; e.g., action of the hamstrings while walking uphill.

Postural hypotension Diminished or low blood pressure due to a sudden change from horizontal to the upright position or from prolonged standing, causing dizziness, faintness, and sometimes temporary unconsciousness.

Prostatectomy Excision or surgical removal of part or all of the prostate gland.

Prostatitis Inflammation of the prostate gland.

Pulse rate Number of pulsations of an artery per minute—normally varies from 50 to 100.

Reliability coefficient   An estimated form of expressing the consistency of measurement; degree of similarity of performance on repetition of a task.

Reminiscence   Recall and review about past life experiences—used as a therapeutic tool to assist the elderly in strengthening coping mechanisms.

Renin   A protein enzyme secreted by the kidneys and associated with the regulation of blood pressure.

Rheumatoid arthritis   A progressive and destructive disease affecting the connective tissues and joint structures—leads to deformities and disabilities.

Rheumatologist   A physician who specializes in rheumatic conditions (disorders of connective tissues and muscles, especially the joints and related structures).

RNA   Ribonucleic acid, found in all living cells, which transmits information from DNA to the protein forming system of the cell.

Saturated fats   Animal fats and dairy products.

Schizophrenia   A group of several emotional disorders characterized by misinterpretation and retreat from reality, delusions, hallucinations, withdrawn, bizarre, or erratic behavior.

Scleroderma   Chronic hardening and shrinking of the connective tissues, including the skin, heart, esophagus, kidney, and lungs.

Senile dementia   A general designation for mental deterioration associated with old age; senile psychosis.

Senile plaques   Neuritic patches or flat areas commonly found in the cortex of the brain among persons with Alzheimer's disease.

Senility   Physical and mental deterioration associated with old age.

Sensorineural hearing loss   Loss caused by impairment of the cochlea or auditory nerve within the internal ear, usually classed under the heading of "nerve deafness."

Spondylitis   An inflammatory disease of the spine.

Static stretching   Holding a stretch position without movement; a nonballistic exercise.

Stereotype   A trite impression or image lacking originality, initiative, or creativeness; an antiquated or obsolete perception.

Steroid   Any of a large group of fat-soluble organic compounds, such as the sterols, bile acids, and sex hormones, including testosterone, adrenosterone, estrogen, and corticosterone.

Stress   A state or group of conditions arising from the external environment or from within the body that demands some form of action to restore normal balance.

Stress incontinence   Loss of urinary retention control due to weakened muscles of the pelvic floor—commonly associated with elderly females.

Stretch reflex   Reflex muscular contraction in response to longitudinal stretching or extending; also called *myotatic reflex*.

Syndrome   A set of symptoms which produce an unhealthy state or disease.

Synovial membrane   Membrane or sheath lining the fibrous capsule of a joint which secretes a lubricating fluid.

Synovitis   Inflammation of the joint articular capsule (synovial membrane)—usually painful, particularly in joint movement.

Systolic pressure The highest level of arterial blood pressure created by heart contraction.

Tachycardia A term used to describe excessive rapidity in heart rate.

Target population A particular subgroup of the older population, such as well-aging, frail elderly, limited ambulatory, or old-old.

Test objectivity The degree to which a test or performance is consistent in measuring what it is supposed to measure when administered or conducted by different testers.

Test reliability Refers to the consistency of the measurement for any given test.

Test validity A state or quality of being sound; a test that measures accurately what it is supposed to measure.

Testosterone A male steroidal hormone (androgen) produced by the testes.

Thrombosis The formation of a blood clot within the heart or blood vessels.

Tinnitus Noise in the ears such as ringing, buzzing, roaring, clicking, or hissing sounds.

Toxicity The quality of being poisonous.

Trabecular bone One of the variously shaped bone formations resembling a small beam or crossbar.

Tranquilizer An agent that acts on the emotional state, quieting or calming the individual.

Tricyclic Drug used in treating depression associated with organic brain syndrome.

Unsaturated fats Fat from vegetable oils and marine oils from fish (e.g., cod-liver oil).

Vagus nerve Tenth cranial nerve, located in the medulla oblongata, which supplies sensory stimulation to the trachea, cardiac, esophageal, and abdominal areas.

Valsalva effect Breath holding during the expiratory effort of exercise with the glottis closed, creating increased intrathoracic pressure.

Vasodilator Agent producing dilation of blood vessels.

Ventricular arrhythmia Irregular rhythmic contractions of the heart ventricle which may interfere with the pumping effectiveness of the heart.

Vertigo Illusions of motion, relating to the sensation of turning or falling, often stemming from a disorder of the inner ear.

VO$_2$ max Refers to the individual's ability to use oxygen within a given time unit (usually one minute).

Well-aging Vigorous and active older persons, well integrated with members of their families and society (*see* well-derly).

Well-derly A subgroup of the older population designated as independent, active, and free of serious disabilities or diseases.

Wolff's law The hypothesis that bone develops the structure most suited to resist the forces acting upon it—bone development reacts to influences of mechanical stresses.

Work Application of force through a distance ($W = f \times d$); e.g., application of five pounds through one foot equals five foot-pounds of work.

Index

450